GENDER AND HEALTH

GENDER AND HEALTH

Major Themes in Health and Social Welfare

Edited by
Kate Hunt and Ellen Annandale

Volume III
Gender and Healthcare

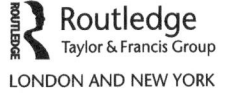

LONDON AND NEW YORK

First published 2012
by Routledge
2 Park Square, Milton Park, Abingdon, Oxon OX14 4RN

Simultaneously published in the USA and Canada
by Routledge
711 Third Avenue, New York, NY 10017

Routledge is an imprint of the Taylor & Francis Group, an informa business

© 2012 Kate Hunt and Ellen Annandale

All rights reserved. No part of this book may be reprinted or reproduced or utilised in any form or by any electronic, mechanical, or other means, now known or hereafter invented, including photocopying and recording, or in any information storage or retrieval system, without permission in writing from the publishers.

Trademark notice: Product or corporate names may be trademarks or registered trademarks, and are used only for identification and explanation without intent to infringe.

British Library Cataloguing in Publication Data
A catalogue record for this book is available from the British Library

Library of Congress Cataloging in Publication Data
Gender and health / edited by Kate Hunt and Ellen Annandale.
   p. ; cm. – (Major themes in health and social welfare)
   Includes bibliographical references and index.
   ISBN 978-0-415-56976-7 (set) – ISBN 978-0-415-56977-4 (v. 1) –
ISBN 978-0-415-56978-1 (v. 2) – ISBN 978-0-415-56979-8 (v. 3) –
ISBN 978-0-415-56980-4 (v. 4) 1. Health–Sex differences.
2. Women–Health and hygiene. 3. Men–Health and hygiene.
I. Hunt, Kate, 1959–   II. Annandale, Ellen.   III. Series: Major themes in health and social welfare.
   [DNLM: 1. Gender Identity–Collected Works. 2. Health Status Disparities–Collected Works. 3. Health Behavior–Collected Works.
4. Men's Health–Collected Works. 5. Sex Factors–Collected Works.
6. Women's Health–Collected Works. WA 300.1]
   RA564.85.G45 2011
   613–dc23
                                                          2011007587

ISBN: 978-0-415-56976-7 (Set)
ISBN: 978-0-415-56979-8 (Volume III)

Typeset in 10/12pt Times NR MT
by Graphicraft Limited, Hong Kong

Publisher's Note
References within each chapter are as they appear in the original complete work

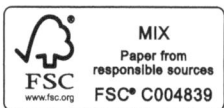

Printed and bound in Great Britain by the MPG Books Group

CONTENTS

VOLUME III GENDER AND HEALTHCARE

Acknowledgements	ix
Introduction	1

PART 10
Policy trends and health system change 9

42 Well women and medicine men: gendering the health policy agenda 11
ANNA COOTE AND LIZ KENDALL

43 Thinking about the production and consumption of long-term care in Britain: does gender still matter? 24
CLARE UNGERSON

44 Gender and equity in health sector reform programmes: a review 45
HILARY STANDING

45 Gender mainstreaming in health: looking back, looking forward 74
T. K. S. RAVINDRAN AND A. KELKAR-KHAMBETE

46 Reforming gendered health care: an assessment of change 99
MARY K. ZIMMERMAN AND SHIRLEY A. HILL

PART 11
The impact of gendered assumptions on health and healthcare — 125

47 A funny thing happened on the way to the orifice: women in gynecology textbooks — 127
DIANA SCULLY AND PAULINE BART

48 Doctor–patient negotiation of cultural assumptions — 133
SUE FISHER AND STEPHEN B. GROCE

49 Women as patients: a problem for sex differences research — 161
KATHY DAVIS

50 Sex differences and the new politics of women's health — 174
STEVEN EPSTEIN

51 Gender and the medicalization of healthcare — 202
SUSAN E. BELL AND ANNE E. FIGERT

52 Gendering the migraine market: do representations of illness matter? — 219
JOANNA KEMPNER

53 The influence of patient and doctor gender on diagnosing coronary heart disease — 239
ANN ADAMS, CHRISTOPHER D. BUCKINGHAM, ANTJE LINDENMEYER, JOHN B. McKINLAY, CAROL LINK, LISA MARCEAU AND SARA ARBER

54 Continuity and change in the gender segregation of the medical profession in Britian and France — 262
ROSEMARY CROMPTON AND NICKY LE FEUVRE

55 The feminization thesis: discourses on gender and medicine — 280
ELIANNE RISKA

PART 12
Accessing and experiencing healthcare — 299

56 Help seeking for cardiac symptoms: beyond the masculine–feminine binary — 301
PAUL M. GALDAS, JOY L. JOHNSON, MYRA E. PERCY AND PAMELA A. RATNER

CONTENTS

57 Gender and help-seeking: towards gender-comparative studies 318
KATE HUNT, JOY ADAMSON AND PAUL GALDAS

58 Gender and access to HIV testing and antiretroviral treatments in Thailand: why do women have more and earlier access? 333
SOPHIE LE CŒUR, INTIRA J. COLLINS, JULIE PANNETIER AND EVA LELIÈVRE

59 Gender, sexuality and embodiment: access to and experience of healthcare by same-sex attracted women in Australia 352
JANE EDWARDS AND HELEN VAN ROEKEL

60 Choosing Cesarean: feminism and the politics of childbirth in the United States 370
KATHERINE BECKETT

61 Doing health, doing gender: teenagers, diabetes and asthma 396
CLARE WILLIAMS

ACKNOWLEDGEMENTS

The publishers would like to thank the following for permission to reprint their material:

JPPR for permission to reprint Coote, A. and Kendall, L. (2000) 'Well women and medicine men: gendering the health policy agenda', pp. 149–60 in A. Coote (ed.), *The New Gender Agenda*, London: IPPR.

Cambridge University Press for permission to reprint Ungerson, C. (2000) 'Thinking about the production and consumption of long-term care in Britain: does gender still matter?' *Journal of Social Policy*, 29, 623–43.

Oxford University Press for permission to reprint Standing, H. (1997) 'Gender and equity in health sector reform programmes: a review', *Health Policy and Planning*, 12 (1): 1–18.

Taylor & Francis for permission to reprint Ravindran, T. K. S. and Kelkar-Khambete, A. (2008) 'Gender mainstreaming in health: looking back, looking forward', *Global Public Health*, 3 (S1): 121–42.

Baywood Publishing for permission to reprint Zimmerman, M. K. and Hill, S. A. (2000) 'Reforming gendered health care: an assessment of change', *International Journal of Health Services*, 30 (4): 771–95.

University of Chicago Press for permission to reprint Scully, D. and Bart, P. (1970) 'A funny thing happened on the way to the orifice: women in gynecology textbooks', *American Journal of Sociology*, 78 (4): 1045–51.

Wiley for permission to reprint Fisher, S. and Groce, S. B. (1985) 'Doctor–patient negotiation of cultural assumptions', *Sociology of Health and Illness*, 7 (3): 342–74.

Elsevier for permission to reprint Davis, K. (1984) 'Women as patients: a problem for sex differences research', *Women's Studies International Forum*, 7 (4): 211–17.

ACKNOWLEDGEMENTS

University of Chicago Press for permission to reprint Epstein, S. (2008) 'Sex differences and the new politics of women's health', pp. 233–57 in S. Epstein, *Inclusion: The Politics of Difference in Medical Research*, Chicago: University of Chicago Press.

Palgrave for permission to reprint Bell, S. E. and Figert, A. E. (2010) 'Gender and the medicalization of healthcare', pp. 107–22 in E. Kuhlmann and E. Annandale (eds), *The Palgrave Handbook of Gender and Healthcare*, London: Palgrave.

Elsevier for permission to reprint Kempner, J. (2006) 'Gendering the migraine market: do representations of illness matter?', *Social Science & Medicine*, 63: 1986–97.

Wiley for permission to reprint Adams, A. *et al.* (2008) 'The influence of patient and doctor gender on diagnosing coronary heart disease', *Sociology of Health and Illness*, 30: 1–18.

Emerald Publishing for permission to reprint Crompton, R. and Le Feuvre, N. (2003) 'Continuity and change in the gender segregation of the medical profession in Britain and France', *International Journal of Sociology and Social Policy*, 23 (4): 36–58.

NORA for permission to reprint Riska, E. (2008) 'The feminization thesis: discourses on gender and medicine', *NORA—Nordic Journal of Feminist and Gender Research*, 16 (1): 3–18.

Elsevier for permission to reprint Galdas, P. M. *et al.* (2010) 'Help seeking for cardiac symptoms: beyond the masculine–feminine binary', *Social Science & Medicine*, 71: 18–24.

Palgrave for permission to reprint Hunt, K., Adamson, J. and Galdas, P. (2010) 'Gender and help-seeking: towards gender-comparative studies', pp. 207–21 in E. Kuhlmann and E. Annandale (eds), *The Palgrave Handbook of Gender and Healthcare*, London: Palgrave.

Elsevier for permission to reprint Le Cœur, S. *et al.* (2009) 'Gender and access to HIV testing and antiretroviral treatments in Thailand: why do women have more and earlier access?', *Social Science & Medicine*, 69: 846–53.

Sage for permission to reprint Edwards, J. and van Roekel, H. (2009) 'Gender, sexuality and embodiment: access to and experience of healthcare by same-sex attracted women in Australia', *Current Sociology*, 57 (2): 193–210.

Sage for permission to reprint Beckett, K. (2006) 'Choosing Cesarean: feminism and the politics of childbirth in the United States', *Feminist Theory*, 6 (3): 251–75.

Elsevier for permission to reprint Williams, C. (2000) 'Doing health, doing gender: teenagers, diabetes and asthma', *Social Science & Medicine*, 50: 387–96.

Disclaimer

The publishers have made every effort to contact authors/copyright holders of works reprinted in *Gender and Health (Major Themes in Health and Social Welfare)*. This has not been possible in every case, however, and we would welcome correspondence from those individuals/companies whom we have been unable to trace.

INTRODUCTION

Kate Hunt and Ellen Annandale

Health systems are being transformed around the world. In many countries, the social relations of gender are also changing. These two developments do not necessarily add up to greater gender-sensitivity in the healthcare that men and women receive; indeed, the reverse is often the case. A highly complex picture emerges from the diversity of settings covered in the articles in this volume. On the one hand there is evidence of hard-set gender disparities. Yet on the other hand, the articles highlight that, be it in relation to the structure of health systems, the configuration of services, the attitudes of healthcare providers, or the help-seeking behaviours of patients, the relationship between gender and healthcare is highly varied. Above all, the combination of papers provide mounting evidence that gender inequalities and gender stereotyping have a damaging effect on the quality of care that individuals receive. This makes the papers in this volume of practical as well as theoretical interest. They are grouped into three overlapping themes: 'policy trends and health system change', 'the impact of gendered assumptions on health and healthcare', and 'accessing and experiencing healthcare'.

Part 10 Policy trends and health system change

The review by Anna Coote and Liz Kendall (**42**) draws attention to many of the themes considered in more detail in the papers that follow and serves as a useful introduction to the volume. With a focus on the UK's national health service (NHS), they look at how ideas about gender and healthcare have changed since the 1970s, raising issues relevant to other countries. It was in the 1970s that the women's movement mounted a forceful challenge to the reigning orthodoxy that 'health was a matter of biology, gender a natural phenomenon and medicine inevitably a male preserve' (**42**). The gender spotlight at this time was on the social construction of women's health and the hazards of being treated within patriarchal health systems. As noted elsewhere in these four volumes, by the mid-1990s, 'gender and health' had expanded to encompass men's health and healthcare (see also Volume I).

Coote and Kendall observe that 'there are significant differences in the ways in which women and men do things and have things done to them' in healthcare contexts. However they also emphasise that 'a one-dimensional or over-simplified view of gender will distort policy and practice' and highlight the need to take account of the 'shifting complexities of gender' (**42**). They point in particular to the dangers for the diagnosis and treatment of men and women of over-simplification and of gender-stereotyping by healthcare professionals. They end with the vital observation that 'gender is embedded in the politics of health', an observation powerfully demonstrated in the articles that follow.

The article by Clare Ungerson (**43**) considers the production of domiciliary care within the 'mixed economy of care', i.e. the marketisation and privatisation of health and social care in Britain with a particular focus upon long-term paid care for the frail elderly and disabled people. Her discussion is situated within a longstanding policy debate about the gendering of care work, which initially centered on women as carers before shifting to encompass the care work that men also undertake (see, for example, Graham 1993). Ungerson points out that women workers predominate in the paid care economy, making the point that 'paid *formal* care is far more gender skewed than unpaid *informal* care' (emphasis in original). She concludes that 'gender remains at the heart' of the care system.

In her review of health sector reform (HSR) and its implications for women's health and gender equity, Hilary Standing (**44**) turns our attention to developing countries. She highlights that, although gender is a major factor that cross-cuts other dimensions of inequality and disadvantage in relation to access to and provision of healthcare, this is not typically to the fore in HSR policies which are usually concerned with 'making more efficient use of available resources through infrastructural reforms' and widening financial options and the range of players who provide healthcare. Drawing on Cassels' framework (1995), Standing considers the gender implications of various key aspects of HSR.

Gender-mainstreaming is a policy objective that is being adopted by many health systems worldwide (see Kuhlmann and Annandale 2010). Ravindran and Kelkar-Khambete (**45**) review experiences of mainstreaming in health internationally and at different levels of care, including national health policies, programme interventions (such as maternal mortality and morbidity, quality of care initiatives), specific health projects, health research, and the training of health providers. They conclude that mainstreaming is often more about form than content and that progress typically gets stalled by such factors as the delinking of gender mainstreaming from wider social justice agendas, the adoption of top-down approaches, and the increased privatisation of healthcare and the retrenchment of the state.

Mary Zimmerman and Shirley Hill's paper (**46**) continues the theme that recent changes in health systems have done relatively little to improve women's healthcare. They analyse the gendering of healthcare in US policies and practices from the late 1960s onwards. They assess how far six broad demands of the early 'feminist consumer model of healthcare' of the late 1960s and early 1970s are met in the current managed care environment of the US. This feminist consumer model stresses: increased control over health decisions and actions; the demedicalisation of women's life events and problems; an emphasis on information, prevention, and less invasive treatment; an atmosphere of respect for women patients and healthcare providers; an emphasis on a sociomedical (rather than biomedical) model of health; and a commitment to healthcare as a right. They conclude that, although there have been some gains, managed care and other US health policies have done little to alter the gender disparity that 'is still firmly embedded in health care' (**46**).

The next selection of papers in the volume draws further attention to how gendered assumptions, either biologically and/or socially framed, can influence how health problems are construed by health professionals and how healthcare is provided.

Part 11 The impact of gendered assumptions on health and healthcare

Diana Scully and Pauline Bart's classic article from the early 1970s attends to how women were portrayed in textbooks (which they describe as the 'primary professionalisation agents for practitioners') between 1943 and 1972 (**47**). The depiction of women as first and foremost mothers, as passive and as frigid, leads them to conclude that gynaecology is an agent of social control of women, as conveyed in a quote provided from a 1968 textbook: 'If like all human beings, he [the gynaecologist] is made in the image of the Almighty, and if he is kind, then his kindness and concern for his patient may provide her with a glimpse of God's image' (Scott 1968, quoted in **47**).

Writing a decade later, Sue Fisher and Stephen Groce analyse medical conversations between women and their doctors in a US resident training programme, to 'shed light on how doctors act as secret apprentices, ferreting from their medical interactions with new women patients cultural assumptions (or norms) about these patients as "good" or "bad" women' (**48**). Kathy Davis (**49**) also explores how women's oppression manifests in the interaction between women patients and their physicians. She takes a feminist standpoint and foreshadows many issues that are still of concern for gender and health research. She laments the abiding focus on men and women as distinct groups and questions the habitual reporting that women use health services more than men and suffer more from ill-defined conditions than men; these, she rightly concludes, threaten to become self-fulfilling prophecies whilst reality is far more complex.

The issues raised so far remain important today but are subject to new twists and turns in gender health politics. Steven Epstein coins the term 'the inclusion-and-difference-paradigm' to depict how the movement for sex-based biology has led to the inclusion of women and men within medical research, but also to a 'proliferation of difference findings' and a kind of sex profiling in medicine (**50**). He argues that this is problematic because biological sex is not an either/or at the anatomic, the hormonal, or the chromosomal levels, echoing issues raised by Lynda Birke (**3**) and Anne Fausto-Sterling (**4**) in Volume I. Epstein (2007) points to several problematic results that might flow from the binary logic of sex-based medicine, such as the risk of improper treatment of a patient who does not conform to the stereotype of his or her group. More generally, in contrast to earlier feminist emphases on the demedicalisation of women's experiences and eschewal of corporate medicine, he points out that the new movement of sex-based medicine extends the scientific scrutiny of women's bodies and seems to embrace corporate ties, particularly to the pharmaceutical industry.

Susan Bell and Anne Figert (**51**) also reflect on medicalisation and bring our thinking up to date in a critical review. They argue that, although the concept of medicalisation is still useful, it tends to rely on outmoded ways of thinking about processes of control, regulation, knowledge, and power in the healthcare arena. Originally tied almost exclusively to women's health, and particularly to the control of women's bodies by a predominantly male medical profession, medicalisation processes are now seen as important in the field of men's health as the medicalisation of their reproductive and sexual health develops apace (Rosenfeld and Faircloth 2006, Conrad 2007). Bell and Figert propose that 'in a world where postmodern forms of knowledge and power circulate, medicalisation as a process is too simple and as a concept too narrow for capturing the gendered circulation of pharmaceuticals, genetics and technoscience' (**51**).

Joanna Kempner (**52**) shows how the pharmaceutical industry portrays women as the prototypical migraine sufferers (see also the paper (**36**) in Volume II on gender and images of heart disease in drug advertising in Scandinavia). While higher prevalence of migraine amongst women than amongst men appears to hold across societies, Kempner asserts this 'does not constitute sufficient evidence for assigning migraine to the exclusive purview of women'. Yet through the use of familiar tropes of femininity and feminine behaviours and the obscuring of male migraineurs, this is precisely what advertising and marketing materials do, exacerbating the existing gender bias in help-seeking, diagnosis and treatment of migraine.

Ann Adams and colleagues (**53**) address the issue of gender bias in the diagnosis and treatment of heart disease (see also, for example, Riska 2010). In order to explore 'patient gender' and 'doctor gender' effects, male and female primary care doctors in the UK and the USA were asked to watch standardised videotaped vignettes of actors portraying patients presenting with classic symptoms of coronary heart disease (CHD); the videos varied by patient age, gender, ethnicity and social class. Female doctors recalled more patient cues and paid more attention to the way that patients presented their verbal histories, particularly when the patient was female. However, they paid less attention to age for women than they did for men. The authors suggest this may mean that 'female doctors have a higher age threshold over which they will recognise potential CHD amongst women compared with men' (**53**), perhaps reflecting wider perceptions of CHD as a 'male' disease (see also paper **37**, Volume II) and a reluctance to accept that women are as prone to CHD as they age as men are.

This section concludes with two discussions of the gender configuration of the medical professional workforce. A topical issue currently is the 'feminisation' of the medical profession in many countries. Rosemary Crompton and Nicky Le Feuvre (**54**) draw on statistical data and narrative interviews with male and female general practitioners in Britain and France. Their analysis shows that it is important to seek to understand gender segregation within the medical profession not in terms of the behaviour of individual women, but rather in terms of the 'variations in professional and domestic architectures' which prevail in each national context. Elianne Riska (**55**) reflects on the meanings given to the term 'feminisation' itself. She identifies three discourses of feminisation; the sociological research discourse, the medical discourse, and the public media discourse. She found three prevalent arguments concerning the impact of women's increase in the medical profession across all three. These were that structural changes in medicine are caused by an influx of women into the profession; a 'vision that nothing can stop women' who are 'taking over medicine'; and the proposition that an older, more 'humane tradition of medicine will be revived with the aid of women'.

Part 12 Accessing and experiencing healthcare

In this final section we turn from health systems and healthcare providers to the relationship between gender and how patients access and negotiate healthcare. Drawing on in-depth interviews with men and women in British Columbia, Paul Galdas and colleagues (**56**) explore the role of gender in help-seeking for acute cardiac symptoms. Although they found that help-seeking was often aligned with stereotypical ideals of 'stoic men' and 'vulnerable accommodating women', 'men's and women's experience were not easily parsed into distinct binary patterns'. Rather, men and women were found to share behaviours typically defined as 'masculine' and 'feminine'. The authors reinforce Epstein's (2007) point that 'gender-sensitive' health promotion messages may actually back-fire as they often rest on misguided gender ideals. Kate Hunt and colleagues (**57**) also question the strongly held belief that men and women behave in intrinsically different ways in their use of health services. They problematise binary assumptions about gender that translate into the belief that men delay their help-seeking longer than women, and that this 'delay' is inherently problematic. They critically analyse published research to challenge the 'universality' of men's 'reluctance' to seek help. They also highlight how little gender-comparative research on help-seeking takes account of underlying morbidity.

The multifaceted and context-sensitive nature of gender and help seeking and provision of treatment is highlighted further in Sophie Le Coeur and colleagues' (**58**) research on gender and access to HIV testing and antiretroviral treatments (ART) in community hospitals in northern Thailand. Unexpectedly they found that, although more men are infected with HIV than women, proportionally more women were receiving ART. In the context of research on gender and healthcare which often points to women's disadvantage, it is instructive to note their conclusion that 'women appear to have a double advantage in both diagnosis and treatment'. The reasons for this are complex, but include factors associated with the 'evolving dynamics of the HIV epidemic, the initial prioritisation of mothers for treatment and earlier access to HIV testing for women' (**58**).

Jane Edwards and Helen van Roekel (**59**) explore the relatively neglected issue of how same-sex attracted women negotiate primary healthcare. Their research, based on in-depth interviews in rural Australia, is a nuanced account of the intricate ways in which women evaluated their general practitioners on 'how well they treat women's bodies'. They show how these same-sex attracted women 'selectively and strategically' employed 'discourses of gender, sexuality and embodiment to structure and evaluate healthcare' (**59**).

Katherine Beckett's (**60**) theoretical deliberation on elective cesarean section also explores the theme of women's assessments about what kind of care is best for them. She continues a longstanding interest in women and childbirth, and problematises both the alternative/natural birth movement position that choosing a cesarean is capitulation to the inappropriate biomedical depiction of birth as high risk and the stance of 'third wave feminist critics' and of medical advocates that this choice can reflect a considered appreciation of high-tech birth.

Clare Williams' paper (**61**) reminds us that healthcare is not solely the dominion of formal health systems; patients themselves can be considered as health workers (Stacey 1988; Olesen 2002). Drawing on interviews in London, she explores how the 'social constructions of femininities and masculinities affect how teenagers live with asthma or diabetes'. Her discussion brings us back to 'doing' health as a form of 'doing gender' (see Volume I and West and Zimmerman 1987, and Volume IV in relation to smoking and drinking). Teenagers in her study managed their illnesses in gendered ways. Girls showed greater adaptation, incorporating their regimens into their daily lives and making them part of their identities. Boys, by contrast, strove to keep asthma and diabetes out of their identities in the manner of 'passing' (Goffman 1963). Williams signals that girls' greater adaptability to their condition could be disadvantageous, as they 'often lowered expectations for themselves', especially when this was combined with the 'detrimental gendered effects of diet and exercise' (**61**). The feeling of control of their bodies and their condition that most boys displayed was often associated with managing well, although a small minority who did not feel in control were unable to 'pass' and suffered disparaged identities.

The articles in this volume are varied in the health issues that they address and the health systems and levels of care that they focus on. Drawn from the 1970s to the early twenty-first century, they conjure a picture of a long road travelled to draw associations between gender and healthcare together. Nonetheless, it is also clear that there is still some long way to go before we reach a full understanding. To return to a point made by Coote and Kendall, 'the evidence suggests a complex and often contradictory picture'; that is, there are differences in men and women's health experiences, but these 'are not always in line with prevailing assumptions about gender differences' (**42**). Researchers and practitioners have only recently begun to appreciate the need to reconcile an awareness that gender matters in healthcare: it can influence how patients seek care and be important in the diagnosis and treatment of health problems; and can also prevent gender-stereotyping and binary thinking which could lead to unsafe care.

References

Cassels, A. (1995) *Health Sector Reform: Key Issues in Less Developed Countries*. WHO Forum on Health Sector Reform, Discussion Paper No. 1 (SHS/NHP/95.4). Geneva: World Health Organisation.

Conrad, P. (2007) *The Medicalization of Society*. Baltimore: Johns Hopkins University Press.

Epstein, S. (2007) *Inclusion: The Politics of Difference in Medical Research*. Chicago: University of Chicago Press.

Goffman, E. (1963) *Stigma*. Englewood Cliffs, NJ: Prentice Hall.

Graham, H. (1993) 'Social divisions in caring', *Women's Studies International Forum* 16: 461–70.

Kuhlmann, E. and Annandale, E. (2010) 'Bringing gender to the heart of health policy, practice and research', pp. 1–17 in E. Kuhlmann and E. Annandale (eds) *The Palgrave Handbook of Gender and Healthcare*. London: Palgrave.

Olesen, V. (2002) 'Resisting "fatal unclutteredness"', pp. 254–66 in G. Bendelow, M. Carpenter, C. Vautier and S. Williams (eds) *Gender, Health and Healing*. London: Routledge.

Riska, E. (2010) 'Coronary heart disease: gendered public health discourses', pp. 154–71 in E. Kuhlmann and E. Annandale (eds) *The Palgrave Handbook of Gender and Healthcare*. London: Palgrave.

Rosenfeld, D. and Faircloth, C. (eds) (2006) *Medicalized Masculinities*. Philadelphia: Temple University Press.

Scott, C. Russell (1968) *The World of a Gynecologist*. London: Oliver & Boyd.

Stacey, M. (1988) *The Sociology of Health and Healing*. London: Unwin Hyman.

West, C. and Zimmerman, P. (1987) 'Doing gender', *Gender and Society* 1: 125–51.

Part 10

POLICY TRENDS AND HEALTH SYSTEM CHANGE

42
WELL WOMEN AND MEDICINE MEN
Gendering the health policy agenda

Anna Coote and Liz Kendall

Source: A. Coote (ed.), *The New Gender Agenda*, London: IPPR, 2000, pp. 149–60.

Health and healthcare are profoundly affected by sex and gender differences. Indeed, there are few aspects of human health or of any conventional healthcare system that are not experienced differently by men and women or shaped by physical or social differences between them.

Right across the spectrum, from bodily functions and personal behaviour, through morbidity and mortality rates, to attitudes to disease and medicine, patterns of demand for services, and employment in health-related professions, there are significant differences in the ways in which women and men do things and have things done to them. But there is nothing simple about this. In strikingly similar ways, gender and health are both products of a complex interplay of biological and shifting social, economic and environmental factors. Public policy is much better informed now than it was – say – ten years ago about the construction of gender and of health. Inevitably, though, understanding has developed in fits and starts and remains unevenly distributed in opinion-forming and policy-making circles. It is still common to hear leading politicians, health care professionals and media commentators conflate health with the National Health Service, as though dealing with the 'crisis in the NHS' were really the only way to solve the nation's health problems. Just as often, similar voices are heard addressing the problem of 'teenage pregnancy' in terms that suggest girls achieve it singlehandedly, or discussing the 'family responsibilities' of employees as though they had nothing to do with men.

The comparison cannot be pushed too far. One important difference is that health – as opposed to health care – has always been on the policy agenda. Its ranking in the hierarchy has varied but only for the last half-century has it been treated as a second order issue. Gender has, until relatively recently, been overlooked or uncontested, except in the margins of political debate. Gender politics run much deeper in society than do the politics of science, clinical autonomy and welfarism that have combined to promote the cause of health services above that of the nation's health and well-being. In both cases, though, there are conflicts of interest and imbalances of power that serve to downplay or disempower one 'side' in favour of the other. And it is gradually becoming more widely recognised that this ultimately has negative consequences for both. If public policy fails adequately to prevent ill-health, to promote better health and to tackle health inequalities between different groups in the population, the National Health Service must pick up the increasingly expensive pieces. If public policy persists in assuming that gender roles are simple and satisfactorily fixed, men as well as women will find their opportunities unfairly limited and their quality of life seriously impaired.

In this chapter we argue, with health as our example, that a one-dimensional or over-simplified view of gender will distort policy and practice. In order to be relevant and effective, decision-making requires a sophisticated understanding of the multiple determinants of health and the shifting complexities of gender, as well as the relationships between health and gender – and how these bear upon the changing dynamics of power within the health sector. We look first at how ideas about gender and health have developed since the 1970s, and at some of the differences between women's and men's health and their relationship with health services. We then consider the lessons for health policy.

Ideas about health and gender

The relationship between gender and health did not become explicit in mainstream political or sociological discourse until the 1970s. The orthodoxy, until then, was that health was a matter of biology, gender a natural phenomenon and medicine inevitably a male preserve. Men of science fought gladiatorial battles against disease within the human body, over which they ranged as if by right. Health was the product of victory in battle and patients – male and female – were the passive beneficiaries. Feminists challenged the orthodoxy, asserting women's ownership of their bodies, the value of their experiential knowledge, the fallibility of the medical establishment, and their right to participate in their own health care on their own terms (Phillips and Rakusen, 1996). The new women's movement campaigned for access to effective birth control, including abortion, and for more female-friendly health care and maternity services.

At the same time, feminist researchers had begun to trace links between women's ill-health and the unequal distribution of power and opportunity between women and men. By the late 1970s a new paradigm had emerged that emphasised the social construction of gender, the impact of gender on health, the differences between men's and women's healthcare requirements, and the need to focus on the specifics of women's health (Hunt and Annandale 1999, Annandale and Hunt, 2000).

Relatively simple connections were made at first between aspects of women's health and their subordination in a patriarchal system. It was argued, for example, that women were disadvantaged by the fact that the male-dominated medical professions overlooked or misunderstood their health problems and/or treated them as second-class patients; if women were treated more like men, they would enjoy better health services and eventually better health.

But over the next two decades a more sophisticated analysis took shape. This was heavily influenced by feminists as well as by proponents of the 'new public health' who insisted on a holistic view of health and its determinants (Ashton and Seymour 1998). Broadly, it sought to understand gender in the context of race, ethnicity and social class, and health as a product of the interplay between biological, psycho-social, economic and environmental factors (Bird and Rieker 1999). It acknowledged shifting patterns of influence – within and between groups, and across the life cycle. It took more interest in gender comparisons, rather than targeting women's health and eventually the specifics of *men*'s health became a new focus of concern. In 1992, the Chief Medical Officer's Annual Report drew attention to differences between male and female morbidity and mortality rates (Department of Health, 1993). In 1994 the Royal College of Nursing established a Men's Health Forum, promoting the case for more and better health services for men.

Men's and women's health

Once the spotlight had shifted, it was hard to imagine how men's health had failed to attract attention. Men were dying, on average, five years younger than women. Boys born in 1996 could expect to live to 75, compared with 80 for women (Equal Opportunities Commission 1998). Between the ages of 20 and 24, vehicle accidents and suicides helped to drive up the male death rate to nearly three times the rate for women. Across the whole of adult life, death rates were higher for men than for women for all the major causes of death, including cancer and cardiovascular disease (Acheson 1998).

Some (notably in the misogynist school of journalism) have argued that, in asserting women's health needs, feminism has distorted the picture and eclipsed the more serious needs of men. A more defensible argument is that the case for men's health would not have been made at all if feminists had not put gender on the policy map. This prompted men (and women) to investigate masculinities and how these are shaped by social and economic circumstances. This, in turn, is beginning to shed some light on why men die younger than women and what might help to safeguard their health.

Gender is now, so to speak, out in the open. But how much is known about the specifics of men's and women's experiences of health and health care, and the differences between them? There is certainly a wealth of information, but it often seems to beg more questions than it answers. Many of the changes in men's and women's lives and life choices are not captured by statistics. All we can do in this short chapter is to offer some visible evidence of the range of contradictions and uncertainties that prevail. Broadly, these fall into four categories: mortality and morbidity rates; health-related behaviours; patterns of health service use and employment and status in the National Health Service.[1]

Mortality and morbidity

- Overall life expectancy has increased for both sexes over the last century and a half, but the gap between them has grown. Between 1841 and 1991, male life expectancy increased from 41 to 73, while female life expectancy increased from 43 to 79. Only recently has the gap begun to narrow very slightly.
- Poverty and ill-health are closely related. Women's income over lifetime is significantly lower than men's. Yet, using the Townsend index as a measure of deprivation, the least well off women have lower mortality rates than the most well off men.
- Boys appear to have higher rates of chronic physical illness in childhood, as well as higher rates of psychological disorder. This pattern is reversed in early-to-mid adolescence, when rates for both are higher for girls.
- Women suffer more from poor mental health, especially from anxiety and depressive disorders. Lone mothers are particularly prone to ill-health, even after controlling for household income, employment status and occupation. However, men are a lot more likely to commit suicide, especially in young adulthood.
- While women can expect to live five years longer than men, their expectation of a healthy life is only 2-3 years longer. Fewer than one in five men over 85 are unable to go out and walk down the road, compared with nearly one in two women in the same age group.
- It has been claimed that 'men and women have different perceptions of their own and each others' health' (Lloyd 1996). While men and women have similar concepts of health, both see men as healthier. Men stress being fit, strong, energetic, physically active and being in control, while women stress not being ill and never seeing a doctor (Saltonstall R). Men are more likely see exercise as more important than food and rest, whilst women see food, rest and then exercise as important (Blaxter 1990).
- Recent research examined the differences among men and among women (rather than between them) in how they rated their own health. When

they were sorted by social class, gender appeared to make no difference. But when education was used instead of class as a measure of socio-economic status, the study found greater inequality among men at age 33 for limiting long-standing illness and respiratory symptoms, but greater inequality among women for poor rated health at age 23 and psychological distress at age 33.

Health related behaviour

- Men appear to take more risks with their health (through sport, through dangerous or violent activities and, classically, through war). Young men are much more likely to die from an accident than young women: 40 per cent of premature deaths among 16–24-year-old men are due to accidents, compared with 24 per cent for women in the same age group. Yet accidental death is associated with lower socio-economic status and, when measured by employment status, as it usually is, low socio-economic status is more common among young women than young men (Colhoun and Prescott-Clarke 1996).
- Men are more likely to drink than women, and to drink more. In 1997 27 per cent of men drank more than 21 units per week, while only 14 per cent of women drank more than 14 units. However, the proportion of 18–24 year old women drinking more than 14 units a week has risen from 15 per cent in 1984 to 24 per cent in 1996. Drinking rates among professional women have also risen during this period.
- The proportion of 15-year-old girls who smoke has risen from 22 per cent in 1988 to 33 per cent in 1996. But overall, men still smoke more than women (30 per cent compared with 27 per cent of women) and smoking rates have recently increased among younger men aged 16 to 34 – from 33 per cent in 1993 to 39 per cent in 1996. (Department of Health, 1998.)
- Men are more likely to be overweight than women, (45 per cent compared with 34 per cent), but women are more likely to be obese (18 per cent compared with 16 per cent). Weight also varies by social class, with men and women in manual occupations more likely to be obese or overweight than those in professional groups.

Patterns of health service use

- Boys are between 30 and 40 per cent more likely than girls to have consulted their GP for a serious condition, but 10 per cent less likely to have done so for a minor illness.
- Women are more likely to consult their GP than men, particularly under the age of 45. In 1996-7, one in five women aged 16–44 had consulted their GP in the fortnight prior to their interview with the General

Household survey, compared with one in 10 men in the same age group. The proportion of men and women consulting their GP has increased since 1971, but the increase has been greater among women.
- It is widely assumed that women are more ready than men to report illness and to seek help. Men – by contrast – are thought to be reluctant visitors to surgeries. So when they do go, their complaints are somehow presumed to have a more serious content. But this is not supported by evidence, according to Professor Sally Macintyre, of the Medical Research Council (MRC) social and public health sciences unit, in Glasgow. Her analysis of data from the MRC's common cold unit has shown that men 'over-rate' their sniffles, sore throats, headaches, and shivers compared with ratings given by clinical observers, while women under-rate their symptoms (McKie 2000).
- Although older women are substantially more likely to experience functional impairment in mobility and personal self-care than men of the same age, there is little difference between women and men in their reporting of self-assessed health and limiting longstanding illness – regardless of marital status, social class, income and housing tenure.
- When a group of 192 doctors examined male and female actors playing the part of patients suffering identically from chest pains and shortness of breath, they were much more likely to arrive at a cardiac diagnosis in men, and to rate women as suffering from emotional problems and recommend psychiatric treatment (McKie 2000).

Employment in health services

- Women account for 33 per cent of hospital doctors, 31 per cent of GPs and 21 per cent of consultants. Their share of jobs in health professions has increased significantly in the last 10 years. In 1998, women accounted for 56 per cent of the new intake into medical school. But they remain under-represented among surgeons (less than five per cent) and among senior consultants in all fields. (Millar 2000)
- Nursing, health visiting, midwifery and community nursing are predominantly female professions.

Lessons for health policy

The evidence suggests a complex and often contradictory picture. Men and women have different health experiences, but these are changing as men's and women's social and economic circumstances change, and are not always in line with prevailing assumptions about gender differences. The causes of health and ill-health clearly need to be sought beneath the surface of official statistics, in the shifting relationships between social change and individual choice. For example, very little of the data about different male and female mortality rates are adequately explained. If policy-makers are serious about tackling inequalities in health, this needs much more careful consideration.

Men and women may react differently – and in ways that may affect their mental or physical health – to different conditions. Adolescence appears to bring more risk of psychological disorder to females more than to males, with consequences for the physical health of young women (Sweeting 1994). There are conventions of masculinity that affect the way men regard their bodies and risk taking, making them more prone to accidents and injury and more careless about the adverse effects of behaviour on their health. 'The ideal male body suffers no pain or weakness, is never ill and never breaks down . . . [but if it does] This experience may even challenge a man's sense of his masculinity . . . In discourses on masculinity it is often suggested that to be a man is to invite, rather than to avoid, risk.' (Petersen and Lupton, 1996)

Unemployment may be more of a blow to self-esteem for men in their early 20s than for women – at least as long as the tradition of men being the family breadwinner persists. Young women can derive a sense of purpose and an adult identity from early parenthood. But young men who don't have jobs (or jobs that mean anything to them) have to earn their rites of passage to adulthood in other ways, often depending more heavily on their peers and on 'proving' themselves through risky or challenging behaviour (Coote 1993).

Michael Marmot's much-quoted Whitehall studies have indicated an important link between health and the extent to which people feel in control of their lives. He found that ill-health had less to do with income or one's place in the workplace hierarchy, than with the relationship between the levels of demand put on individuals and how far they can control their own work and its outcomes (van Rossum *et al.* 2000). Power and control are available to men and women – and hold meaning for them – in different ways. Not just at work, but in the rest of life too. This affects the distribution of resources which, in turn, may affect the quality of individuals' lives and their sense of well-being.

So in understanding the causes of ill-health, we need to consider how social and economic change affects gender and how changing gender roles affect health. As paid employment becomes more significant to the identity of women, will that mean that unemployment carries a greater health risk for them? If men play a greater role in parenting, deriving from it an enhanced sense of purpose and identity, could that mean that they would find it easier to cope with spells of unemployment? As lone parenthood becomes more commonplace and less stigmatised, is it less likely to be correlated with ill-health in women? Or is the fact that lone mothers are considered a deviant social model less detrimental to health than the burden of bringing up children alone?

These are all things that need to be better understood in order to tackle inequalities in health and to improve the health of men and women. There are now some experimental health improvement strategies that are designed to reach men through their masculinity. 'Alive and Kicking', for example, is a Midlands-based health outreach project organised around amateur football teams. The aim is to raise awareness of health issues with young men, and help them develop healthier lifestyles, using a multi-agency approach.

But there are dangers in oversimplifying the picture. One danger is that health improvement strategies will entrench gender stereotyping (for example, underscoring the message that competitive sport is a 'manly' pursuit). Another danger is that the differences *among* men and *among* women will be overlooked. That is why we need a complex understanding not only of the multiple determinants of health, and of the multiple components of gender – but also of the interaction between gender and other factors, including ethnicity, education, employment, income and environment.

As Macintyre and others have commented, the view that women experience more ill health but on average die later than men has become so well-entrenched that 'over-generalisation has become the norm, with inconsistencies and complexities in patterns of gender differences in health being overlooked. In the face of an apparently clear pattern, there has been a tendency to downplay (or maybe not even to report) data that conflict with rather than confirm the general pattern'. (Macintyre, Hunt and Sweeting, 1999).

This complex analysis is important not only for understanding why men and women get ill and how they might improve their health, but also, as we have seen, for accurate diagnosis and treatment. If clinicians make stereotyped assumptions about the diseases to which men and women are prone, or about male and female patterns of interpreting and reporting symptoms, they could do more harm than good. Women suffering from heart disease are evidently vulnerable to misdiagnosis. More generally, if the notion of women as neurotic or hysterical complainers persists, then it is more likely that their complaints will be underrated by clinicians.

Equally important is the relationship between patterns of employment of men and women in the health service and the character and quality of treatment and care – and health policy more generally. There is still a significant gender divide within the health services and there is some evidence that this affects health outcomes. One study showed that general practices with female doctors, young doctors or more practice nurses had lower rates of teenage pregnancy (Hippisley-Cox *et al.* 2000). The attitudes of clinicians and the quality of their relationships with service users are likely to be influenced by gender, age and ethnicity because their professional behaviour and judgements inevitably draw on their personal experience as well as their training. Their attitudes and relationships can, in turn, elicit a more or less positive response from service users, making their interventions more, or less, effective.

Most of the leading positions in the NHS are occupied by men. By and large they control the Department of Health, the NHS Executive, the major hospitals, most health authorities, almost all of the prestige specialist units in acute care and the all-important Royal Colleges, except the Royal College of Nursing. The President of one of the Royal Colleges was heard at a London seminar in 2000 to refer to the Minister for Public Health (Yvette Cooper) as 'What's her name – that little girl.'[2] We should not become so dazzled by the shifting nature of gender relations that we overlook the way in which male hegemony and an unreconstructed masculine view of the world prevail in the upper echelons of health policy and health care. Men still rule and it is *not* okay.

Traditional structures outlive the circumstances that created them: they defend sectional interests by helping to stave off the adjustments that are needed to work constructively with change. This may help to explain why it has been so difficult to shift priorities away from the 'battle against disease' towards a more holistic approach which puts health improvement, prevention, mental health and care of long-tem chronic conditions higher up the agenda. It may help to explain why power and the lion's share of resources, remain – in spite of much political rhetoric to the contrary – with the traditionally prestigious areas of acute healthcare. It certainly helps to explain why it has taken so long for nurses to play a bigger role in general practice. And why informal carers (usually grandmothers, mothers or daughters) – who in fact provide the backbone of healthcare – have been having such a hard time gaining recognition and a voice in shaping services.

Arguably, it also helps to explain why New Labour's public health agenda is so fixated on disease-based targets. Traditional forms of audit and evaluation, such as epidemiological studies and randomised control trials are a product and property of the traditional scientific establishment. They belong at the top of a 'hierarchy of evidence' by which other methods (such as observation, narrative and the views of service users) are judged inferior. Though invaluable for some purposes, they are less helpful in appraising strategies aimed at influencing the subtler, long-term developments in culture and social relations that are needed to address the root causes of ill health and inequality. At a time of diminishing confidence in scientific expertise, a strong focus on controlled evaluation can help to fend off public distrust. But traditional methodologies exert a powerful restraint on innovation and change. Policies that cannot be tested in a controlled environment, or that otherwise fail to produce easily measurable results, are regarded with suspicion. Decision-makers committed to 'evidence based medicine' and 'evidence based' policies would rather focus on what can be counted – such as the numbers of 'preventable deaths' from specific causes. This is one reason why the goal of developing 'healthy neighbourhoods' set out in New Labour's public health Green Paper *Our Healthier Nation*, gave way to goals aimed at reducing mortality rates in the subsequent White Paper, *Saving Lives*. The latter keeps health policy safely inside the traditional territory of professional medicine. The former is a messier objective, with multiple components, no scientific methods to rely upon and far less predictable outcomes. It requires the involvement of communities – and that means devolving power. As Bea Campbell has pointed out, women play a central role in communities, especially in deprived areas (Campbell, 1993). If the goal of healthier neighbourhoods is to be pursued, public sector institutions, including the NHS, need to understand the way women experience the world, in order to engage effectively with them. And they must be prepared to share power with them – not as patients but as partners in the production of better health. There are some promising examples of women leading innovations in local health improvement – such as the 'community mothers' scheme in Sparkbrook, Birmingham. But so far these are marginal to government health policy, which remains preoccupied with successive crises in acute care.

It would be facile to suggest that change is being resisted because men still dominate health policy-making. Many defenders of tradition in the health sector are female. Many advocates of the new health agenda are male. More to the point, the same historical factors that encouraged the emergence of feminism in the latter 20th century have undermined the orthodoxies of the medical world. The infallibility of science, the plausibility of a paternalistic, cradle-to-grave welfare state and the Victorian model of gender relations have all been challenged over the same period. Each challenge has a different dynamic, but all reflect – and owe their potency to – the same interplay of social and economic developments. Broadly, they arise because society has become more individualised and commodified, and because men and women are better educated, have a wider range of choices in how they live and are more inclined to want to decide for themselves, rather than be told what to do. As communications technologies and economic power become increasingly globalised, there is a growing awareness of risks affecting individuals, organisations, nations and the entire planet, which traditional political and professional institutions are manifestly ill-equipped to manage. All this has profound implications for the way decisions are made and implemented, in health and in other sectors. Individuals and organisations are having to negotiate new ways of living with uncertainty and change. Consequently, relations are changing between doctors and patients, between policy-makers and citizens and between men and women.

The same forces that have enabled women – and, more recently, men – to challenge assumptions about gender roles also impel them to question received wisdom about medicine and government, and to distrust experts and politicians who claim to know what is best for them. This is not a temporary blip in human behaviour, but a sea-change in the way society works and how it seeks and accommodates change. Policy makers must work with new patterns of attitude and behaviour. Traditional lines of authority are frayed to breaking point. Top-down instruction will have to give way to dialogue and reciprocal learning, with the internet playing an increasingly significant role. New weight must be given to the 'lay expertise' of those who experience illnesses, therapies and health services at first hand. Responsibility for change and attendant risks must be shared between individuals, community-level groups and organisations, and different layers of government.

Strikingly, both the green paper *Our Healthier Nation* and the subsequent white paper, *Saving Lives*, have called for a new, three-way 'contract' between the individual, the 'community' and national government – an approach that appears characteristic of 'third way' thinking. If any such 'contract' is to be effective, then the partners must have a clear view of each others' strengths and weaknesses, and how they can contribute, separately and together, to health improvement. Government will need to open itself up so that it can be better understood. It must acknowledge the complex ways in which social and economic circumstances, as well as gender, age and ethnicity, influence the behaviour of individuals and groups. It must use the resources of the state to build the capacity of individuals and groups to play their part to the full. And it must be prepared to share power with those it cannot directly control.

However, more traditional currents inside national government and the NHS are pulling in contrary directions. These favour professional hierarchies, cling to assumptions about medicine as a magic bullet and seek safety in policies that have measurable outputs. Their protagonists want change – a 'modern, dependable' NHS – but see change as best achieved by consolidating power at the centre, giving local leadership to one kind of doctor (general practitioners) at the expense of others (hospital consultants), and improving systems of management to speed up treatment, use beds more efficiently and reduce waiting lists. They are lukewarm about empowering patients and citizens because that cuts across their desire to centralise control. They are generally at ease in a system run by white middle class men and find the politics of gender and difference uncongenial. Traditional reformers of this kind are more powerful in Blairite circles than the more radical proponents of power-sharing and health strategies built from the bottom up. The 'third way' is sufficiently elastic to accommodate them, but they act as a brake on progress towards health improvement and greater health equality because they insist on the primacy of the NHS agenda, which is more about illness than health. Thus, while men are not responsible as such for resisting change, gender is an important part of the picture. More men than women derive power and status from the health system as it stands and therefore have an interest in defending the status quo. Paradoxically, it does not appear to be doing them any favours in terms of their life expectancy. A shift away from tradition, towards a broader and more innovative agenda, may be good for their health as well as for women's.

Conclusion

We set out to consider why gender should be of interest to those involved in health policy. First and foremost, it matters for reasons of equity in health.

If health policy-makers are committed to reducing inequalities, then the fact that men die younger than women must be taken into account. There is an urgent need to know more about why people are healthy and why they get ill and how the health of men and women are affected differently by their different (and similar) life experiences.

Secondly, if policy-makers are committed to making health care more appropriate and effective, then they must take account of the different needs of men and women that are due to biological as well as social-economic factors, and to the ways in which the attitudes and behaviour of healthcare practitioners and their relationships with patients are influenced by gender.

Thirdly, gender is embedded in the politics of health. Those trying to change priorities – for example, by shifting resources towards tackling the root causes of illness – need to understand why change is required (or, indeed, inevitable) and why it is resisted. On both counts, a gendered analysis is helpful.

That said, a great deal depends on how gender is taken into account in each of these fields of interest. A stereotyped view of gender is as likely to distort policy and practice as is the more traditional tendency of 'gender-blindness'. What matters is acknowledging the complexities of gender and how roles and identities change over time – and how, in turn, these affect health, its determinants, health care and health policy.

Notes

1 Except where specifically referenced, data in the rest of this section are taken from Acheson, 1998; Equal Opportunities 1998 and *Social Science & Medicine* (48), 1999.
2 Author's observation.

References

Acheson D. (1998) *Report of the Independent Inquiry into Inequalities in Health* London: Stationery Office.
Annandale E. and Hunt K. (2000) *Gender Inequalities and Health* Buckingham: Oxford University Press.
Ashton J. and Seymour H. (1998) *The New Public Health* Oxford University Press, Oxford.
Bird C. E. and Rieker P. P. (1999) 'Gender matters: an integrated model for understanding men's and women's health' in *Social Science & Medicine* 48, 745–755.
Blaxter M. (1990) *Health and Lifestyles* London: Tavistock/Routledge.
Campbell B. (1993) *Goliath* London: Methuen.
Colhoun H. and Prescott-Clarke P. (1996) in Department of Health, *Health Survey for England, 1994* London: Stationery Office.
Coote A. (ed) (1993) *Families, Children and Crime* London: IPPR.
Department of Health (1993) *On the State of the Public Health 1992: The Annual Report of the Chief Medical Officer* London: Stationery Office.

Equal Opportunities Commission (1998) *Social Focus on Women and Men* Office for National Statistics, London: Stationery Office.

Hippisley-Cox J. *et al.* (2000) 'Association between teenage pregnancy rates and the age and sex of general practitioners: cross sectional survey in Trent 1994–7) *British Medical Journal* 320, 842–5.

Hunt K. and Annandale E. (1999) 'Relocating gender and morbidity: examining men's and women's health in contemporary Western societies' in *Social Science & Medicine* 48, 1–5.

Lloyd T. (1996) *Men's Health Review.* Prepared on behalf of the Men's Health Forum, Royal College of Nursing.

Macintyre S., Hunt K. and Sweeting H. (1996) 'Gender differences in health: are things really as simple as they seem?' in *Social Science & Medicine* 42, 617–642.

McKie R. (2000) 'Moaning men push women to back of the health queue' *Observer* 7 May, 8.

Millar B. (2000) 'Not there yet' *Health Service Journal* 17 February, 24–7.

Petersen A. and Lupton D. (1996) *The new public health: health and self in the age of risk* London: Sage.

Phillips A. and Rakusen J. (1996, revised edition) *The New Our Bodies Ourselves* (British edition) London: Penguin.

Saltonstall R. (1993) 'Healthy Bodies, Social Bodies: Men's and Women's Concepts and Practices of Health in Everyday Life' *Social Science & Medicine* 36 (1), 7–14.

Social Science & Medicine (Special Edition) 48, 1999.

Sweeting H. (1994) 'Reversals of fortune? Sex differences in health in childhood and adolescence' in *Social Science & Medicine* 40, 77–90.

van Rossum C. T. M., Shipley M. J., van de Mheen H., Grobbee D. E., Marmot M. G. (2000) 'Employment grade differences in cause specific mortality. A 25-year follow up of civil servants from the first Whitehall study' *Journal of Epidemiology and Community Health* 54, 178–184.

43
THINKING ABOUT THE PRODUCTION AND CONSUMPTION OF LONG-TERM CARE IN BRITAIN
Does gender still matter?

Clare Ungerson

Source: *Journal of Social Policy*, 29 (2000), 623–43.

Abstract

This article suggests that the literature on care, which originally was heavily influenced by a gendered perspective, has now taken on other important variables. However, it is argued that if we look at the particular impact of the marketisation and privatisation of long-term care, we can see that gender is still a useful perspective on the production of care, especially paid care. The reordering of the delivery of domiciliary care within the 'mixed economy of welfare' is having important effects on the labour market for care and is likely to lead to further inequalities between women, both now and in old age. The article proceeds to look at the impact of these inequalities on the consumption of care in old age, particularly by elderly women and considers factors that may provide women with the resources to purchase care and/or pay charges for care. The article argues that gender does still matter, but that its impact has to be understood within a context of growing inequalities between women, and an analysis that takes account of wider social and economic relations within kin networks and between generations.

The modern literature on 'care' has its foundations in a gendered perspective on the operations of the welfare state, and owes a great deal to the pioneering work of British feminist writers coming from within social policy (Finch and Groves, 1980; Land, 1978; Finch and Groves, 1983). Over the past ten years, as one might expect given the general trends of social science analysis, the caring literature has slowly moved away from the emphasis on gender towards a critique which reflects the growing interest in diversity and difference. In a series of articles in the early 1990s (1991; 1993; 1997), Hilary Graham suggested that feminist perspectives on care had 'become fixed in the form in which they developed in the early 1980s' (Graham, 1997:124). She pleaded for a more 'fluid and open-ended framework' that could take class and race as well as gender into account in the caring literature. Since she began to write in this vein, there has been a growth of literature on care which has looked at care and 'race', notably Askham *et al.* (1995) who consider the allocation of social service resources to black elders, and Ahmad and Atkin (1996) who have collected together a number of wide-ranging essays concerning general issues embedded in 'race' and community care. Class and care has been investigated by Arber and Ginn (1992) who use the General Household Survey data set to argue that resources are an important determinant of informal care since those with higher incomes are less likely to be involved in co-resident care and are more able to maintain 'intimacy at a distance'.

The original focus on women as carers has also, in the British literature, been reconfigured within a gendered perspective to focus on men as carers (Arber and Gilbert, 1989; Bytheway, 1987; Fisher, 1994). The series of General Household Surveys (1985, 1990, 1995) which looked at informal care has now established the comparably high proportion of men who claim to be informal carers – in the most recent 1995 survey, 11 per cent of men said they were carers compared to 14 per cent of women (Rowlands, 1998, Table 1). This evidence, plus the secondary data analysis of Parker and Lawton (1991), has established the new category of 'spouse care' which most men carers are engaged in. It is now clear that the early feminist literature had overemphasised the inter-generational aspects of care at the cost of ignoring care between spouses. Finally, the third stream of literature, and the one that has probably had the greatest impact, has been that taken by disabled writers such as Jenny Morris and Lois Keith. In their work, dating from the early 1990s, they have been critical of the feminist literature's assumption that the care relationship consists of 'carer' and 'dependant' and that disabled people are without agency (Keith, 1992; Morris, 1991; 1996). In that sense these commentators have used the original ideas of second wave feminism to make claims for visibility in social analysis in exactly the same way as feminists in the 1960s and 1970s did. This critique has been very successful in shifting the gendered analysis of care away from a dichotomous discussion of 'carer' and 'dependant' towards a commentary that recognises the value of independent living for all disabled people.

The purpose of this article is to recover gender, and, most particularly, a focus on women, as a way of understanding the production of care for frail elderly and disabled people. In doing so, it looks particularly at *paid* care. Paid care of elderly people is a growing phenomenon in Britain. Data from the Labour Force Survey, analysed by Yeandle (1999), demonstrates that paid care work (in the form of 'assistant nurses and auxiliaries' and 'care assistants and attendants') grew between 1992 and 1998 by 34 per cent to a total of 652,880 jobs in 1998. Moreover, what is particularly striking about these jobs is their gendered nature. In 1998, 91 per cent of these employees were female (although, as Yeandle points out (p. 13) there has been a slight increase in the proportion of men employed in paid care, largely due to rapid entry of men into the growing sector of care assistance and attendance). Such predominance of women in this sector means that, in effect, paid *formal* care is far more gender skewed than unpaid *informal* care. Thus a focus on paid care has to be analysed within a gendered perspective. This article considers the way in which the new community care system put in place in Britain in the early 1990s, with its emphasis on marketisation and privatisation of care provision, is impacting on and is likely to continue to affect, the labour market for care. In turn, it suggests that the reorganisation of the production of care will impact on the consumption of long-term care, especially in old age, and that there are gendered implications. However, it should also become clear that 'gender' pure and simple is not an altogether satisfactory way of understanding social divisions and care; income inequalities and the opportunity to acquire social rights during a working life are equally important and point to ways in which 'gender' is increasingly cross-cut by income and labour market inequality, both between women and men, and between women.

The immediacy of the need to consider whether gender still matters arises out of the recent publication of the Royal Commission on Long Term Care (1999). This lengthy document, complete with three volumes of research papers, mentions sex and gender hardly at all, except within a discussion of the future supply of informal, unpaid care (pp. 15–18). Throughout the report and the research volumes, those in need of care are referred to using the gender-free term of 'elderly people'. This is despite the fact that the need for long-term care is highly sex specific. Wittenberg *et al.* (1998) demonstrate that, particularly at ages 80+, women are considerably more likely than men to have slight to substantial 'dependency rates'. At age 85+ the differences are most marked: 31.1 per cent of women aged 85+ compared to 17.3 per cent of men of that age have 'substantial' problems (Table 6.3, p. 50). Using a model which the Royal Commissioners themselves recommend (Royal Commission on Long Term Care, 1999, p. 8), the same team also estimated numbers resident in institutional care up to 2031. Women are currently, and are expected to continue to be, residents of care institutions in a ratio to men of approximately 3:1 (my calculations based on Wittenberg *et al.*, 1998, Table 10.4). This reminder as to the gender of 'elderly people' in need of care is not a new point and indeed it is one that has been much explored in the literature (Arber and Ginn, 1991). The purpose of reiterating it here is to remind ourselves that we have to consider the social and economic relations of these elderly men and women, and, especially if we are to understand their position as consumers of care within a privatised and marketised system, the way in which their personal biographies and social networks affect their ability to pay for care.

At the core of the Royal Commission Report is the central issue of keeping costs down in the labour intensive industry of long-term care production while, at the same time, ensuring that those who need care are able to access it, either through use of their own resources or through state subsidy. There are very occasional mentions of the costs of caring labour, and they are made with a certain nervousness, pointing to the implications of the national minimum wage (p. 19). Only Laing and Saper, in *Research Volume 3*, recognise the sex of the care-workers involved, and use an index of women's hourly wage rates to demonstrate their concerns about staff wage inflation in care homes and to estimate, at an aggregate cost of £100 million, the effects on care home costs of the introduction of the national minimum wage (Laing and Saper, 1999, p. 93). What is missing from the report as a whole, though, is any sense of the dynamic relationship between wages of care workers, the huge majority of whom are women, and the ability of the gender-free category of 'elderly people' to act as consumers in the care system. It is this dynamic that is explored in this paper.

Gender and the mixed economy of care

There have been two paradigm shifts in the organisation of care services for the elderly in the past twenty years. The first concerns policies for decarceration, reflecting the research of Goffman and others critical of institutional care of all kinds (Goffman, 1961; Jones and Fowles, 1984). Indeed it was the growing emphasis on policies for 'community care' in the late 1970s, alongside the rapid development of a feminist critique of family and community life (e.g., example, Barrett and McIntosh, 1982), which underlay the first stage of feminist analysis of 'care' (Finch and Groves, 1980). The second paradigm shift began in the 1980s and culminated in the National Health Service and Community Care Act, 1990. It concerns the idea of a 'mixed economy of welfare' with the core notion of an internal market based on a purchaser/provider split. 'Choice' for the newly empowered consumer of the 1990s is ultimately best served by the market, brokered by a local authority care manager if necessary, but nevertheless consisting of alternatives between which the care customer can choose.

However, the market, in combination with domiciliary services, cannot resolve all problems without some radical inventiveness. Despite the strong critique of the destructive elements of residential care, its outstanding advantage is that it stretches over twenty-four hours. In that sense it provides continuous surveillance and hence management of risk. Residential care can also respond to urgent and unpredicted need. (These points assume of course that there are no risks that arise directly out of residential care, such as abuse by staff and by other inmates, and that residential care staff will effectively respond as needs arise.) If home care is to replicate this important feature of 'round the clock' care but on an individual basis, then methods have to be found which produce domiciliary services which in some way copy but do not exactly reproduce the features of twenty-four hour care, and do so within carefully costed limits. Obviously, informal care, which is traditionally unpaid, is the primary method of replication of twenty-four hour care, especially when it is provided by co-resident informal carers. As one would expect, all the documentation surrounding the introduction of marketised and privatised community care in Britain stressed the importance of informal care as the 'lynch pin' of the new system (Griffiths, 1988). If, in this article, I were to concentrate on the production of informal care as part of the 'new' British community care system, there is little I could add to what has already been said: the advent of the new system of domiciliary care appears so far to have made little difference to gender differentials in informal care (Parker, 1998) and it is proving very difficult to say with certainty how the new system has affected the production and resources of informal care overall (Parker, 1999). More fruitful is a consideration of the impact of these reorganisations on the production of paid care. I will concentrate on how the state and the market have developed inventive ways of marshalling paid and volunteer carers, able to deliver care at all hours of the day and night, and willing to do so at a price both state and individual consumers are able to pay. It is here that the nub of the argument of this article lies. I will argue that the way in which these inventive replications have worked in combination with the introduction of marketisation and privatisation means that the system that is emerging is profoundly gendered and is, in both the long and the short run, disadvantageous to many women.

The three features of replicated twenty-four hour care which particularly affect women are as follows: the reconfiguration of the tasks of care and their consequent deskilling and – paradoxically – reskilling; the construction of the tasks of 'care' as a hybrid of love and instrumentality that persuades people to work beyond contract; and, in a contracting out system where private agencies are involved in marshalling labour, a source of employment particularly suited to women who are paid very low wages and who wish to fit employment around their own domestic lives but which, at the same time, allows very limited opportunities for the acquisition of social rights. I shall tackle each of these aspects in turn.

The reconfiguration of tasks follows from two aspects of the attempt to replicate twenty-four hour care without actually providing it. First, it is essential that people who are living in their own homes are able to get the advantage of being at home in the sense that they can move around within it and even beyond it, and can generally survive without total care. After all, if they are not able to move beyond their beds then the additional expense of caring for each individual *at* home rather than *in* a home is hardly justified. Thus care tasks must involve ensuring that individuals are out of bed in the morning, in bed at night, regularly fed, bathed etc. Second, it is also essential that, in a 'needs led' system which is also supposed to reflect personal preferences, users of services are not helped in and out of bed before or after they want, and that, above all, they receive reliably punctual services. As a result of these two features of home care, the tasks of care are fragmented into smaller and smaller units so that they can be delivered at speed. This in turn alters the content of the occupation of caring. If there are fifteen people in a neighbourhood who need to be helped out of bed punctually within a period of two hours then the emotional content of care, and the particular attentiveness which generally takes time, have to be withdrawn – only the instrumentality of the task remains. The same is obviously true of meal delivery, bathing, shopping and helping someone back to bed. In a recent study of the impact of domiciliary care developments on demand for caring labour, Ford *et al.* (1998) found that workers were unhappy with the deskilled nature of their new style jobs and were themselves inventing ways of reintroducing more labour intensive methods of work:

> The growing trend of reducing the period for the delivery of certain kinds of services (sometimes to as little as 15 minutes) created less favourable employment conditions for workers. The more fleeting pattern of contact could in itself be unrewarding and unsatisfactory and this was a development that both contractors and providers also acknowledged as a potentially exploitative one as care workers might then provide additional services in their own time.
> (Ford, *et al.*, 1998, 28–9)

The times at which many of these services have to be delivered are outside 'normal' working hours. Hence, if the labour that provides these fragmented tasks has to be cheap despite being at the 'expensive' ends of the day, the tasks have to be construed as essentially unskilled and easily undertaken by the untrained, uncredentialised and unlucky. Moreover, they are tasks that can easily be allied to the experience of the instrumental tasks of mothering. Thus women's labour seems 'natural' for these deskilled and fragmented activities. In the study by Ford *et al.*, which included a survey of care workers, 96 per cent of their respondents were women, reflecting female predominance of care work at national level (Ford *et al.*, 1998, 30).

Paradoxically, there are also pressures to 're-skill' care work. This arises out of the aspect of the shift of the mixed economy of care that involves targetting of domiciliary services on those who in previous decades would, through their frailty, have been obvious candidates for residential or hospital care.

The result is that domiciliary care-work delivered by or purchased by the state sector involves dealing with very sick people, many of whom will be mentally infirm as well as have physical problems. For them, the rapid delivery of fragmented tasks is inappropriate. It is noticeable, therefore, that the conventional amount of time spent with individual households by home helps and home carers is moving rapidly upwards – from an average of 3.2 hours per week in 1992 to 5.1 hours per week in 1996 (Department of Health, 1997). Over the same period, the number of households in England receiving home help and home care services *dropped* by 19 per cent but the number of hours delivered *increased* by 50 per cent. The study by Ford *et al.* indicates how these changes were influencing the nature of the occupation of home carer:

> Some of those previously providing the home help service were not really up to the new job. In particular, people had to be able to make decisions, liaise with other agencies and handle a more dependent set of clients. *The authority was trying to professionalise the service more and more.*
>
> (Ford *et al.*, 1998: 42, my emphasis)

Ford *et al.* are clear as to what is happening to the labour markets for domiciliary care as a result. Two segmented markets are developing: one that contains women workers on very low wages with poor working conditions, producing standardised services on a care production line, and most often employed by a private sector company or finding work through a private agency. The other market is located within local authorities and a few specialist voluntary organisations. They are delivering more complex care services for which the workers are increasingly specially and comprehensively trained and where both wages, which are still low, and working conditions, are considerably better than in the private and agency sector. Thus the replication of the twenty-four hour feature of residential care is developing into a bifurcated domiciliary care labour market where *both* fragmentation and consolidation are taking place. Both labour markets are heavily dominated by women workers.

The second method that is used to replicate but not reproduce twenty-four hour care is to recruit workers who can easily be persuaded to work beyond contract – so long as they have the time to do so. There are ways of presenting the work of care so that it particularly appeals to those who seek out intimacy at work. If the care work can be organised so that there is an opportunity to develop a relationship over a long period of time with a particular individual and where the caregiver can act relatively autonomously, then the work can rapidly acquire non-pecuniary benefits for the worker and the relationship between the two people can expand so that the problem of fragmented care resolves itself into continuous care. In Britain, 'community care helpers' have been recruited to care for single individuals within their neighbourhoods and paid symbolically to do so (Qureshi *et al.*, 1989). Schemes of this kind, which essentially present the work of care as a 'labour of love', have been very successful, both in recruiting workers who have time on their hands and no great desire to earn conventionally sized wages, and in satisfying the needs of very frail elderly people (Leat with Ungerson, 1993; Blacksell and Phillips, 1994). It has also been argued that part of the purpose of these schemes, and part of their success, is to introduce *feeling* into the relationship such that the workers behave increasingly like informal carers and involve their own families in the provision of total care (Davies and Challis, 1986). What these schemes essentially do is profile the 'nurturing' aspect of motherhood (as opposed to the instrumentality of mothering referred to above).

The third method of replicating but not reproducing the merits of residential care is to find methods of recruiting labour which do not entail high administrative costs or the possibility of unionisation and which reduce the wages of the workers involved. The contracting out culture which has come through marketisation has proved, in the British context, to be a very successful means of encouraging both the growth of private firms and voluntary organisations which provide caring labour on a casual and task orientated basis, and also of reducing its costs. As Table 1 indicates, over a third of home help and home care is now provided by the private sector and this is on an upward trajectory.

Research on early forms of privatisation conducted by the Equal Opportunities Commission in the early 1990s demonstrated that the total number of jobs in local authorities was reduced particularly in the occupations dominated by women and particularly in part-time jobs. For example, there was a 13 per cent drop in employment in community care in the case study local authorities, an increased use of temporary staff, and 'overtime opportunities and unsocial hours payments for evening and weekend work have also been severely restricted under contract' (EOC, 1995:16). The private sector paid considerably less than the local authorities, very rarely had

Table 1 Contact hours of home helps and home care per 10,000 households, by sector of provider, 1994–1996.

England	1994		1995		1996	
	number	index	number	index	number	index
All sectors	1,180	100	1,277	108	1,451	123
Local authority	952	100	900	95	924	97
Voluntary	33	100	42	127	56	167
Private 1994 = 100	195	100	335	172	471	242

Source: Department of Health, *Community Care Statistics*, England 1996, Table 1.7.

maternity leave and sick pay schemes, and some private contractors also had managed to avoid paying towards contributory benefits by 'a combination of employing people on low hours and paying lower wage rates' (EOC, 1995:19). Thus, the work involved in the delivery of care has literally been cheapened. As the provision of care switches from local authority employed workers to private sector workers it is to be expected that, for many workers, wages and working conditions will take a turn for the worse. It is this point, and its implications, that provides the context for the later discussion of the gendering of care consumption.

Paid care work and the effects on resources in old age

In the previous section the changes that have taken place in the organisation of long-term care were explored in terms of their impact on the labour market for care, and the prospects for care workers. What is happening here is that the tasks of 'front-line' care are being reconfigured so that new fractions of task are emerging such that some are moving towards 'core' parts of the labour market, and others are moving further towards the periphery. On the one hand, a 'core' labour market is emerging, particularly for care workers who manage to retain their jobs with local authorities, where the shift to domiciliary care means that front-line care work is developing in complexity and is likely therefore to lead to increasing credentialism and career ladders. Although much of this work will remain part time, the particular 'flexibility' that will be demanded will be 'adaptive flexibility' whereby well-trained and trusted workers will be allowed to acquire relative autonomy to practise a variety of skills in relation to the varied needs of care recipients with high and complex needs. At the same time, opportunities are developing for individuals, who will obviously include women, to enter self-employment in the care sector and, assuming that they are successful in winning competitive tenders for contracted out care, lay the basis for growth into the world of for-profit enterprise. In contrast, some care tasks will be increasingly routinised and standardised so that they can be undertaken by untrained and classically flexible labour working at 'unsocial hours' and for short shifts and casual contracts. The overall gendered impact of these trends may mean that some women will succeed whereas others will remain impoverished in terms of both money and time. What we are seeing here are the embryonic beginnings of divisions between women engaged in front-line and hands-on social care work, parallel to the growing inequalities between women already visible in the British labour market as a whole. These divisions will manifest themselves both in terms of income and of status as some occupations within domiciliary care which are currently regarded as unskilled become credentialised, and as opportunities for profit in care develop.

The knock-on effects into old age are obvious. The low waged and the 'atypically' employed are profoundly disadvantaged when it comes to the accumulation of social security rights both to cover exigencies such as sickness and unemployment during the working lifetime, and, more particularly, to provide pensions on retirement. This disadvantage is a feature of the British social security system which means that those on very low wages do not participate in the otherwise compulsory national insurance scheme (McKnight *et al.*, 1998). Discussion of the recent Green Paper on pensions reform (DSS, 1998) has so far suggested that the mooted State Second Pension will be largely a women's pension, and constitutes a 'missed opportunity' to shift effectively 'the institutional features that contribute most to the perpetuation of economic disadvantage experienced during the working life' (Falkingham and Rake, 1999). Hence, although the pensions situation of low-paid workers may be improved a little by the proposed replacement of SERPS by the State Second Pension (Agulnik, 1999), it remains highly probable that the provision of *paid* care during a working life will entail poverty in old age. That poverty will in turn impact on the consumption of care. Such an argument is a variant of the usual argument linking women's working lives with their subsequent poverty in old age (Joshi, 1992; Walker, 1992; Groves, 1992). Those arguments are commonly couched within the framework of the impact of *unpaid* care, particularly for normal children, on the labour market opportunities of British women. What is being suggested here is that the way in which the new systems of care are being developed, with their core search for cheap but exhaustive methods of care service delivery, means that *intrinsic* to the system itself is a basic element of gendered exclusion. Many of the workers within the system will become impoverished consumers within it – unless methods are adopted, both endogenous and exogenous to the community care system, which attempt to ameliorate the impact of paid care provision on ultimate care consumption.

Gender and the costs of care consumption

The impact on the need for care and the costs entailed by women's greater morbidity in old age is considerable. Glennerster found that for all ages over 60, the expected lifetime public expenditure on long-term care services is about two and a half times as much for women as for men (my calculations based on estimates in Glennerster, 1996, p. 14). Burchardt (1997) estimated, using models of incapacity based on the British Household Panel Survey, and assuming that an insurance benefit of £15,000 per annum becomes payable on failure of three 'activities of daily living', that the lump sum premium payable by men at age 65 would be £19,000 compared to £37,200 for women of the same age. The actual premia payable to PPP (a private health insurance company operating in the UK) for various types of long-term care insurance are reproduced in *Research Volume One of the Report of the Royal Commission on Long Term Care*: they too indicate considerable differences between the costs for men and for women, with women only approaching the lower costs for men when the benefits are at their most restricted (Royal Commission on Long Term Care, 1999).

The conundrum that emerges is as follows: the poorer members of the population – namely women – have the most expensive long-term care needs. As a result of their poverty, they have very considerable difficulty in providing for their own care needs, even at very low cost for a minimal service. In terms of income, 23 per cent of all pensioner households are dependent on State Retirement Pension plus Income Support only, with a somewhat higher proportion (38 per cent) of those aged 85 or over, who are likely to be the most frail, similarly reliant on the very low British pension arrangement (Department of Social Security, 1997). While the above data is not presented by gender, work by Dulcie Groves, using data from various surveys in the late 1980s and early 1990s, indicates that on all counts – state pensions, occupational pensions, earnings and investment income – women of pensionable age are considerably worse off than male pensioners (Groves, 1995). Given the low levels of income represented by the state pension plus income support on which nearly 40 per cent of very elderly pensioners depend, it is also the case that they will have very limited resources to pay for small amounts of domiciliary care even at the low rates of pay that prevail in that sector (over 56 per cent of female 'care assistants and attendants' earned less than £4 70p per hour in 1997 (New Earnings Survey, 1998: Table D10)). Chetwynd and Ritchie (1996), in a study of local authority charging policies found that pensioners, some of whose incomes were well *above* the state pension level, were having to make considerable sacrifices in their 'normal' consumption in order to pay even very low charges for their 'care packages'. Almond *et al.* (1999), in an overview of the correlation between poverty, disability and the receipt of long-term care services, conclude that those on income support are deterred from using publicly subsidised services because of user charges. In terms of capital assets (apart from their accommodation), it is also the case that only a minority of pensioners have any form of cushioning such that they could afford, for example, to purchase long-term care insurance with a lump sum premium. According to the British Family Resources Survey, 20 per cent of pensioner couples and 34 per cent of single pensioners have *no savings*. Altogether 41 per cent of pensioner couples and 60 per cent of single pensioners have total savings of less than £3,000 (Department of Social Security, 1997: Table 5.10). They clearly cannot possibly afford the kinds of premia that Burchardt suggests and PPP demand, especially if they are women.

Care cost cushions for women consumers?

There are two ways in which this very bleak picture of a mass of impoverished elderly women in need of care but facing a targeted and very carefully rationed social care sector may improve – exogenously to changes within the care system itself. The first concerns the impact of the expansion of owner-occupation, and the second concerns trends in the labour market as far as 'women's work' is concerned. Owner-occupation has been widely regarded as the means by which ownership of capital assets would become widespread across social classes, and there is no doubt that its impact has been to equalise wealth holding a little. In 1988–89, Hamnett's data indicates that the total value of property left by dead married people to their spouses was £3.66 billion, of which £3 billion was left by married men to their widows (Hamnett, 1995:171). Such acquisitions may well represent problems, in the form of expensive maintenance and repair bills, but they also represent very considerable capital assets made available to generally elderly women. Moreover the expansion of owner-occupation will have considerable effects on the assets of old age well into the next century: over 50 per cent of people aged 80 years or more are now owner-occupiers, and this group will increase as lower cohorts with even higher rates (up to 77 per cent for those presently in their forties) move into old age (Family Resources Survey, 1997: Table 4.3). Such ownership represents a possible route into the purchase of care which has considerable potential for those who are otherwise very poor. Hancock (1998), using data from the Family Expenditure Survey, argues that about one-fifth of owner occupiers aged over 80 can be classified as 'income poor but housing rich'. Moreover, she found that, for those aged 80+, women were 10 per cent more likely than men to be income poor but housing rich and suggests that 'the potential for equity release schemes to supplement low incomes is of special significance for older women' (Hancock, 1998: 29). She concludes that housing equity could be used to fund the cheaper forms of long-term care – in particular, the charges for domiciliary care.

However, there are two problems about this kind of analysis. The first is that there is a large gap between arguing what *could* happen from what *will* happen. The study of the potential of equity release schemes generally ignores the social relations of inheritance, and the way in which decisions about the uses of equity are embedded in the social processes of kinship. One study of attitudes to saving by Rowlingson *et al.* (1998) does throw some light on this question. They found deep resistance among the majority of their respondents to using housing equity to fund long-term care and suggest that the desire to leave assets to children is very closely bound up with owner-occupation. As these authors put it, 'housing wealth was ring-fenced for bequests and financial wealth was considered available for spending in old age' (*ibid.*, 1999, p. 81). The second problem is that, despite the expansion of owner-occupation, there will nevertheless remain some one-quarter of the population to whom such additional resources will never be available and for whom no cushioning of any kind, whether from their accommodation or from other savings, will be of assistance. For them it will be a matter of family biography and structural determinants of social mobility as to whether other members of their kin network – their adult children, for example – are in a position to help them financially, and it will be a matter of personal psychology and of culture as to whether such assistance is welcomed by elderly parents.

The second factor which may ameliorate the bleakness of poverty in old age, particularly for women, concerns changes in the labour market especially in 'women's occupations'. As we have already seen, the care labour market is showing distinct signs of bi-polarising. Similar bi-polarisation is taking place in the labour market for women as a whole, with some women, especially those with high levels of qualification, beginning to generate working histories and working conditions that look much more like those traditionally located in men's occupations (Sly *et al.*, 1998). These inequalities that are developing between women are likely to generate a politics of care provision and pensioner protection which do not have gender at their heart, but rather social class. It is interesting to note that alongside the mass of elderly poor there is also a significant minority of elderly people, particularly those who are still married, who are relatively well off (Rowlingson *et al.*, 1999). For example, 31 per cent of pensioner couples have savings of £20,000 or more, and 15 per cent of single pensioners are that affluent (Family Resources Survey, 1997: Table 5:10). But if attention drifts towards the affluence of what remains a minority of British pensioners, and the polity is mesmerised by the potential of owner-occupation to act as a resource for up to three-quarters of the populace, the eye can move away from the fundamental point: that there will, as a result of labour market trends, remain a significant minority of elderly pensioners, most of whom are women, whose work histories – many of them, ironically, one time paid care workers – will guarantee an old age characterised by ill health and financial dependency and an inability to enter the world of care consumerism.

Discussion: the implications of growing income and wealth inequalities

Thus it can be argued that gender remains at the heart of the new care system. Women are caught in a vicious circle: as carers of their own children they are seriously disadvantaged in the labour market. In addition, 'care' jobs assume a lack of skill in care tasks because they bear such a close resemblance to the practices based on the experience of mothering and hence are construed as 'natural' aptitudes of women. For these reasons employers of caring labour are likely to continue to seek out women as care workers. Despite the low pay prevailing in the care sector, it is also likely that care occupations will remain attractive to women with few qualifications but who also seek intimacy at work and the special satisfactions that arise out of the delivery of nurturing service (Ungerson, 1999). In material terms too, the fragmentation of care and the attempt to replicate features of twenty-four-hour care by extending the working day renders such paid work particularly flexible and amenable to delivery over short shifts which can be fitted around other domestically based responsibilities. Yet in the long run such occupations offer little in terms of acquisition of savings or pension rights and hence underwrite an insecure old age. However, it is also the case that this stark story is complicated, particularly by the phenomenon of growing inequalities between elderly people and especially between elderly women, both in terms of income and their access to housing equity. In the discussion that follows, the well-established 'welfare triangle' of state, family and market (Evers and Wintersberger, 1986) provides the framework within which I speculate on the way in which inequalities will differentially impact on care consumption.

At the heart of the 'family' is the question of the determinants and nature of intergenerational transfer, for it is within the 'family' that assets in the form of wealth and other resources such as labour are located, and where the potential for exchange, negotiation over and transfer of these assets exists. There is a growing literature which considers the importance of intergenerational transfers and how far money flows and instrumental help are both part of the same system of exchange (Finch *et al.*, 1996; Künemund and Rein, 1999; Kohli, 1999). Amongst the findings are that intergenerational cash transfers are much more common from older generation to younger generation than the other way round. Künemund and Rein (1999) argue that this partially reflects the level of income which some older people, in some welfare regimes, enjoy. Unfortunately the data is not analysed in such a way as to allow for an understanding of the way that inequalities both within and between families might impact on these cash and care flows. Thus, while this literature points to something that can be characterised as a 'family welfare system', it is not at all clear how those family welfare systems work at a micro level and vary across income inequalities. There are also likely to be differences between the social relations of cash transfers *inter vivos*, and the social relations of inheritance. It may be the case that ideas about what constitutes appropriate cash transfer, and its direction, are more amenable to change than ideas about inheritance, which in Britain appear relatively inflexible, with an idea of equal treatment among siblings (rather than desert or need) at their core (Finch *et al.*, 1996) and, as we have seen, a deep attachment to the idea of keeping the equity of the owner-occupied home intact to allow for eventual transfer down the generations.

However, one thing is clear: social care, as a set of tasks, can be easily substituted between family and household on the one hand, and the market on the other (Yeandle *et al.*, 1999). The context for decision-making as to how a kin network's resources for care – whether in terms of assets, income or labour – should be marshalled and expended lies in the interaction of the affective and material base of family and kin network relations. A combination of income poverty with ownership of a capital asset in the form of the accommodation occupied by the elderly person means that there may be contradictory pressures both to use up the current capital resource to fund care and, at the same time, to preserve it for future generations. In family networks where, given lack of social mobility, the marginal utility of even a low-value house is high, it is likely that there will be considerable pressure, from those expecting to inherit, on individuals within the network to provide informal care rather than use housing equity to purchase care. These kinds of pressures will be particularly heavy within poorer family networks and in this sense gender and social class cross-cut and intereact. Unless there are other forms of intervention, particularly from the state, and very cheap forms of purchasable care develop within the market, the family welfare system especially amongst the poor will have to grow. Again, the likely involvement of female kin in the younger generation in the provision of informal care will store up problems for those women when they reach their own old age.

One means whereby the impact of providing unpaid informal care for members of the older generation may be obviated is through *state* intervention, particularly in the organisation of pension rights. If informal care is recognised as a form of work which can legitimately lay claim to pension contributions, then the impact of absence from the formal labour market on incomes in old age will be ameliorated to some extent. Similarly, pension rights can be organised in such a way that those with chequered work histories or those who have worked 'atypically' in low-paid part-time occupations (for example, in paid care work) are not plunged into considerable poverty on retirement from paid work. The very recent introduction of a minimum wage in Britain should lead to higher wages within the paid care sector which in turn may mean that care workers have a small opportunity to save for the exigencies of retirement. However, the evidence as to whether they will or not is mixed. Walker *et al.* (1989) suggest that there is an 'occupational pensions trap' whereby means tested pension entitlement creates a disincentive to save. Rowlingson *et al.* (1999) argue that saving attitudes are subject to a range of determinants, from personal biography, through opportunity to save, to life events which trigger an interest in saving. Hence higher wages in paid care create an opportunity but one which only a few are likely to use. Nevertheless, such contextual factors help determine the effective demand for privatised and marketised care, but they are exogenous to the care system as a whole.

There are also ways in which the state can intervene to break the impact of low-paid work on the purchase of long-term care which are *endogenous* to the care system. The most obvious is the rapid development of means tested charges for care services which in turn are heavily targeted, particularly to those living on their own and those assessed by care managers as having 'high' needs. If women recipients of care packages are relatively poor and, as is likely given their longevity, living alone, then the combination of means testing and targeting will mean that they will, in the short run, be immediate beneficiaries of subsidised services. Indeed, one can argue that means tested and targeted service delivery is likely to constitute institutionalised gendering of the long-term care system since so many of those in need who are on low incomes will be women rather than men. Hence one can suggest that in the prevailing British social and economic structure, where there are growing inequalities between rich and poor and growing divisions, in paid work, between core and periphery, selectivity and targeting towards the very poor is the obvious ameliorative policy solution to the consumption problems entailed by women's poverty in old age. However, this leads to the classic question about selectivity. While selectivity may resolve problems in the short run (assuming that means testing does not immediately depress take-up of services) the long run problems surrounding selectivity involve loss of political support for state funded services, with subsequent tightening of resources and increasing emphasis on the merits of self-provisioning. The fact that poor, elderly women would be the major consumers of selectively allocated and subsidised services may add to the residualisation process.

Alternatives to such drift towards residualisation involve some pressing choices. On the one hand, it is possible to envisage promotion of market-based consumption through, for example, state organised and subsidised long-term care insurance as is currently part of the German welfare system; on the other hand, it is possible to envisage social care which is free at the point of consumption where funding is based on taxation revenues. In both cases, gender remains problematic. Long-term care insurance will have similar problems to social security insurance based schemes in that it is particularly difficult to see how an adequate system of benefits for all can include those who, due to low and irregular income, are able to make only very low contributions during their working lives. The Royal Commission on Long-Term Care decided against long-term care insurance and has recommended that the care element in long-term care should be free and funded from general taxation, while means tested charges should be put in place for other elements of care such as accommodation, meals etc. But the Commission was aware that such a system would have very strong tendencies to withhold allocation of free social care where there is the presence of a carer. It is highly likely that such tendencies to allocate free social care only where there is no 'obvious' informal carer will be gendered. The Commission recommended 'that the Government ensure services become increasingly "carer blind" when allocating support services to users of care' (Royal Commission on Long-Term Care, 1999: 90). The looseness of the wording – the word 'increasingly' is a giveaway here – indicates how difficult (but necessary) it is to avoid the problem of what can be named as 'gendered subsidiarity'.

As far as the *market* is concerned, there are a number of issues which have gendered implications and which also reflect growing inequalities between elderly people. One factor is the extent to which different types of market for care services will develop across space. For example, the development of private sector care, particularly of residential care, has had very clear spatial elements to it, with heavy concentrations of for-profit residential care homes in the south of Britain and in towns and cities, such as at the seaside, where there already existed a housing stock that was both cheap and suitable for conversion into multiple occupation (Audit Commission, 1986). As far as markets for domiciliary care are concerned the structure of the British community care system is such that the spatial concentration of markets for care may be less heavily skewed. All local authorities were, in the first two years of the implementation of the new community care system, obliged to contract out up to 85 per cent of their domiciliary care services. Hence one would expect that there would be tendencies towards less spatial concentration of for-profit enterprise. However, private sector domiciliary care firms cannot rely on a continuous flow of contracts for care from local authorities (Laing and Saper, 1999) and will need to be reassured that there is, in the areas where they operate, sufficient effective demand from private consumers to support their services. Thus one might expect the skewed development of well-organised and quality audited domiciliary care enterprise in areas where there are concentrations of middle-class, middle and upper income elderly owner-occupiers. In contrast, where there are concentrations of poor elderly people (for example, on social housing estates or inner cities) one would expect there to be little in the way of an organised market for domiciliary care. In these areas, the market for domiciliary care will exist but it may have a very different feel to it – it may constitute part of the largely invisible system of informal economic activity whereby neighbours provide each other with services at very low cost (for examples, see Baldock and Ungerson, 1994) or payments for care develop within families and kin networks (Ungerson, 1997).

Conclusion

It is clear that changes in the production of care will generate new forms of gendered inequality which in turn will impact on gendered patterns and exigencies of consumption of care. The reorganisation of care work entails the reproduction of a minority of very poor elderly women who will be unable to enter a private market for care, and will have considerable difficulty in accessing even quite heavily subsidised but nevertheless charged-for care. This argument points to two main conclusions. First, it is essential to consider, with any policy innovation, but most particularly in those areas of the welfare state such as social care which are heavily labour intensive, the impact of that policy *as a whole* – not only on consumers but also on *producers*. In the particular case of social care, there is an internal dynamic linked to a cohort effect. Low-paid care work leads to lack of resources to consume care in old age; this in turn drives a dependence on the substitute of informal care, and the dynamic of low-income production leading to highly constrained consumption is once again repeated. The second conclusion concerns how this cycle is to be broken: both exogenous factors to do with the remuneration of low-paid care work and the acquisition of social rights in old age, and endogenous factors to do with the financing of long-term care for those with a range of needs and *with a range of incomes*, need to be placed high on the agenda. Policy changes in the delivery and organisation of long-term care are themselves having profound knock-on effects. We are at the cusp of decision-making where, unless other policies are introduced to deal with these effects, we will make no progress whatsoever in resolving gendered inequality amongst the elderly.

References

Agulnik, P. (1999), 'The proposed State Second Pension and National Insurance', in *Partnership in Pensions? Responses to the Pensions Green Paper*, CASEpaper 24, Centre for Analysis of Social Exclusion, London School of Economics, London.

Ahmad, W. and K. Atkin (eds.), (1996), *'Race' and community care*, Open University Press, Buckingham,

Almond, S., A. Bebbington, K. Judge, R. Mangalore, O. O'Donnell (1999), 'Poverty, disability and the use of long-term care services', *Research Volume One* of the report of the Royal Commission on Long-Term Care.

Arber, S. and N. Gilbert (1989), 'Men: the forgotten carers', *Sociology*, 23: 1, 111–118.

Arber, S. and J. Ginn (1991), *Gender and Later Life*, Sage, London.

Arber, S. and J. Ginn (1992), 'Class and caring: a forgotten dimension', *Sociology*, 26, 4.

Askham, J., L. Henshaw, M. Tarpey (1995), *Social and Health Authority Services for Elderly People from Black and Minority Ethnic Communities*, HMSO, London.

Audit Commission (1986), *Making a Reality of Community Care*, HMSO, London.

Baldock, J. and C. Ungerson (1994), *Becoming Consumers of Community Care: households and the mixed economy of welfare*, Joseph Rowntree Foundation, York.

Barrett, M. and M. McIntosh (1982), *Women's Oppression Today*, Verso, London.

Blacksell, S. and D. R. Phillips (1994), *Paid to Volunteer: the extent of paying volunteers in the 1990s*, The Volunteer Centre, London.

Burchardt, T. (1997), *What Price Security?*, WSP/129, The Welfare State Programme, London School of Economics, London.

Bytheway, B. (1987), *Informal Care Systems: an exploratory study within the families of older steel workers in South Wales*, Joseph Rowntree Memorial Trust, York.

Chetwynd, M. and J. Ritchie (1996), *The Cost of Care: the impact of charging policy on the lives of disabled people*, The Policy Press, Bristol.

Davies, B. and D. Challis (1986), *Matching Resources to Needs in Community Care: an evaluated demonstration of a long-term care model*, Gower, Aldershot.

Department of Health (1997), *Community Care Statistics, England 1996*, HMSO, London.

Department of Social Security (1997), *Family Resources Survey Great Britain 1995–96*, HMSO, London.

Department of Social Security (1998), *A New Contract for Welfare: partnership in pensions*. Cm 4179. HMSO, London.

Equal Opportunities Commission (1995), *The Gender Impact of CCT in Local Government: summary report*, EOC, Manchester.

Evers, A. and H. Wintersberger (1986), *Shifts in the Welfare Mix*, European Centre for Social Welfare Training and Research, Vienna.

Falkingham, J. and K. Rake (1999), 'Partnership in pensions': delivering a secure retirement for women?', in *Partnership in Pensions? Responses to the Pensions Green Paper*, CASEpaper 24, Centre for Analysis of Social Exclusion, London School of Economics, London.

Finch, J. and D. Groves (1980), 'Community care and the family: a case for equal opportunities?', *Journal of Social Policy*, 9: 4, 487–511.

Finch, J. and D. Groves (eds.) (1983), *A Labour of Love; women, work and caring*, RKP, London.

Finch, J., L. Hayes, J. Mason, J. Masson, L. Wallis (1996), *Wills, Inheritance and Families*, Oxford University Press, Oxford.

Fisher, M (1994), 'Man-made care: community care and older male workers', *British Journal of Social Work*, 24: 59–80.

Ford, J., D. Quilgars and J. Rugg (1998), *Creating Jobs? The employment potential of domiciliary care*, The Policy Press and Joseph Rowntree Foundation, Bristol.

Glennerster, H. (1996). *Caring for the Very Old: public and private solutions*, WSP/126, The Welfare State Programme, London School of Economics, London.

Goffman, E. (1961), *Asylums: essays on the social situation of mental patients and other inmates*, Anchor Books, Ganden City, NY.

Graham, H. (1991), 'The concept of caring in feminist research – the case of domestic service', *Sociology*, 25: 1, 61–78.

Graham, H. (1993), 'Social divisions in caring', *Women's Studies International Forum*, 16: 5, 461–70.

Graham, H. (1997), 'Feminist perspectives in caring', in J. Bornat *et al.* (eds.), *Community Care – a reader*, 2nd edn, Macmillan, Basingstoke.

Griffiths, R. (1988), *Community Care: Agenda for Action*, HMSO, London.

Groves, D. (1992), 'Occupational pension provision and women's poverty in old age' in C. Glendinning and J. Millar (eds.), *Women and Poverty in Britain, the 1990s*, Harvester Wheatsheaf, Hemel Hempstead.

Groves, D. (1995), 'Costing a fortune? Pensioners' financial resources in the context of community care', in I. Allen and E. Perkins (eds.), *The Future of Family Care for Older People*, HMSO, London.

Hamnett, C. (1995), 'Housing equity release and inheritiance', in I. Allen and E. Perkins (eds.), *The Future of Family Care for Older People*, HMSO, London.

Hancock, R. (1998), 'Housing wealth, income and financial wealth of older people in Britain', *Ageing and Society*, 18: 5–33.

Jones, K. and A. J. Fowles (1984), *Ideas on Institutions: analysing the literature on long-term care and custody*, Routledge Kegan Paul, London.

Joshi, H. (1992), 'The labour market and unpaid caring: conflict and compromise', in I. Allen and E. Perkins (eds.), *The Future of Family Care for Older People*, HMSO, London.

Keith, L. (1992), 'Who cares wins? Women, caring and disability', *Disability, Handicap and Society*, 7: 2, 167–75.

Kohli, M. (1999), 'Private and public transfers between generations: linking the family and the state', *European Societies*, 1: 1, 81–104.

Künemund, H. and M. Rein (1999), 'There is more to receiving than needing: theoretical arguments and empirical explorations of crowding in and crowding out', *Ageing and Society*, 19, 93–121.

Laing, W. and P. Saper (1999), 'Promoting the development of a flourishing independent sector alongside good quality public services', in *Research Volume Three* of the report of the Royal Commission on Long-Term Care, 87–102.

Land, H. (1978), 'Who cares for the family?', *Journal of Social Policy*, 7: 3, 257–84.

Leat, D. with C. Ungerson (1993), *Creating Care at the Boundaries: issues in the supply and management of domiciliary care*, Department of Social Policy, University of Kent, Canterbury.

McKnight, A., P. Elias, R. Wilson (1998), *Low Pay and the National Insurance System: a statistical picture*, EOC, Manchester.

Morris, J. (1991), *Pride against Prejudice: transforming attitudes to disability*, The Women's Press, London.

Morris, J. (ed.) (1996), *Encounters with Strangers: feminism and disability*, The Women's Press, London.

New Earnings Survey (1998), HMSO, London.

Parker, G. (1998), 'Trends in caring 1985–1995', Part 2 of O. Rowlands, (1998), 39–48.

Parker, G. (1999), 'Impact of the NHS and Community Care Act (1990) on informal carers', in *Research Volume 3* of *With Respect to Old Age*, a report by the Royal Commission on Long-Term Care, 51–67.

Parker, G. and D. Lawton (1991), *Further Analysis of the 1985 General Household Survey: Data on Informal Care, Report 4: Male Carers*, DHSS 849 10/91, Social Policy Research Unit, University of York. York.

Qureshi, H., D. Challis and B. Davies (1989), *Helpers in Case-managed Community Care*, Gower, Aldershot.

Rowlands, O. (1998), *Informal Carers*, The Stationery Office, London.

Rowlingson, K., C. Whyley and T. Warren (1999), *Wealth in Britain: a lifecycle perspective*, Policy Studies Institute, University of Westminster, London.

Royal Commission on Long-Term Care (1999), *With Respect to Old Age*, Stationery Office, London.

Sly, R., T. Thair and A. Risdon (1998). 'Women in the labour market: results from the spring 1997 Labour Force Survey', *Labour Market Trends*, HMSO, March.

Ungerson, C. (1997), 'Social politics and the commodification of care', *Social Politics*, Fall, 362–81.

Ungerson, C. (1999), 'Personal assistants and disabled people: an examination of a hybrid form of work and care', *Work, Employment & Society*, 13: 4, 583–600.

Walker, A. (1992), 'The poor relation: poverty amongst older women', in C. Glendinning and J. Millar (eds.), *Women and Poverty in Britain, the 1990s*, Harvester Wheatsheaf, Hemel Hempstead.

Walker, R., G. Hardman and S. Hutton (1989), 'The occupational pension trap: towards a preliminary empirical specification', *Journal of Social Policy*, 19, 4.

Wittenberg, R., L. Pickard, A. Comas-Herrera, B. Davies and R. Darton (1998), *Demand for Long-Term Care: projections of long-term care finance for elderly people*, PSSRU, London School of Economics, London.

Yeandle, S. (1999), 'Supporting employed carers: new jobs, new services?', paper presented to Seminar 3, ESRC Seminar Series on 'The interface between public policy and gender equality', Centre for Regional Economic and Social Research, Sheffield Hallam University, Sheffield.

Yeandle, S., T. Gore, H. Pickford and B. Stiell (1999), *Employment, Family and Community Activities: a new balance for women and men*, UK National Report on Employment in Household Services, European Foundation for the Improvement of Living and Working Conditions, Dublin.

44
GENDER AND EQUITY IN HEALTH SECTOR REFORM PROGRAMMES
A review

Hilary Standing

Source: *Health Policy and Planning*, 12:1 (1997), 1–18.

This paper reviews current literature and debates about Health Sector Reform (HSR) in developing countries in the context of its possible implications for women's health and for gender equity. It points out that gender is a significant marker of social and economic vulnerability which is manifest in inequalities of access to health care and in women's and men's different positioning as users and producers of health care. Any analysis of equity must therefore include a consideration of gender issues. Two main approaches to thinking about gender issues in health care are distinguished – a 'women's health' approach, and a 'gender inequality' approach. The framework developed by Cassels (1995), highlighting six main components of HSR, is used to try to pinpoint the implications of HSR in relation to both of these approaches. This review makes no claim to sociological or geographical comprehensiveness. It attempts instead to provide an analysis of the gender and women's health issues most likely to be associated with each of the major elements of HSR and to outline an agenda for further research. It points out that there is a severe paucity of information on the actual impact of HSR from a gender point of view and in relation to substantive forms of vulnerability (e.g. particular categories of women, specific age groups). The use of generic categories, such as 'the poor' or 'very poor', leads to insufficient disaggregation of the impact of changes in the terms on which health care is provided. This suggests the need for more carefully focused data collection and empirical research.

Introduction

The drive to reform the health sectors of developing countries has stimulated much debate about the impact of such reforms on the poorest sections of their populations. Of particular concern have been the implications of cost recovery for the poor. Other important dimensions of vulnerability, notably gender, have received comparatively little attention. Similarly, other important aspects of health sector reform agendas, such as restructuring health service employment, have not been considered from the viewpoint of their possible impact on the gender composition of the workforce.

This discussion seeks to address some of the empirical and conceptual gaps in the debate about health sector reform (HSR), with particular reference to gender and women's health.[1] Its premise is that gender is a significant indicator of inequality and disadvantage in relation to health care in most developing country contexts, which may cut across poverty indicators.[2] It follows, therefore, that gender should be a major consideration in measuring equity in health care. However, to the extent that gender interacts with other inequalities deriving from age, class, ethnicity etc., it is important to contextualize its significance.

In thinking about gender in relation to health sector reform, it is useful to distinguish between two approaches to vulnerability among women which are found in the literature on health care:

- women's health needs,
- gender inequality.

A women's health needs approach is concerned with the implications for women of differences in the epidemiological profile between the sexes. This approach highlights the specific health needs of women and girls as a consequence particularly (although not exclusively) of the biology of reproduction. Two broad stances derive from this approach. One stresses the need to provide specific, women focused health care interventions as a basic right in order to address the imbalance of need. The other stresses the cost-effectiveness of interventions which target women and girls (particularly reproductive health interventions), both in comparison to other types of intervention and as a means to improve the health of infants in particular.

Women's health and nutrition have become an increasing focus of international concern, which is well exemplified in a recent World Bank publication (1994). This stance is then part of the wider theme of 'investing in women' to reduce the burden of poverty, in which women have increasingly become seen as the most effective conduit to improving household welfare, and particularly the welfare of children.

A gender inequality approach to health is concerned with the role of gender relations in the production of vulnerability to ill health or disadvantage within health care systems and particularly the conditions which promote inequality between the sexes in relation to access and utilization of services. It is thus more centrally concerned with power relations and the ways in which health may also be a site of gender conflict.

One of the most important features of a gender approach is its emphasis on the need to examine resource allocation *within* households, rather than treating the household as the most minimum focus of intervention. Another important feature is the emphasis on the relationship between formal and informal domains. Thus, policies which have an impact on health care staffing levels will simultaneously affect the extent of the informal care burden carried predominantly by women.

Gender is an important pointer to vulnerability in two senses. First, women are found disproportionately among the most vulnerable population groups. They tend to be poorer than men on average, to have less access to income earning opportunities and other resources, including health care, and to be more dependent on others for their longer term security. In terms of absolute vulnerability, therefore, being female can be one of the most important predisposing factors. Vulnerability is also relative. Urban women and girls generally have better access to health care than their rural counterparts. However, the access of women and girls to household resources for health expenditure in both rural and urban areas has been found in many instances to be less than that of men and boys (Timyan et al. 1993).

Second, access to and utilization of health services are importantly influenced by cultural and ideological factors, such as embargoes on consulting male practitioners, lack of freedom to act without permission from husbands or senior kin and low valuation of the health needs of women and girls compared to that of men and boys (Key 1987; Stock 1983; Tipping and Segall 1995).

A gender approach also highlights the ways in which women and men are positioned differently in relation to health care services. There are two especially critical aspects to this in the context of HSR. First, women generally carry more of the care burden in relation to sick household and family members. Thus, adverse health impacts on children, for example, are more likely to affect mothers than other immediate adults. The household division of labour also tends to place greater burdens on women's time, resulting in higher opportunity costs for women in seeking treatment (Leslie et al. 1988; Leslie 1992).

Second, both formal and informal health care systems are gender differentiated in terms of their divisions of labour and associated hierarchies. Women are important health care producers as well as consumers, but they tend to be concentrated in particular segments of the health care labour force (Butter et al. 1987; Bloom 1991; Holden and Littlewood 1991).

These two approaches raise somewhat different questions in relation to HSR. From a women's health needs point of view, the question is how far HSR affects or takes into account women's different health needs. The current debate about minimum health care or essential clinical packages (World Development Report 1993) is important from this perspective. First, how far does the proposed *content* reflect these needs? Second, what is the likelihood of their acceptance and implementation in resource poor countries? Similarly, debates about cost recovery are important from a women's health point of view. Does cost recovery have a more adverse impact on women's capacity to utilize services than on that of men, leading to a neglect of their specific health needs?

From a gender perspective, HSR raises questions about both the consumption and the production of health services. How does HSR affect existing imbalances in gender relations? For example, in terms of differential access to health care resources, does it worsen or improve them, or create no changes? In the context of women's roles as health care producers, what are the consequences of changing human resources policies on staffing levels and mix for those segments of the health care system traditionally staffed by women?

Health care, gender and equity

The concept of equity is a troublesome one to pin down. An analysis of its use in a range of literature on the health sector reveals multiple meanings and points of reference for measurement (see e.g. Vogel 1988). Mooney (1987) has reviewed the various social theories underlying different stances on equity and shown how they lead to sometimes profoundly different ways of conceptualizing it. From the point of view of this discussion, the most important relevant distinction is between measures of equity which relate to *access* (which tend to be allied to concepts of health need, i.e. improving access for those with the greatest needs) and measures which relate to *outcomes* (such as health status or consumption of health goods).

Access measures of equity appear to be used more commonly than outcome measures, perhaps because the WHO has long used improved access by disadvantaged groups as its touchstone for equity (Kutzin 1995). Improving access also implies an outcome goal of improving health status. Access is undoubtedly a very useful and relatively straightforward way of operationalizing equity which lends itself to measurement through factors such as utilization rates. It is also a helpful measure from the point of view of a gender approach to health care, which emphasizes problems of access and under-utilization for women. However, in linking it to gender disadvantage, it also begs some questions.

First, if women do have additional, specific health needs which derive from biology and reproductive health risks, then improved access is not of itself a sufficient condition for achieving equity in terms of health status. It is also necessary to consider the mix of services on offer, including possible needs to switch scarce resources into services which will more directly advantage women.

Second, the notion of a disadvantaged group has tended to be a broad brush related to poverty or to regional indicators. Currently, in health systems writing, there is almost no disaggregation of data by gender. Thus, it is not possible to say whether improved access for 'the poor' or for disadvantaged regions translates into equal improvement for women (and children) as for men. Given the weight of evidence on gender inequality in health care access referred to already, there are grounds for concern that this may not always be so. It is possible that measures to improve access for broadly drawn disadvantaged population groups may result either in no increase in access for women or a smaller increase for women than for men, thus widening gender disparities. An aggregate improvement in the level of access to health care may still therefore disguise significant sectional inequalities. Unfortunately, we lack the appropriate data with which to tackle these questions.

Another important equity issue concerns the distribution of the burden of cost and its relationship to the ability to pay, either indirectly through systems of taxation or insurance, or through direct payment for services received (see e.g. Dave 1991). Again, although much has been written on issues such as the equity implications of different forms of taxation for health expenditure (see WHO 1993), and the impact of cost recovery on the poorer sections of populations (for a summary see McPake 1993), very little data is available on the gender dimensions of the burden of cost.

Clearly, equity can mean a number of things. For countries struggling simultaneously to achieve health sector objectives of expenditure control, service quality improvement, increased utilization and equity, definitions of equity have at best to be pragmatic. Thus, Zambia's approach to equity within an HSR framework 'refers to the extent to which no group or individual receives less than a minimum benefit level or (more than) a maximum cost level of health care' (Kalumba 1994:17). This leaves those who can afford a higher level of health care free to make that choice. This consumption based approach to equity would not satisfy several of the more common social theories of equity (notably, it lacks a redistributive element). However, the Zambian emphasis on the role of minimum health care packages in achieving its equity objectives, and the definition of their content in terms of greatest health need, mean that women and children could be net beneficiaries of this approach to equity.

From a gender perspective, therefore, different approaches to equity may be associated with a range of outcomes which are not predictable from first principles and which require empirical investigation.

A framework for health sector reform

As Kutzin (1995) points out, HSR is not a new development. In its broader sense, it has been happening for many years in many countries. However, in its more recent usage, it is associated with a set of fairly focused activities and objectives which are being considered or implemented by countries across the developing world and the political spectrum. These are particularly addressed to financing, resource allocation and management issues, although the precise mix and emphasis of HSR policies varies. It should also be noted that in some contexts, the rhetoric of HSR is significantly greater than the reality.

Most developing countries implementing HSR are doing so against a background of serious economic pressures and the need to constrain health sector costs. At the same time, the goal of universal coverage appears as elusive as ever but remains a principle to which most governments are abstractly committed. HSR policies are thus addressed particularly to making more efficient use of available resources through institutional reforms and to widening the range of financing options and institutional players who provide health care. Allied to these major concerns, there is also a growing debate about the quality of service provision and its relationship to utilization, notably in the context of moves towards cost recovery.

Cassels (1995) provides a helpful map of the current territory of HSR. He sees the underlying principles of HSR as institutional. First, they concern the development of a managerial rather than a provider led culture, with associated changes in accountability. Second, they involve the clear setting of priorities, objectives and standards of performance, the monitoring of outputs and outcomes and the tracking of human and financial resource use. Third, they entail a clearer distinction between the institutional relationships of service commissioning and service provision. These may be summarized further as a general move (at least in theory) towards a contract based rather than a bureaucratic model of health systems functioning.

He also suggests that HSR may be understood in terms of both content and process. While content understandings focus on specific activities and goals (e.g. decentralizing health systems management, broadening financing options), process understandings are concerned with the relationships between institutional actors and the way these define, react to or are affected by HSR activities. He points out that process approaches to HSR have been relatively neglected and that much more research is needed on the institutional processes and outcomes of HSR.

This theme is echoed by Walt (1995), for whom HSR is essentially about the restructuring of relationships between, for instance, public and private sectors and users and providers. The emphasis on process and relationships is very important from a gender perspective, as gender is itself a relational concept. Such an approach allows us to ask critical questions about how HSR may restructure social and economic relationships in which gender is a significant marker. Unfortunately, until some more gender aware empirical research is done, these will remain questions.

The six main components of HSR programmes outlined by Cassels (1995) are used as a framework to consider the possible gender implications of

HSR. These six components, together with the main issues which they raise, are first summarized briefly here:

1. Improving the performance of the civil service (e.g. reducing staff numbers, changing pay, grading and appraisal systems, and reworking job descriptions)

Gender issues – the impact on the gender balance and composition of staffing at different levels, effects of human resources policies on relations between predominantly 'male' and female' health service professions.

2. Decentralization (management systems/health care provision devolved to local government or other agencies closer to local populations)

Gender issues – under what circumstances do decentralized systems improve access or further marginalize vulnerable groups?

3. Improving the functioning of national ministries of health (organizational restructuring to improve human and financial resource management, monitoring performance, defining priorities and cost-effective interventions)

Gender issues – in defining priorities, what criteria are used to determine health needs within the wider population? What criteria are being used to determine cost-effectiveness? Human resource policies also raise gender issues (see under 1).

4. Broadening health financing options (introduction of user fees, community financing mechanisms, social and private insurance schemes, voucher systems)

Gender issues – what are the gender implications of different modes of payment? Are poor women affected differently than poor men? How does cost recovery affect access to services by gender?

5. Introducing managed competition (promoting competition between health service providers/multiple purchasers)

Gender issues – how does managed competition affect equity and access for the most vulnerable?

6. Working with the private sector (establishing systems for regulating, contracting with, or franchising providers in the private sector)

Gender issues – are vulnerable groups more or less likely to be appropriately served by different parts of the private sector? Are women's health needs more or less likely to be met in a mixed economy of health care?

Although this provides a useful framework for developing these issues, there are large areas of overlap between these components, in particular, between 1, 2 and 3, 2 and 4, and 5 and 6.

1. Improving the performance of the civil service

This refers to a range of institutional reforms which are broadly human resource based and which link in both with attempted reforms at ministry of health level and with moves towards decentralization. In terms of formal sector employment in health care systems, many LDCs inherited structures put in place by departing colonial powers. This applies particularly to the professional hierarchies of medicine and the training of health professionals. This legacy has remained despite the growth of primary health care (PHC) which has generally been superimposed onto existing hierarchies, with tensions resulting from the clash of logics. Most low-income country health systems remain biased in terms of resources and personnel towards urban, hospital based health care, despite a professed commitment to PHC. Professional status reflects this bias, with doctors monopolizing the most senior positions.

Gender maps onto this in complex ways. There is a broad correlation between status (which in turn determines career structure, rewards and right to private practice) and gender. Front-line health workers are often disproportionately female. Senior positions are held disproportionately by men. However, women have made some important inroads into this structure, notably through the nursing profession. As Bloom (1991) points out, the nursing profession has become an important power base for women in a number of African countries (see also Marks 1995).

The politics of reform in the public sector are thus also complex. On the one hand, resistance to reforms may be expected to come from key professional interest groups, such as the medical profession, which are dominated by men, particularly at senior levels. This will be particularly strong where reforms challenge professional boundaries and internal professional demarcations by, for example, widening the range of people who can carry out certain tasks. Such a change could potentially open up more possibilities for women who are at the lower end of the hierarchy. On the other hand, women in professions such as nursing also have a strong interest in the maintenance of existing professional boundaries and career structures, particularly where there are so few areas of formal sector employment in which they have achieved any comparable collective power.

The political dynamics of such attempted reforms have received very little attention so far, but two brief examples illustrate some of the potential dilemmas. Bloom (1991) notes that in Zimbabwe, an attempt by a reforming Minister of Health to change the structure of nurse promotions brought about his political downfall. There, senior nursing staff, as well as being powerful in their own right as part of a professional lobbying group, had important familial and social links with senior politicians and civil servants.

Cassels and Janovsky (1994) comment on the impact on some professional interest groups of introducing general management into the health sector in Ghana. Before the reforms, management was functionally based, which meant that control over postings, transfers and promotions was retained within the professions. The move to separate management functions, including a human resources function, has, not surprisingly, upset the professions. However, it appears to have upset the nurses and pharmacists most. Under the new system, all management positions are theoretically open to all health professionals with management experience. In practice, they have been dominated by doctors who have monopolized the relevant training opportunities at the expense of nurses and pharmacists.

At the same time, the few nurses with graduate training have experienced problems when posted to management positions. Their training sets them apart from the rest of the nursing community and they are subject to envy and mistrust. Cassels and Janovsky see this primarily in terms of the struggle for legitimacy between two competing concepts of seniority – one based on length of service and the other on merit based preferment. However, it seems likely that gender is also an important factor in the political contests that are being fought out on the terrain of general management.

It is likely that more women were represented in senior positions, at least in the nursing profession, when management functions were retained within professional groups. The subsequent monopoly of management roles by doctors suggests a worsening of sex ratios, given the prevalence of men at senior levels of the medical profession. Nurses may thus have double grounds for complaint over their loss of status. Similarly, there may be a gender dimension to the problems experienced by those nurses in management positions, as female managers face resistance connected both to occupational status and to hostility to female superiors (which may come from both men and women). Cassels and Janovsky rightly draw attention to the need to develop equal opportunities for those groups which are losing out. However, account also needs to be taken of the equal opportunities implications of low numbers of – and inadvertent further reduction in – women in management positions.

The interlinking and reinforcing nature of gender, class and professional status in health sector employment patterns is well demonstrated in these examples, and means that gender cannot be analyzed in isolation from these other factors. From a gender and equity perspective, however, two crucial questions may be posed. First, given the high degree of gender segmentation in health sector employment, how do specific health sector reforms affect those sectors dominated by women? Second, are reforms likely to affect female health sector employees in a similar way to or differently from male employees of comparable status?

Recent reviews of human resources issues in the context of HSR throw little light on these questions.[3] However, Hornby (1995) notes the need to explore the opportunities for changes in skill mix in order to increase the number of lower skilled staff and reduce the need for higher skilled, more expensive staff. Such a policy, if it were able to be implemented against certain opposition from powerful professional groups, could be advantageous to the great numbers of women employed at the lower levels of the health service who would benefit from multi-skilling, and would thus improve gender equity in employment.

The reality in many countries labouring under severe economic constraints is of significant layoffs of public sector personnel at all levels, and declining real wages. It is as or more likely that reductions in personnel will fall on the less powerful groups of employees, more of whom will be women. Another possible scenario is that some health care tasks which currently form part of the role of paid front-line health staff will increasingly drop out of the formal system and devolve onto unremunerated 'community' workers (also frequently women), and, less directly, onto female carers within households.

As Bloom (1991) points out, restructuring health sector employment raises a number of issues relevant to gender. As we have already seen, the question of control over senior posts has an important gender dimension and is one aspect of a broader issue about reforming career structures and their associated rewards throughout the health sector, which will require attention in terms of their effects on both gender balance of staffing and equity of treatment between the sexes.

A related issue concerns access to private practice in a climate where there is increasing emphasis on the role of the private sector in delivering health care. Historical differences in access to private practice between the various health professions have helped to institutionalize a division between a disproportionately 'female' public sector and a disproportionately 'male' (formal) private sector. Changing the balance between these will have important implications for women's roles and status as health professionals.

Summary of issues

There are a number of compelling reasons to take the question of gender equity in health sector employment seriously. First, there are grounds for concern that women's employment in this sector is particularly vulnerable to any significant reduction in staffing levels, given their preponderance at lower levels and in specific occupations. Second, evidence from many developing countries suggests that female users of health services are more likely to, or in some cases will only, utilize certain services if the service provider is female. Maintenance of appropriate levels of female staffing is thus important for the delivery of such services. Third, human resources policies tend to be couched in gender neutral language, yet in situations where there are major imbalances in the gender composition of the workforce, their effects may not be neutral.

2. Decentralization

The concept of decentralization has been the subject of considerable debate (see Mills 1990; Kutzin 1995; Bossert 1995; Collins 1995). The most commonly used definition sees it as a transfer of resources, functions and authority from the centre to the periphery; that is, reserving its use for devolution within the public sector. The discussion which follows concentrates on the potential gender and equity outcomes of devolution from the centre to the periphery of the public infrastructure, including to community based structures such as local health committees (Bossert's 'regulated market model', 1995, p.2). The possible implications of decentralization for gender inequality have received almost no attention.

The main equity concern which has been raised is that of regional inequity. Kutzin (1995) suggests three ways in which regional equity may be reduced by decentralization. First, inter-regional inequalities can arise when wealthier districts are able to raise more funds than poorer ones and offer better staff conditions. An example of this occurred in Zambia, where the original draft of the reform programme suggested that district and hospital boards would be able to set their own levels of fees and decide locally on terms for the staff. This would have meant that hospitals in wealthier areas which could have raised the most income would have been able to draw key staff away from the less wealthy areas by offering them better terms and conditions.

Such examples point to the tensions inherent in the decentralization process – what is the precise tradeoff between decentralization and the centralized revenue allocation required to offset such inequalities? In raising this question, McPake (1993) points to the need to develop measures of equity and relate them to the basis for allocating resources to the appropriate decentralized units. Measures do, however, need to be designed to take account of social (including gender) vulnerability. One possibility would be to develop a vulnerability index for regions or districts which could incorporate contextually specific indicators of vulnerability such as the proportion of female-supported households.

Second, decentralization may simply result in the transfer of power from the centre to regional elites, thus producing an adverse impact on *intra-regional* equity. This points to the importance of the organizational framework within which decentralization is pursued. Where decentralization becomes defined primarily as a battle for resources between different types of elite, those without any access to local or national power structures will almost certainly lose out.

Third, decentralization might 'serve as an excuse by central government authorities to transfer the burden of financing development to the local community' (Kutzin 1995, p.30), with adverse effects on poverty alleviation. This raises the broader questions of the link with cost recovery and the use of decentralization as a tool for greater community level participation in health care delivery.

The issue of community involvement is not a new one. However, recent interest in the context of HSR has focused much more directly on the pragmatics of financing and managing PHC (and to some extent district hospitals) in more efficient and self-sustaining ways. Community participation is thus more of a means to an end than an end in itself. There is no doubt that communities (whether as sets of individuals or as collectivities) are increasingly being required to raise more resources towards their own health care. At the same time, decentralization may enable them, through vehicles such as local health committees (LHCs), to acquire greater control over the disposal of centrally allocated funds, the type of services available, and the health personnel who provide them.

The implications of this form of decentralization for equity and for allocational decision making are as yet little researched. Two sets of issues are relevant. The first concerns the organizational framework of such bodies and their capacity to act effectively. The second concerns the kinds of allocational decisions which LHCs actually make.

Effective local management of community based structures appears to be intrinsically tied to wider organizational decisions about financing mechanisms and about bureaucratic and political control. In terms of current interest in decentralization involving LHCs, the issue is also linked to cost recovery in the context of whether money raised through user charges at PHC level is retained locally and there is sufficient capacity to translate this revenue into improved service quality, which *may* in turn have a compensatory effect on utilization rates. (See also next section.)

The WHO's Second Evaluation, for the Africa region, of the 'Health for All' Global Strategy (WHO 1994) does not paint a very optimistic picture of community involvement through LHCs. It suggests that they are often set up solely to mobilize for centrally determined programmes, that participation is low and that inter-sectoral coordination is often weak. This theme is echoed by Hanson and McPake (1993, and see also McPake et al. 1993) in their evaluation of the Bamako Initiative.

In terms of the politics of local control, the degree to which LHCs represent, and are accountable to, their local communities is unclear. Hanson and McPake (1993) found a notable absence of women on LHCs, despite the emphasis in Bamako on promoting the health of women and children. The accountability of community based health staff is also often confused: to what extent are they answerable to bureaucratic control from regional and central structures, and to what extent to the communities themselves?

These broad organizational issues have two main implications for equity. First, in terms of financing mechanisms, without a clear framework for resource allocation and management at local level, the efforts of LHCs and their equivalents will be at best ad hoc and contingent, possibly resulting in wide variations or fluctuations (both intra- and inter-community) in what services get provided and their quality. In terms of bureaucratic and political control, without appropriate mechanisms for accountability both up and down the structure, it is unlikely that the interests of the more vulnerable sections of the population will find representation.

The second major issue concerns the allocational decisions which LHCs and other community based bodies make. Very little is known about this aspect of community involvement, and the concept of 'community' is often a taken for granted one in which predominantly male leaders are assumed to 'speak for' the community as a whole. There is, perhaps, a tendency to assume that if organizational and resource problems are resolved, then communities will automatically operate in the best interests of all their members. Yet no studies appear to have looked systematically at the question of how health related priorities are decided at local level in contexts where such bodies operate.[4] There is certainly evidence to suggest that local preferences may favour curative services, especially those involving high rates of drug dispensing (see LaFond 1995; Tipping and Segall 1995). This may be to the neglect of the less locality specific, longer term gains from preventive and public health interventions.

In this context, it is instructive to note the list of essential health service needs for women suggested by the World Bank in its recent publication on women's health and nutritional needs (World Bank 1994). These fall substantially into the category of preventive and health promotional measures (e.g. the prevention of nutritional discrimination against women and girls and of violence against women). It is not at all clear, therefore, that measures which could have a major impact on women's health will be considered priorities for the communities in which they live, particularly where they involve challenging entrenched behaviours.

At present, there are only snippets of evidence on what communities regard as priorities and how community based forms of decentralized decision-making operate. In a study in rural and urban Tanzania, Abel-Smith and Rawal (1992) asked people (gender not specified) which services they would be prepared to pay for. The most frequent response was drugs, followed by in-patient services. When asked what they should not be charged for, the most specific answers were MCH services.

This encouraging response may be compared with the actual experience of the long running Pikine urban PHC project in Senegal, described by Carrin (1992) in which very high levels of political, financial and managerial devolution to community health committees were achieved. Children's service fees were initially set at half adult fees and cross-subsidized by flat rate fees for adults. However, over a 15 year period, the cost of pre-natal checks rose by half as much as the increase in other adult fees, and the cost of maternal deliveries rose by twice as much.

Thus, while in the early years, the project effected a major increase in the numbers of women obtaining access to MCH services, a survey 15 years on, found health service utilization substantially reduced among 22% of mothers and 23% of infants. It is not clear what decision-making processes took place at community level, but the fee increases seem to have been ad hoc responses to financial pressures. This suggests that even highly devolved and comparatively participatory structures may sacrifice equity considerations when confronted by other kinds of pressures.

Summary of issues

So far the debates about decentralization have focused largely on the issue of interregional inequalities. The argument has thus been about the balance of decision making between central and regional (local) structures and to what extent central authorities should intervene to reallocate resources. While many commentators have stressed the importance of community participation as a means to improve service quality and utilization, little attention has been paid to what happens within communities, in terms of how resource allocation decisions are made and which groups benefit from them, how existing intracommunity inequalities can be addressed, and what are the organizational support needs for more community devolved structures, including developing greater participation by under-represented groups such as women.

3. Improving the functioning of national ministries of health, monitoring performance, defining priorities and cost-effective interventions

There are obvious links between this aspect of HSR and the reform of the civil service in terms of the issues raised for equal opportunities in the context of staffing structures and composition, so these will not be discussed further here (see section 1). The relationship between attempts to change the institutional culture within which health systems function, and access and health status outcomes on the ground has not really been researched. This is partly because it is more of a normative issue at present. Reform is aimed ultimately at creating a health care system which is more contractually than bureaucratically driven and thus more responsive to users, but there is limited experience of such institutional change so far.

Where equity concerns most obviously arise is in the definition of priorities and cost-effective interventions. Zambia provides an interesting example of a country attempting to implement a programme of HSR in which this issue is prominent. The centrepiece is an integrated Health Care Package designed for each service level and incorporating a combination of priority curative and preventive services and organizational interventions to support these services. Such packages cut across conventional vertical programme structures and entail quite far reaching changes in financial and human resource management. The HSR programme in Zambia is a very bold attempt to change the behaviour both of providers, in terms of how they deliver services, and users, in terms of producing more 'appropriate' health seeking behaviours (e.g. in drug use and referral). It is coupled with a commitment to monitor outcomes using a range of indicators, including health status.

Summary of issues

A critical question for programmes of this kind is whether and to what extent equity and affordability can co-exist. How far, for instance, can such integrated packages (which have to be costed within very modest parameters in the poorest countries) take account of the specific health needs of women or other groups with particular health needs? By what process are priorities defined? What considerations are involved in determining cost-effectiveness? What will be the response if, amid an overall improvement in health systems functioning and health status, equity worsens for particular groups such as rural women?

4. Broadening health financing options

Although this component of HSR covers a wide range of issues concerned with the financing of national health care systems, it is notable that far more has been written on cost recovery from the direct user, mainly at point of service, than on any other aspect of HSR. This perhaps indicates the extent to which 'user charges' have become synonymous with HSR. It is also the one issue where considerable, if rather narrowly focused, attention has been paid to equity, mainly because of concern with the impact of cost recovery on the poor.[5]

Much has already been written on the impact of user charges on the poor (see Creese 1991; Creese and Kutzin 1994; Huber 1993; McPake 1993; McPake et al. 1993; Yoder 1989). This discussion focuses mainly on gender as a relatively neglected aspect of the debate. However, some key issues arising from this literature need noting.

First, one of the consistent arguments in defence of user charges has been that poorer sections of the population in most LDCs do spend substantial amounts on private sector health care.[6] This is considered to be partly because public sector services are often of poor quality and partly because, although 'free', in practice they carry hidden and not so hidden costs (drugs may be unavailable, staff may expect payment, time is lost through waiting etc.). The evidence on the comparative costs of resort to the private, as opposed to the public, sector is conflicting and subject to different interpretations depending on how costs are defined. More comprehensive interpretations of cost include time spent waiting and on travelling to purchase drugs which should have been available at the public facility. They may also include the opportunity costs of women's time.

However, we still know little about how (and with what degree of elasticity) these non-monetary costs are commensurated by the poor themselves (both men and women), and this will be a major factor in an already complex household decision-making process (see Leslie 1992).[7] This is important in the context of Kutzin's argument that the overall effect of an increase in fees must be to lower the costs facing potential users in gaining access to effective care (Kutzin 1995).

Second, the debate is dogged by methodological problems. There is a lack of comparability between case study methodologies, making it difficult to compare one concept of the 'poor' with another.[8] Generalizations (for instance about the link between service quality and utilization rates) have been made confidently, based on single or non-comparable cases. Part of the difficulty has been the concentration on a generic category such as the poor or very poor, rather than on more substantive indicators of vulnerability. This has often meant a lack of disaggregation of data in terms of important markers such as gender, age or location.

Studies of the impact of user charges which have provided more disaggregation include Creese (1991) who found that following the introduction of user charges, the largest drop in utilization was among children under 14 and adults over 45. Waddington and Enyimayew (1989, 1990) found major differences between rural and urban areas in Ghana: three years after the introduction of user charges, utilization rates recovered to their pre-charge levels in urban health centres, but in rural ones the downward trend continued. They also found that the proportion of female users declined significantly.

The impact of user charges on health status has received little systematic attention, but there are some suggestive studies in relation to the impact of user charges on women's health. Kutzin (1995) points out that in Zimbabwe, the greater enforcement of user charges in the early 1990s may have harmed maternal health, as the use of MCH services declined by 30% and the number of babies born before their mothers reached hospital increased by 4%.

A study in Nigeria suggests that maternal mortality rates (MMR) could provide a suitable proxy for monitoring changes in health status in the context of cost recovery. It was noted that between 1983 and 1988, when fees were introduced for most aspects of health care, maternal deaths in the Zaria region increased by 56%. This coincided with a decline of 46% in the number of deliveries in the main hospital and a threefold increase in obstetric complications. The interval between admission and surgery increased 'strikingly' as relatives often spent a long time looking for money (Ekwempu et al. 1990).

From a gender and equity perspective, two themes need to be explored. First, *exactly which groups suffer most from the levying of user charges?* Second, *what has been the impact of the various measures, such as exemptions and cross subsidies, which have been used to ameliorate the effects on the most vulnerable?*

On the basis of analyses of utilization rates, a fairly consistent answer has emerged that the poor are the losers. The poor are, however, a large category from the point of view of policy. Is it possible to be more specific about degrees of vulnerability? Unfortunately, data on utilization rates have their limitations. The first problem is that they tell us only about trends among those who have been users at some time. Although this will include most of the population, other data from studies of health seeking behaviour suggest that the poor are both more likely to fall sick and less likely to seek treatment (McPake 1993a; Huber 1993). Thus, the groups being compared are not fully comparable in terms of their health seeking behaviour.

A second problem with data on utilization is that it is not possible to extrapolate how health expenditures become redistributed within the populations affected by user charges. For instance, does a change in overall utilization rates disguise other changes in who, within a household, gets access to health care, or the kind of care they get? Such data would be essential to understanding the allocation of scarce resources between the generations and across the genders.

A third, and related problem, as McPake et al. (1993) point out, is that utilization does not capture the impact of health expenditure on other household expenditures. Does more spent on health, whether through preference or necessity, mean less spent on education, for instance? And which categories of individuals gain or lose? This question is linked to the importance of understanding the trade-offs which households and individuals make between health and other public goods, especially where user charges are being introduced or increased in several sectors at once.

One of the few studies to take gender as a variable in examining the impact of user fees on service utilization is Moses et al. (1992), which looked at attendance at a sexually transmitted diseases referral clinic in Kenya. This found that before the introduction of user charges, smaller numbers of women attended the clinic than men. However, after charges were introduced, male attendance dropped by more than that of women. After charges were abandoned, men's attendance rose to only two thirds of its pre-charge level, whereas women's attendance rose to 22% above its earlier level. Without more understanding of the *rationales* behind men's and women's health seeking behaviour in relation to STDs, it is difficult to draw any wider conclusions from this study other than to make the obvious point that introducing charges for STD services is probably counter-productive for both sexes and for public health generally.

To return to the question of whether it is possible to be more specific about vulnerability, there are a number of pointers to this. First, data on utilization trends suggest that the rural poor are more vulnerable to the imposition of user charges than the urban poor (Waddington and Enyimayew 1989, 1990; see also Vogel 1993). Within the rural poor, known indicators of greatest vulnerability are being a woman or a child in a female headed or supported household in an area of high economic deprivation, and/or being without kin who are able or prepared to offer support at critical times (Vogel 1993; McPake et al. 1993; Musowe 1995). Widows are disproportionately found in this category, but elderly men with attenuated kinship links, those with disabilities, and orphaned children and adolescents are also highly vulnerable. What may be noted is that these are as much social as economic categories. This has an important bearing on the question of how to ameliorate the impact of user charges.

The adverse effects of user charges on the economically vulnerable have been sought to be reduced mainly through various exemption mechanisms. The most systematic reviews so far have focused on 'community financing'. This links user payments to the retention and management of the income at community level, and has been suggested as an effective way of reducing inequities in health service utilization (WHO 1993). This again depends on the assumption that, if able to raise additional resources for health care, communities will make more equitable decisions than planners or health personnel.

McPake (1993), McPake et al. (1993) and Hanson and McPake (1993) look at the experience of the Bamako Initiative (BI) from the point of view of its effects on equity in selected BI countries. Bamako particularly emphasizes the promotion of the health of women and children (see also Jarrett and Ofosu-Amah 1992). In general, they find that Bamako has brought about a relative improvement in most of the countries studied in terms of its effect on access and quality of health services. They also find that on *relative* affordability criteria, BI initiatives compare favourably with other alternatives. However, *absolute* affordability problems remain: BI has neither improved nor worsened the position of the most marginalized groups, including categories such as widows, who remain without access. In terms of equity, therefore, the unenviable trade-off seems to be relative improvement for the majority against no change for the most vulnerable minority. In strict terms, this implies a decrease in overall equity.

This lack of improvement for the minority can be linked both to inadequacies in the way exemption mechanisms work and to problems with the concept of community participation already discussed in the last section, but particularly the lack of representation of those most vulnerable to charges for health care.

Exemption mechanisms operate in a variety of ways but a number seem to be based on an approximate assessment of patients' incomes. These assessments may be made at the point of service delivery by staff, or at community level by influential members or by LHCs (Bennett and Ngalande-Banda 1994; Huber 1993). Those made by staff in particular are often done in a somewhat ad hoc way, may be open to abuse, and are of no benefit to those who do not seek health care in the first place because of fear of cost. While all exemption schemes tend to embody some unfairness (especially to those who fall just above the specified minimum level), income based exemptions in the context of poor rural economies are notoriously difficult to operationalize in a fair way. The resources of both the rural poor, and the not so poor, tend to be a complex and ever-changing patchwork of the tangible (e.g. seasonal cash, land) and the intangible (e.g. gifts, informal credit). Commensurating these into a notional income is fraught with pitfalls.

Some alternatives to the fruitless search for a more refined income-based criterion have been emerging. Dawson (n.d.) describes a method to develop more context specific indicators of socioeconomic status by involving rural households in developing their own wealth ranking criteria. Whether this will provide a more generalizable tool for local communities is yet to be tested. Where community based exemptions have been set up, it is interesting to note in the context of conceptualizing vulnerability that they seem to be based more on social categories. McPake (1993) found that LHCs may define exemption criteria quite narrowly (e.g. victims of natural disasters, abandoned women). In Carrin's account of the Pikine PHC Project, initiated in the 1970s in Senegal (1992), which bears many similarities to more recent Bamako approaches, exemptions covered the blind, 'indigent' and widowed. These categories, while narrow, may well accord better with people's own perception of vulnerability as a social phenomenon, and thus be more implementable at a community level.

This again returns us to the question of what kinds of community based structures produce what kinds of decisions and health outcomes for different groups. It also raises similar questions to those already discussed in relation to decentralization. Involving communities in these kinds of decisions may produce outcomes which health professionals and planners may not see as optimal in terms of equity. What kinds of trade-offs between community involvement and wider goals of equity (such as positively discriminating in favour of women's health needs, or regions with high levels of economic deprivation) are going to be acceptable, and who will arbitrate/decide?

There is some evidence to suggest that access and utilization by vulnerable groups are affected by different modes of payment. It is well established that most existing health insurance schemes in developing countries are partial, disproportionately benefiting middle class urban populations and designated groups such as public sector workers (Vogel 1993).

More recent experiments with different models of community based health insurance schemes, mainly in Francophone Africa (see Bennett and Ngalande-Banda 1994), would repay systematic evaluation from an equity and utilization point of view. Such schemes have to tread a delicate balance to maintain commitment by households from diverse socioeconomic backgrounds. Charging a flat rate to all members may create major problems for poor households in paying regular contributions. Yet concessions to the poor on amount, type or timing may alienate wealthier households or render the scheme unviable. Carrin (1992, Pikine Project) noted that pre-payment schemes were less popular than fee for service as people worried about their ability to pay and perhaps did not trust the scheme to deliver on its promises.

Arhin (1994) provides some evidence that pre-payment schemes may be more helpful to women. Her study in Burundi found that women could more readily utilize health services with a pre-payment card as – having little access to cash – they could attend the clinic without seeking permission and money from their husbands. The beneficiaries of this appeared to be the children rather than the women, and it would be premature to draw the conclusion that pre-payment schemes benefit women per se.

Lack of access to cash for women is a general feature of rural African economies. Where women experience a high degree of dependency on male kin for such access, a pre-payment system may improve their situation. Where they are unsupported, it may have the opposite effect, unless ways are found to enable women to build up their own system of credits. Again, more systematic research is needed on the question of how modes of payment affect particular social groups, what is likely to be acceptable and what these imply for developing viable community level insurance schemes. For instance, literacy levels are generally lower among women than men and they often have less access to information sources. This may affect women's capacity to participate in such schemes.

Summary of issues

The debate about the impact of cost recovery on vulnerable groups has been marked by a) a rather piecemeal approach in which sometimes conflicting generalizations have been based on a limited number of methodologically non-comparable studies, and b) an insufficient level of disaggregation of categories such as 'the poor' to produce well informed and imaginative policy responses. This points to a more general need to collect data which are methodologically and conceptually comparable and which are sufficiently disaggregated to enable the groups most affected to be pinpointed more precisely and the precise effects of different aspects of cost recovery understood more clearly.

5. Introducing managed competition *and*
6. Working with the private sector

These two aspects of the Cassels framework are considered together as they raise similar issues in relation to gender and equity. Their implications in these areas have also been little explored as yet, and there is little information to draw upon. The introduction of managed competition generally refers to the promotion of competition between multiple providers in some kind of 'managed market' arrangement involving both public and private providers (including NGOs and potentially 'traditional' practitioners as well). Working with the private sector entails the establishment of regulatory and contractual regimes to govern relations between purchaser and provider and to lay down standards of service provision.

While the first raises the more general question of whether the introduction of competition into the health sector may increase or detract from equity, the answer is to a large degree dependent on the second – that is, what are the specific outcomes of the contractual arrangements which are made and how can they be made sensitive to equity concerns? It follows that any answers given are likely to be context specific.[9]

Before considering the possible impact on gender and equity of managed competition and the involvement of the private sector, note must be taken of the de facto situation in many developing countries, where private health provision, loosely defined, already constitutes a significant proportion of total health care expenditure. Tipping and Segall (1995: 18–19) note some of the factors involved. There are cases of private practitioners being preferred because they offer a more accessible, convenient and flexible service (which is particularly important to women who suffer greater time and other constraints), are perceived to offer better quality services (particularly in the area of interpersonal skills), and may be cheaper in the case of traditional practitioners and when indirect as well as direct costs are taken into account. In addition, substantial use is made of private pharmacies, both for over-the-counter drug sales and for medical advice and sometimes actual interventions.

The private sector, in all its diversity, has thus always been an important provider of services to poorer households and to women, as well as being generally the first resort of the wealthiest sections of the population. Women in particular have always been major users of traditional practitioners. Additionally, the contracting out of services to non-government providers, such as mission hospitals in sub-Saharan Africa, has a long history.

A mixed market in health care provision has thus been a reality for most developing countries. Advocates of managed competition seek both to acknowledge and to build on this reality, and to use competition as a means to improve the technical efficiency of services in the public sector by establishing more transparent cost, quality and efficiency standards across both public and private sectors, and enforcing them contractually (see Bennett and Ngalande-Banda 1994). In this context, the question of equity becomes particularly complex. It should also perhaps encompass the issue of whether managed competition is an improvement over existing forms of unregulated competition in increasing access and service quality for vulnerable groups.

A further issue concerns the extent to which the private sector can be harnessed to the provision of preventive health care services and the achievement of public health objectives, given strong prevailing biases towards curative services, on the part of both practitioners and patients. Public health and preventive services have important gender implications. Women absorb much of the additional burden imposed by, for example, high rates of chronic diarrhoeal infections in children and other environmentally induced health problems.

Two problems hinder analysis of these questions. One is the absence of any systematic empirical data on the impact of these two aspects of HSR on the type of service provided, on access and on utilization. The other is the eclectic nature of the private sector itself. The case studies of health seeking behaviour referred to above are difficult to compare as they examine, variously, resort to a range of traditional practitioners (who are in themselves a highly diverse group), to practitioners trained in other orthodoxies than bio-medicine, to NGO and charitable providers and to private bio-medically qualified/unqualified practitioners.

From an equity point of view, it is particularly difficult, therefore, to disentangle issues of choice within a pluralistic medical system from issues of resource (i.e. income and time) and other constraints. In the case of women's health seeking behaviour, existing studies could be used to support two completely contrasting interpretations. Women's greater use of traditional practitioners and other locally based, non-biomedically qualified providers could be harnessed to support the view that this expresses a genuine preference for such providers. From a woman's point of view, they may be more convenient and flexible, closer to women's own understandings of their health needs, and more of them may be female. Managed competition should therefore include a systematic effort to involve them in service provision with women's health needs specifically in mind.

Alternatively, such patterns of usage could be seen as evidence of entrenched discrimination against women (and frequently children as well). The same studies often show that men are more likely than women to consult qualified bio-medical practitioners and to travel to health centres and hospitals. South Asian studies show that at primary care level, men and boys consume more of a household's total health expenditure than women and girls.[10] A strategy of involving traditional and non-biomedically qualified practitioners could thus be seen as encouraging the institutionalization of a two-tier system between the sexes.[11] More attention needs to be paid to the complexity of the factors underlying the different choices of health provider which are made at household level.

This example illustrates the methodological problems of determining what is an equitable strategy in relation to private sector involvement in health care when it is not at all obvious what are the equity goals to be pursued (and who is to determine them). For the most part so far, contracting out of services to the private sector has been aimed at improving coverage. Examples are the contracting of private practitioners in Namibia to provide surgical services in remote areas, and the provision of subsidies to non-governmental providers to fill gaps in health provision (see Kutzin 1995). Contractual arrangements for managing private sector involvement have focused particularly on quality. However, little attention has been paid to equity issues, nor has there been any significant debate about what equity might mean in the context of managed competition and how it can best be measured.

Arguably, increasing both coverage and quality of services could have a positive effect on equity in that they are likely to increase utilization rates. However, as was seen in relation to cost recovery, an overall increase in utilization can disguise significant differential usage within the population. If one of the primary reasons for women's greater use of private sector practitioners is their lower cost, then regulatory arrangements which result in an increase in their cost to the patient may have a detrimental impact on utilization by women, and by the very poor in general.

Introducing managed competition embodies a possibly heroic assumption that costs can be driven down by introducing more 'efficient' providers, while quality of care can be driven up. However, this in turn depends on there being more efficient providers around (as opposed simply to cheaper ones), and that some way can be found to commensurate the services of these very diverse providers. Further, while not all aspects of quality improvement carry major cost implications (e.g. treating patients more respectfully), some, such as training or technical improvements in laboratory services, undoubtedly do. The pertinent question then is are these costs to be borne by governments (or donors), by practitioners, by redistributive mechanisms such as general taxation or insurance schemes, by targeted measures such as voucher schemes, by the direct user, or by a combination of these? Each mode is likely to have different gender implications.

Summary of issues

This issue clearly raises some very large questions about the goals, scope and direction of policies to involve the private sector in all its variety through a process of managed competition. However, a number of important intermediate level questions are also raised which, if addressed empirically, would give a clearer indication of the implications of such policies for addressing gender based health inequalities. These questions relate particularly to the extent to which contractual frameworks can be devised to improve equity or to counter existing or potential inequalities in provision, such as by explicitly addressing women's health needs or inequalities of access through the contracting process.

Priorities for research on gender issues and HSR

The above analysis suggests that the following issues and questions need particular consideration in reforming countries. In this context, it may be noted that the Platform for Action of the Fourth World Conference on Women (1996) has called for support and funding for research on gender based inequalities in health, support for health systems research to strengthen access and improve service quality, and for the collection of more appropriately disaggregated statistics, including by sex and age.[12]

Improving the performance of the civil service

- What is the current structure and balance of staffing at different levels of the health care delivery system, broken down by gender?
- What is/will be the impact on the gender composition of staff, at different levels, of policies or proposals to restructure and/or reduce formal employment in the health sector?
- Has the introduction of general management functions, payment and grading systems affected the career structures of female employees at different levels of the health care system differently from equivalent male employees?
- What is the political terrain which has to be negotiated, and how can gender equity considerations be incorporated into policy making at the level of human resources policies?

Decentralization

- In addressing the problem of intra-regional inequalities in access to services through differential weighting of resources between areas, what kinds of indices can be developed which are sensitive to social vulnerability?
- What equity indicators are most appropriate for judging the outcomes of different models of decentralization? Are some more conducive to equity than others?
- How do community based structures, such as LHCs, make decisions, who or which groups do they represent, and what are the implications for women's health needs and for gender equity of their allocational decisions? What is the appropriate balance between central objectives to direct more resources to the most vulnerable, and devolution of resource allocation decisions to local structures?
- Where financial and managerial control is being devolved to community based structures, what are their needs in terms of organizational support, training and information, and what mechanisms of inclusion of women (and in particular poorer women) can be developed?

Improving the functioning of national ministries of health

- What kinds of consultation process with stakeholders, including users from different sections of the population, can be cost-effectively undertaken to help determine priorities?
- What process and outcome indicators are most appropriate for monitoring the impact of changes on the health of women and on gender based inequalities?

Broadening health financing options

- Data on health seeking behaviour and health service utilization should be gender and age disaggregated at minimum. Local concepts of vulnerability need to be taken more seriously in research and policy making.
- Longitudinal household level studies are needed to chart the impact of user charges on the allocation of intra-household resources by sector and by category of household member.
- More attention needs to be paid to health outcomes for different groups where cost recovery is operating. Which key indicators are most appropriate for monitoring this?
- How and under what circumstances (financially and politically) can service based exemptions be used to address the specific health needs of women and children?
- In community based health financing programmes, how can participation by the most disadvantaged be developed or strengthened to prevent further widening of the gap between users and non-users of services? For example, can women and other vulnerable groups be assisted to build up credits for PHC and tertiary care?
- Using consistent measures of equity, how do different models of community based health insurance compare?

Introducing health financing options/working with the private sector

- What kinds of incentives to private providers and associated contractual requirements are most likely to ensure that women's health needs are appropriately addressed?
- What kinds of incentives to private providers and associated contractual requirements would be most likely to improve access to services by women and girls?
- How can public health and preventive services be given appropriate weight within a managed competition framework?
- How might contracting out to the private sector be used to increase women's access to and choice of female practitioners?
- Given the ambiguity in interpreting the meaning of women's utilization of private sector providers, what strategies can be developed to involve women in debate about their health needs and preferences?
- How are patterns of health service utilization among women changing with the introduction of managed competition?

Acknowledgements

This is a revised version of a concept paper written for the Health Systems Development Group, Liverpool School of Tropical Medicine, as part of the

UK ODA-funded Health Sector Reform Research Work Programme. I thank Dr Dave Haran for facilitating its production, and two anonymous referees for additional comments. The financial support of the Health and Population Division of the ODA is gratefully acknowledged. The facts presented and views expressed in this paper are those of the author and do not necessarily reflect the policies of the Overseas Development Administration.

Notes

1 Concern here is limited to the health sector and no attempt is made to address the broader debate and substantial literature about the impact of structural adjustment policies (SAPs) on vulnerable groups, or their possible interactions with HSR, as this would require another paper. Work which considers the gender implications of SAPs includes Elson (1993) and Vivian (1995).
2 For an accessible and recent account of gender and development approaches, see Kabeer (1995).
3 Dr Tom Hall, of the University of California School of Medicine, who is preparing a Human Resources for Health Toolkit for the WHO, tells me that he has not come across a single reference on the gender implications of HSR policies.
4 On a recent consultancy visit to West Bengal, where democratically elected local bodies have substantial control over community development funds, it was found that priority always went to 'hard infrastructure' projects such as roads and tube wells. Anecdotally, there was evidence that community level priorities had a gender dimension – while men favoured these kinds of projects, some women at least would have liked resources to go into health service improvements.
5 Cost recovery and user charges are not synonymous. The former concerns the different mechanisms through which health care costs may be recouped from users; the latter focuses on the recovery of costs at or very close to the point of service. Equity aspects of cost recovery relate to whether particular systems or mixes have greater or less equity disposing effects across the population. Equity aspects of user charges usually focus on whether they provide a deterrent to utilization of services by the poor and whether this can be offset by using the recovered costs to improve the quality of services (see Nolan and Turbat 1993).
6 A number of studies report heavy borrowing and significant indebtedness as a consequence of the need to pay for medical treatment (McPake 1993; WHO 1993; Abel-Smith and Rawal 1992).
7 In this context, Abel-Smith and Rawal (1992) provide a lot of data on issues such as waiting time and choice of facility but none of it is broken down by gender, including the 'heads of household' who provided the data. Recent World Bank sponsored studies of household coping strategies in relation to HIV/AIDS should provide a clearer picture of gender differentials in household expenditure allocation.
8 Compare, for example, Abel-Smith and Rawal's findings (1992) on who uses mission hospitals with those of Bloom and Segall (1993).
9 I am aware that this gloss on the question tends to sidestep the wider political debate about the desirability of contracting out a 'public good', such as health care, to private (and especially for-profit) providers, at least part of which is about equity in the wider sense. This is the province of a different paper. It may be noted, however, that the 1993 WHO evaluation of changes in health sector financing pointed out that a longer term concern about private sector involvement is the potential for the creation of a two-tier system. As the private sector expands it may take the wealthier part of the population with it, resulting in (further) erosion

of support for a nationally funded health system. Critics of this view from a developing country perspective would probably argue that a two-tier system exists in most of them already.
10 A review of Indian evidence can be found in Chatterjee (1990).
11 This has echoes in an earlier debate between Claquin (1981) and Feldman (1983) concerning the role of private health care providers in Bangladesh. Claquin argued that, given the prevalence and high level of use of private providers in rural Bangladesh, they should be involved in the implementation of government health programmes. Feldman, in taking issue with this, suggested that the gender and political composition of these providers would further decrease the quality of health care for the rural poor and particularly women (summarized in Tipping and Segall 1995).
12 See 'Strategic Objectives and Actions', para C, *Women and Health* (particularly objective C.4).

References

Abel-Smith B., Rawal P. 1992. Can the poor afford 'free' health services? A case study of Tanzania. *Health Policy and Planning* 7 (4): 329–41.

Arhin D. 1994. The health card insurance scheme in Burundi: a social asset or a non-viable venture? *Social Science & Medicine* 39 (6): 861–70.

Bennett S., Ngalande-Banda E. 1994. Public and private roles in health: A review and analysis of experience in sub-Saharan Africa. *Current Concerns SHS Paper no. 6*. World Health Organization, Geneva.

Bloom G. 1991. Gender and the Production of Health Care Services. Presentation to the Gender and Health Workshop, Institute of Development Studies, University of Sussex, UK.

Bloom G., Segall M. 1993. Expenditure and Financing of the Health Sector in Kenya. Commissioned Study no. 9. Institute of Development Studies, University of Sussex, UK.

Bossert T. 1995. Decentralisation. WHO Ad Hoc Health R & D Review. World Health Organization, Geneva. Draft.

Butter I. et al. 1987. Gender hierarchies in the health labor force. *International Journal of Health Services* 17 (1): 133–49.

Carrin G. 1992. *Strategies for Health Care Finance in Developing Countries*. Basingstoke and London: Macmillan.

Cassels A. 1995. Health Sector Reform: Key Issues in Less Developed Countries. WHO Forum on Health Sector Reform, Discussion Paper No. 1 (SHS/NHP/95.4). World Health Organization, Geneva.

Cassels A., Janovsky K. 1994. Ghana. Report on a Field Visit, 20 February–9 March. ODA/Liverpool School of Tropical Medicine, UK.

Chatterjee M. 1990. Indian Women: Their Health and Productivity. *World Bank Discussion Papers* no. 109. Washington DC: IBRD.

Collins C. 1995. Decentralisation. WHO Ad Hoc Health R & D Review. World Health Organization, Geneva. Draft.

Creese A. 1991. User charges for health care: a review of recent experience. *Health Policy and Planning* 6 (4): 309–19.

Creese A., Kutzin J. 1994. *Health Sector Reform – Report of the Second Consultation*. Geneva: World Health Organization.

Dave P. 1991. Community and self-financing in voluntary health programmes in India. *Health Policy and Planning* **6** (1): 20–31.

Dawson S. (n.d.) How do we measure equity if we can't identify the poor? Health Systems Development Group, Liverpool School of Tropical Medicine, UK.

Ekwempu et al. 1990. Structural adjustment and health in Africa. *The Lancet* (letter) **336:** 56–7.

Elson D. 1993. Structural Adjustment with Gender Awareness. Vulnerable Groups: Gender Based Distortions and Male Bias. Gender Analysis and Development Economics Working Paper no. 2, University of Manchester, UK.

Griffin C. 1992. Welfare gains from user charges for government health services. *Health Policy and Planning* **7** (2): 177–80.

Hanson K., McPake B. 1993. The Bamako Initiative: Where is it going? *Health Policy and Planning* **8** (3): 267–4.

Holden P., Littlewood J. 1991. *Anthropology and Nursing*. London: Routledge.

Hornby P. 1995. Human Resource Policies and Systems. WHO Ad Hoc Health R & D Review. World Health Organization, Geneva. Draft.

Huber J. 1993. Ensuring access to health care with the introduction of user fees: a Kenyan example. *Social Science & Medicine* **36** (4): 485–94.

Jarrett S. W., Ofasu-Amaah A. 1992. Strengthening health services for MCH in Africa: the first four years of the Bamako Initiative. *Health Policy and Planning* **7** (2): 164–76.

Kabeer N. 1994. *Reversed Realities*. London: Verso.

Kalumba K. 1994. Towards an Equity Oriented Policy of Decentralisation in Health Systems Under Conditions of Turbulence. Paper presented to The Forum on Health Sector Reform, Third Meeting, Brussels, 20–21 September.

Key P. 1987. Women, health and development, with special reference to Indian women. *Health Policy and Planning* **2** (1): 58–69.

Kutzin J. 1995. Experience with Organizational and Financing Reform of the Health Sector. *Current Concerns SHS paper No. 8* (SHS/CC/94.3). Geneva: World Health Organization.

LaFond A. 1995. *Sustaining Primary Health Care*. London: Save the Children/Earthscan Publications.

Leslie J., Lycette M., Buvinic M. 1988. Weathering economic crisis: the crucial role of women in health. In: Bell D. et al. (eds). *Health, Nutrition and Economic Crises: Approaches to Policy in the Third World*. Dover, Mass.: Auburn House Publishing Company.

Leslie J. 1992. Women's time and the use of health services. *IDS Bulletin* **23** (1): 4–7.

McPake B. 1993. User charges for health services in developing countries: a review of the economic literature. *Social Science & Medicine* **36** (11): 1397–405.

McPake B., Hanson K., Mills A. 1993. Community financing of health care in Africa: an evaluation of the Bamako Initiative. *Social Science & Medicine* **36** (11): 1383–95.

Marks S. 1995. *Divided Sisterhood: Race, Class and Gender in the South African Nursing Profession*. New York: Saint Martin's Press.

Mills A. et al. 1990. *Health Systems Decentralisation: Concepts, Issues and Country Experience*. Geneva: World Health Organization.

Mooney G. 1987. What does equity in health mean? *World Health Statistics Quarterly* **40**: 296–303.

Moses S. et al. 1992. Impact of user fees on attendance at a referral centre for sexually transmitted diseases in Kenya. *The Lancet* **340**: 463–6.

Musowe V. 1995. Health Reforms Conceptual Framework. Republic of Zambia: Ministry of Health, Planning and Management Unit. Draft.

Nolan B., Turbat V. 1993. *Cost Recovery in Health Services in sub-Saharan Africa.* Washington DC: The World Bank.

Platform for Action and the Beijing Declaration. 1996. *Fourth World Conference on Women, Beijing, China, 4–15 September 1995.* New York: United Nations Department of Public Information.

Stock R. 1983. Distance and the utilization of facilities in rural Nigeria. *Social Science & Medicine* **17** (9): 563–70.

Timyan J. et al. 1993. Access to care: more than a problem of distance. In: Koblinsky M., Timyan J., Gay S. (eds). *The Health of Women: A Global Perspective.* Westview Press.

Tipping G., Segall M. 1995. Health care seeking behaviour in developing countries: an annotated bibliography and literature review. *Development Bibliography 12.* Brighton: Institute of Development Studies.

Vivian J. (ed). 1995. *Adjustment and Social Sector Restructuring.* London: Frank Cass, in association with EADI/UNRISD.

Vogel R. J. 1988. Cost recovery in the health sector: selected country studies in West Africa. *World Bank Technical Paper no. 82.* Washington DC: The World Bank.

Vogel R. J. 1993. *Financing Health Care in sub-Saharan Africa.* Westport, Conn: Greenwood Press.

Waddington C., Enyimayew K. 1989. A Price to Pay: The impact of user charges in Ashanti-Akim District, Ghana. *International Journal of Health Planning and Management* **4** (1): 17–47.

Waddington C., Enyimayew K. 1990. A Price to Pay, Part 2: The impact of user charges in the Volta Region of Ghana. *International Journal of Health Planning and Management* **5** (4): 287–312.

Walt G. 1995. The Policy Process. WHO Ad Hoc Health R & D Review. World Health Organization, Geneva. Draft.

WHO. 1993. Evaluation of Recent Changes in the Financing of Health Services. *Technical Report Series 829.* Geneva: World Health Organization.

WHO. 1994. Implementation of the Global Strategy for Health for All by the Year 2000. *Eighth Report on the World Health Situation.* Vol. 2: African Region. Brazzaville: World Health Organization Regional Office for Africa.

World Bank. 1987. *Financing Health Services in Developing Countries: An Agenda for Reform.* Washington DC: World Bank.

World Bank. 1994. *A New Agenda for Women's Health and Nutrition.* Development in Practice Series. Washington DC: World Bank.

World Bank. 1993. *World Development Report 1993: Investing in Health.* New York: Oxford University Press, for the World Bank.

Yoder R. A. 1989. Are people willing and able to pay for health services? *Social Science & Medicine* **29** (1): 35–42.

45
GENDER MAINSTREAMING IN HEALTH
Looking back, looking forward

T. K. S. Ravindran and A. Kelkar-Khambete

Source: *Global Public Health*, 3:S1 (2008), 121–42.

Abstract

This paper reviews published literature on experiences in mainstreaming gender within the health sector since the 1990s. Although much has been written about the need for mainstreaming gender, and on how to go about it, the gap between intention and practice is palpable. National health policies and programmes that have gender integrally woven into their objectives and activities are rare. Health research to generate gender and sex-specific data, and integrating gender in health provider training, have received scarce attention. Mainstreaming gender within institutions has remained superficial, investing more on form than on content. The apparent lack of progress in mainstreaming gender in health may be attributed to: depoliticization and delinking of gender mainstreaming from social transformation and social justice agendas; adoption of top-down approaches to mainstreaming; growing hostility within the global policy environment to justice and equity concerns; and increasing privatization and retraction of the state's role in health. This paper suggests that the way forward would be to frame gender concerns in the language of equity, rights, and justice; to set agendas which consider gender inequity within the context of inequities by caste, class, ethnicity, and other sources of health inequalities; and to work alongside other movements for social justice.

Gender mainstreaming in health: definitions and concepts

Background

The concept of 'gender mainstreaming' evolved from attempts to improve women's share of the gains of development in the early 1970s. In the years following the International Conference on Population and Development (ICPD) in 1994, and the Fourth World Conference on Women in Beijing in 1995, the agenda shifted from an exclusive focus on women to 'mainstreaming', or integrating, gender into the mainstream in all sectors. This was in response to the realization that the approach of the earlier decades had led to the 'ghettoization' of women's projects, and to the mere addition of a few services, without fundamental changes in the way programmes are formulated and service is delivered.

This paper is an attempt to draw on recent (since 1995) experiences in gender mainstreaming in health across regions and at various levels, in order to understand what has been achieved, what the challenges have been, and to discuss how we may move the agenda forward. The paper is constrained by the limited availability of information. The authors were able to use only published work in English. Literature search was mainly web-based. The search yielded less than a hundred articles and publications dealing with gender mainstreaming in health. All, except a very small number (less than 10), were either how-to manuals, descriptions of projects, or reflections by implementers on barriers to gender mainstreaming. Information on the process of implementation, and evaluations of gender mainstreaming efforts, was very limited. Consequently, this paper depends much on perspectives of implementers and on the authors' own experiences to formulate tentative hypotheses on the reasons for the apparently limited progress of gender mainstreaming efforts in health.

The paper is structured as follows. This first section introduces concepts related to gender mainstreaming in health. The second section presents an overview of examples of 'operational' gender mainstreaming: mainstreaming gender in health policies, programmes, and projects; in health research; and training of health providers. Experiences with 'institutional' mainstreaming, both within the national health sector and within international organizations, are presented in section three. Section four presents the summary, and raises some questions on how we may move the agenda forward on gender mainstreaming.

Definitions and concepts

The most widely known and used definition of gender mainstreaming[1] is from the UN Economic and Social Council:

> Mainstreaming a gender perspective is the process of assessing the implications for women and men of any planned action, including legislation, policies or programmes, in all areas and at all levels. It is a strategy for making women's as well as men's concerns and experiences an integral dimension of the design, implementation, monitoring and evaluation of policies and programmes in all political,

economic and societal spheres so that women and men benefit equally and inequality is not perpetuated. The ultimate aim is to achieve gender equality.

(UNECOSOC 1997)

The World Health Organization's Gender Policy, states that the goal of gender mainstreaming in health is to contribute to better health for both men and women, through health research, policies, and programmes which give due attention to gender considerations and promote equity and equality between women and men. Gender mainstreaming is expected to increase coverage, effectiveness, and efficiency of all interventions. Further, gender mainstreaming aims to promote equity and equality between women and men throughout the life course and, at the least, ensure that interventions do not promote or perpetuate inequitable gender roles and relations (WHO 2002).

According to Gomez-Gomez (2002), gender mainstreaming in health rests on four key concepts: health as a human right; equity in health grounded in principles of social justice and human rights; gender, seen as the social relations of inequality between women and men intersecting with other sources of inequalities, such as class, race, and ethnicity; and democratic participation, as necessary for meeting the 'objectives of equity, social justice and health rights defence effectively and sustainably' (Gomez-Gomez 2002: 7–9). According to this interpretation, gender mainstreaming in health cannot be a top-down agenda, or focus only on gender-based inequities, without attention to other sources of inequities in health.

Two dimensions of gender mainstreaming have been emphasized in the literature on this subject:

- 'Operational mainstreaming', which refers to the integration of equality concerns into the content of policies, programmes, and projects to ensure that these have a positive impact on women and reduce gender inequalities.
- 'Institutional mainstreaming', which involves addressing the internal dynamics of formal (and informal) institutions, such as their goals, agenda setting, governance structures, and procedures related to day-to-day functioning, so that these support and promote gender equality (UN 2000).

Both of these aspects of gender mainstreaming are closely interrelated. The process of operational mainstreaming depends on the institutional support provided by various structures, starting from formal agencies to family and community units and, hence, the need for institutional gender mainstreaming. It must be noted that mainstreaming gender in health calls for a dual focus: addressing gender-based differences and inequalities in all health initiatives; and implementing initiatives addressing women's specific health needs that are a result either of biological differences between women and men (e.g. maternal health) or of gender-based discrimination in society (e.g. gender-based violence, poor access to health services). Both of these are essential for achieving health equity, which is the ultimate goal of gender mainstreaming.

Initiatives in operational gender mainstreaming

In this section, we examine examples of mainstreaming gender in:

- health policies;
- health programmes/projects;
- health research;
- health providers' training.

Mainstreaming gender in health policies

Sweden is perhaps the only available example of a country with a gender-integrated public health policy. There have, however, been several attempts at gender analysis of national health policies, intended perhaps as first steps towards mainstreaming gender within policies. Sweden's new public health policy, which came into force in 2003, has integrated gender within the framework of an equity-oriented public health policy. This policy is unique in many ways. Unlike most public health policies, in which objectives are based on diseases or health problems, Sweden's public health policy addresses the broader social determinants of health, including gender (Ostlin and Diderichsen 2003). The policy was developed over a 3-year period, which was spent on gathering sound scientific evidence, including gender-based inequalities in health. The policy document specifically highlights its commitment to a gender perspective, and to reducing gender-based inequalities in health (Gunnar 2003), alongside reductions in inequalities by socio-economic groups, ethnic groups, and geographic regions. Gender would thus be a crosscutting category within other dimensions of inequalities that the policy seeks to redress.

In Kenya, a Gender and HIV/AIDS Technical Sub Committee, formed in 2002, undertook the task of engendering the National HIV/AIDS Strategic Plan (National AIDS Control Council 2002). The Sub Committee carried out gender analysis of the Strategic Plan, to identify areas where gender differences had not been given due consideration. The gender analysis found that:

- In the area of prevention, there was not enough attention on gender-based violence, rape, and incest as pathways to HIV infection; health education materials did not address gender-specific concerns; and female condom had not been prioritized.

- With respect to treatment, the National Strategic Plan had not mentioned setting up rape/incest crisis centres, counselling, and post-rape STI/HIV/contraceptive prophylaxis. The Plan was silent on nutritional needs of women and men living with HIV/AIDS, and on the special needs of women who cared for HIV positive persons, but had no information on their own seropositivity.
- Collection of sex-disaggregated data had not been emphasized and no attempt had been made to develop gender-sensitive indicators for monitoring and evaluation of interventions.

Based on this analysis, the Gender and HIV/AIDS Sub Committee outlined, within each of the priority areas of the Plan, activities which would pay specific attention to differences between women and men in health needs and access to treatment, care, and support. These were published as a report on which this summary is based

Systematic efforts to integrate gender considerations into health sector reform efforts were facilitated in the Latin American and Caribbean Region by the Pan-American Health Organization (PAHO) (Gomez-Gomez 2002). PAHO's strategy, implemented initially in Chile and Peru, consisted of: helping countries in documenting the implications of health policies for gender inequities in health; disseminating evidence to empower advocates to inform policy makers; and assisting relevant stakeholders and civil society to institutionalize and monitor gender equity priorities into national policies.[2] As part of this project, an observatory of Gender Equity in Health has been set up in Chile to document and disseminate information on gender equity in health (PAHO 2007).

Mainstreaming gender in health reforms was also attempted in Ghana's Sector Wide Approach. The Ministry of Health carried out gender analysis, and held consultations with stakeholders, to develop a draft health sector gender policy to readdress gender gaps as part of the SWAp (Theobald et al. 2004). Timely intervention, through a content analysis-study of Ireland's Cardiovascular Health Strategy document carried out by WHO/EURO, helped identify a number of gender gaps. For example, despite considerable data, presented on differential gender experiences among men and women in the context of cardiovascular diseases, as well as the health services, there were no references to gender considerations in the recommendations made, wherein the emphasis was on inequalities by geographic regions. This study has triggered a lot of research in the area of gender and health in Ireland, and drew attention to the importance of including gender in the cardiovascular health policy at the level of the European Union Council of ministers, paving the way for further action to mainstream gender into the Irish cardiovascular health policy (Women's Health Council and WHO/EURO n.d.). Salmon et al. (2006) have carried out gender analysis of Canada's Mental Health and Addictions Policy, and outlined directions for integrating sex and gender into the policy. The report demonstrates how the application of sex and gender analyses would be useful in refining the health policy in Canada in terms of treatment protocols, accessibility to care, quality of programmes, quality of prevention activity, and help in promotion of good mental health for all Canadians.

The above policy interventions are among the few attempts at mainstreaming gender in the content of health policies. The impact of Sweden's public health policy on bridging gender-gaps in health does not appear to have been assessed as yet. It is not clear if attempts at gender analysis of specific health policies, and of advocacy for integrating gender considerations in health sector reform policies, were translated into policy changes on the ground.

Gender mainstreaming in programme interventions

Mainstreaming gender within community-based NGO health interventions. In this section, we examine 27 community-based NGO health interventions that have mainstreamed gender. These include 22 interventions found in *The 'So What' Report* (IGWG 2004), and five interventions from the Commonwealth report (Commonwealth Secretariat 2002). All of the interventions are donor-funded and community-based, and all aim at improving reproductive health, although the entry points for some of the interventions have been through education or economic development.

The interventions have been classified into four main areas: maternal mortality and morbidity; unintended pregnancies; quality of care initiatives; and STIs/HIV/AIDS. The following framework from *The 'So What' Report* has been used to assess the gender-sensitivity of interventions:

- Gender exploitative interventions: those that exploit gender inequalities for the purpose of gaining reproductive or family planning targets.
- Gender accommodative interventions: those that make it easier for women to perform their gender roles or duties ascribed to them without changing or questioning the inequalities between the roles of men and women in the society.
- Gender transformative interventions: changes that challenge gender equalities between men and women

Table 1 summarizes these 27 reproductive health interventions by nature of problem addressed, level of gender-sensitivity, and reproductive and gender outcomes achieved according to the assessment. The following are some significant findings:

- The vast majority of the interventions (21 of 27) consist mainly of training and education activities. Interventions mainstreaming gender in clinical

Table 1 An analysis of selected 'gender-mainstreamed' reproductive health interventions.

Characteristics	Number of interventions
Area of reproductive health addressed	
Unintended pregnancies	9
Maternal mortality and morbidity	3
STIs and HIV/AIDS	12
Quality of reproductive health care	3
Target group	
Female	15
Male	2
Female and male	10
Nature of interventions	
Education and training	21
Counselling and social support	2
Clinical services	2
Savings and credit	1
Other	1
Gender sensitivity	
Gender accommodating	11
Gender transformative	16
Reproductive health outcomes[3]	
Improved knowledge of RH issues	13
Changes towards positive attitudes	3
Increase in condom use	5
Increase in use of contraception	7
Better self care	2
Increase in utilization of RH services	7
Improved quality of RH services	2
Improved health outcomes	6
Gender outcomes	
Improvement in gender-relations between partners; improvement in communication and gender equitable behaviour	11
Increased empowerment of women	8
Increased awareness of gender issues	1
No improvement	1
Gender outcomes not measured	6

Sources: Commonwealth Secretariat 2002, IGWG 2004.

or psychosocial interventions are rare, irrespective of the reproductive health issue under consideration.
- Many of the interventions (11 of 27) are 'gender-accommodating': that is, they cater to women's and men's different needs without acknowledging or challenging unequal gender power relations.
- In all 27 interventions, there was more than one positive reproductive health outcome, many of these were tangible changes in behaviour, in utilization of services, or in health outcomes.
- Improved gender-outcomes were also noted in 20 of 21 interventions that examined this aspect.

These case studies constitute an important source of evidence on the impact of mainstreaming gender within health interventions. However, the quality of this evidence is compromised by methodological limitations. Comparison of baseline data collected before the intervention, with the achievements after the intervention, has been possible in only a small number of interventions. Gender-mainstreamed interventions are not evaluated against a comparison-group of interventions that do not integrate gender considerations. There is no documentation of the processes and steps through which mainstreaming gender may have brought about the desired health outcomes. The evidence provided does not clarify whether the positive outcomes were a result of a change towards more equitable gender-power equations or simply the result of better access to services. In terms of gender outcomes, many of the conclusions are based on participants reporting that there has been improvement. Questions remain as to whether these gains would be sustained in the long term, and whether women will be able to address and overcome the gender-based barriers they experience in their everyday lives after the short-duration gender interventions.

Mainstreaming gender within government health programmes

The Women-Centred Health Project of the Mumbai Municipal Corporation (WCHP), India, was a collaborative project between the Bombay Municipal Corporation (BMC), SAHAJ, a non-governmental organization, and the Royal Tropical Institute, Amsterdam. The Project was implemented in two wards of Mumbai, covering a population of approximately 1 million (Khanna et al. 2002). The objectives of the project included, among others:

- Implementation of women-centred reproductive health services closer to women, that is, at the health post and dispensary levels, by increasing the range of services on priority reproductive health problems; involving men in ways that will not increase their control over women; and improving information, education and counselling by responding to women's needs and in ways that enhance their control over their bodies.

- Establishment and implementation of quality assurance mechanisms, including better provider–client communication, treatment procedures that respect women and are woman-friendly, and improved referral links.

There were three major categories of project activities: action research, training, and health interventions. The project succeeded in improving both reproductive health and gender outcomes. It put in place 'reproductive health clinics' one day a week in 10 Family Welfare Centres within the project area, and ensured availability of a woman physician, good clinical quality, and availability of relevant drugs. Aspects of quality of care, such as privacy for examining women and respectful and empathetic provider–client communication, were successfully implemented in all health facilities within the project area. In terms of gender outcomes, health providers and senior managers reported that they found gender-sensitization workshops to be informative and thought-provoking, and helped them to make changes in their day-to-day work.

The effects of the project spilled beyond the project area. For example, a gender module developed by the WCHP was incorporated successfully in all training provided in BMC. WCHP's training modules on Gender, Men's Involvement, IEC, Provider–Client Communication, and quality of care were incorporated into the final training schedule for Mumbai's Reproductive and Child Health (RCH) Programme.

The project faced numerous implementation challenges. The bureaucratic and hierarchical nature of a large public system, such as BMC, did not find it easy to accommodate the participatory, bottom-up approach in planning and execution of gender-mainstreaming activities adopted by WCHP. The officers and health care providers did not have much patience for process-oriented approaches which made heavy demands on their time, and were far more comfortable with top-down orders that could be implemented mechanistically.

Acting on gender mainstreaming priorities identified by the project also proved to be very difficult. For example, changing the timings at health facilities to suit men's work schedules could not be implemented. Starting crèches for BMC employees and increasing the number of toilets for women with sanitary bins on BMC premises were identified as needs, but implementing these was fraught with difficulties. It took enormous time and energy, and much patience and optimism, to achieve any substantive change. The biggest challenge for this project has been sustaining the initiatives after the project period. Within a year of the project ending, some of the activities initiated were discontinued, including those that did not involve commitment of additional resources (Khanna et al. 2002).

The WCHP appears to be an example of successful 'operational' mainstreaming, which could not be sustained because the institutional structures within which it was functioning (that of the BMC) had not concurrently engaged in gender mainstreaming, but continued to be hierarchical and gender-blind. The institution treated WCHP as one of its many short-term projects rather than as an attempt to make fundamental changes in the way in which the health services were organized and run. Nevertheless, the contributions of WCHP in terms of gender-sensitization of staff, at all levels, is likely to have brought about at least a few changes in provider attitudes and behaviour.

Another example of mainstreaming gender within Government departments is in Hong Kong. As a result of application of gender analysis to the planning and provision of public toilet facilities in the country, the Food and Environmental Hygiene Department (FEHD) found that females needed to spend a longer time in toilets than males, and it was very common to see queues outside female toilets. Therefore, FEHD increased the WC compartment ratio (female to male) from 1.5:1 to 2:1 since April 2004, as a general guideline in planning FEHD public toilet facilities, and included racks, hangers, baby changing counters, and emergency call bells in the toilets (Health, Welfare and Food Bureau 2006a). Further, Hong Kong's Electrical and Mechanical Services Department (EMSD) has arranged talks in hospitals, planned for afternoon TV information slots, and posted and distributed materials at public places to make information on the safety of electrical and mechanical gadgets used in households more accessible to women (Health, Welfare and Food Bureau 2006b). Both of these are examples of gender-accommodative interventions, which cater to the varying needs of women and men without challenging their gender roles: for example, the intervention of EMSD did not challenge the gender division of domestic work.

Mainstreaming gender in health research

Gender mainstreaming in health research implies consideration of gender at all stages of the research process, from defining the research questions to developing the study design and data collection tools, the process of data collection, and interpretation and dissemination of results. In this section, we present three examples of gender mainstreaming health research. The first is on the experience of National Institute of Health in the USA. The second is a summary of a review of experiences in Latin American and Caribbean countries, and the third is an example of a country-level initiative by a School of Public Health in India.

NIH gender policy in health research

The National Institute of Health (NIH) in the USA set up its Office of Research on Women's Health (ORWH) in 1990. Its mandate included:

ensuring that research conducted and supported by the NIH adequately addressed issues regarding women's health; ensuring that women are appropriately represented in biomedical and bio behavioural research studies supported by the NIH; and supporting research on women's health issues and activities related to career advancement of women in biomedical careers (Caron 2003). An evaluation of the NIH funded studies by the Gender Accounting Office (GAO) in 2000[4] concluded that, although the inclusion of women had been achieved in research processes, the analysis of data did not expose whether there were sex or gender differences in the impact of interventions. It was also found that grant applicants were not informed that research studies had to include an analysis of sex-based differences (Caron 2003). An independent evaluation of the NIH policy, through an analysis of published material by Harris and Douglas (2000) as quoted in Caron (2003), found that efforts to include women in the clinical trials did moderately increase as a result of ORWH policy. However, closer examination found that the representation of women increased only in large trials that were restricted to women. The under-representation of women in areas such as cardiovascular diseases continued unchanged (Caron 2003).

Integrating gender in health research

The Latin American Experience (LACWHN 2002)

There exists a substantive body of 'gendered' research in health in the Latin American region, carried out by feminist researchers, either NGO or university-based, most of which have been individual work not guided by a cohesive agenda. The broad areas of gendered research have been violence against women; sexual and reproductive health and rights; access to health services and quality of care; and mental health. According to the review by the Latin American and Caribbean Women's Health Network (LACWHN 2002), few governments in the region have set an agenda or developed explicit strategy to integrate gender considerations in health research. Although a number of countries in this region have a commitment to equity in health, this is usually framed in terms of socio-economic, ethnic, and geographic regions, leaving gender out of the equation. Gendered research does not feature in government funding policies anywhere in the region. The scenario is one of considerable initiative by feminists and women researchers not backed by policy commitment. Nevertheless, gendered research has had some impact on policy making, especially in the areas of violence against women and sexual and reproductive health. More importantly, such research has contributed to a deepening of understanding of the nature and dimensions of gender inequalities in health by articulating women's experiences.

The Small Grants Programme on Gender and Social Issues in Reproductive Health Research, India[5] (Ravindran 2005)

This was a modest initiative to build capacity among researchers in sexual and reproductive health to undertake 'gendered' research. A small grant programme offered 11 research grants for undertaking research focusing on gender and social dimensions of sexual and reproductive health issues in India. Each grantee was teamed up with a 'mentor' who reviewed the final proposal, provided critical inputs to the development of data-collection instruments, collection, analysis, and interpretation of data, and inputs to the final report. Training workshops for all grantees were conducted at crucial junctures during the research process. The initiative produced 11 research reports on sexual and reproductive health issues, which are good examples of gender-mainstreamed research. Not only the 11 grantees but the 10 mentors also learned first-hand about implementing gender mainstreaming in health research.

There are several such examples of small-scale initiatives. But overall, not enough has been done to change policies that enable the systematic integration of gender considerations in health research in all academic and research settings, and to generate gender and sex-specific data as part of routine data collection. This is one important bottleneck hampering the identification of priority areas and of monitoring progress towards gender equality.

Mainstreaming gender in health providers' training

A large number of efforts have focused on in-service training of health professionals on gender issues. Some of the well-known international efforts include: WHO's training on Gender and Rights in Reproductive Health; Pan American Health Organization's training course on Gender, Health, and Development; and WHO-Western Pacific Regional Office's (WPRO) publication of resource guides in gender, poverty, and health for mainstreaming gender in medical education. Such initiatives are numerous and have yet to be evaluated for their impact.

This section, therefore, focuses on pre-service training of health professionals, and is based on a recent review on integrating gender into the curricula for health professionals (Ravindran 2006). Much of the work on integrating gender into the curricula of health professionals has been done in relation to the undergraduate medical curriculum, and in the area of women's health specialty, especially in the USA. Attempts to integrate gender (rather than women's health) into the medical curriculum are more recent. There are only three known examples of curriculum development and course implementation. Monash University has integrated gender into the curriculum in the 5 years of its new problem-based and patient-centred curriculum. The Medical School at Chulalungkorn University in Thailand has also made a similar attempt. The Gender and Health Collaborative Curriculum Project in Canada has developed web-based modules that are resources for faculty who wish to integrate gender into their teaching, and may also be used by interested students. In contrast, many public health programmes offer optional courses on gender (Ravindran 2006).

Other efforts at integrating gender into the curricula have focused on creating an enabling environment, and in capacity building of medical educators. For example, an initiative in India has been training medical educators from six Indian states on the need and strategies for gender mainstreaming the medical curriculum, with a view to creating change agents within the system who would advocate for gender mainstreaming. A similar initiative is being implemented in Southern Africa, among schools of public health. Advocacy with senior policy makers is also being undertaken in various settings.

Three factors appear to facilitate the process of mainstreaming gender in medical curricula. The first is the window of opportunity provided by larger curricular changes, such as introduction of problem-based and patient-centred learning, and introduction of new courses. The second is the presence of dynamic leadership committed to mainstreaming gender. The third factor is the extensive preparatory work carried out by such leaders: well thought-out and sustained advocacy with decision-makers; capacity-building and introductory workshops for medical educators and students; and devising ways of integrating gender without overloading the existing curriculum.

Some of the major challenges reported by initiatives include institutional resistance and difficulties of involving key faculty and male colleagues in this process. Another issue is that there are very few faculty members in each institution who have the expertise to teach gender and women's health issues. The limited research on gender issues in health and women's health is another blockage hampering the extent to which evidence-based teaching on gender and health is possible (Ravindran 2006).

Institutional gender mainstreaming

Operational gender mainstreaming needs structures, mechanisms, and processes that will catalyse, initiate, and sustain gender-mainstreaming efforts. In the first section, we describe mainstreaming efforts within national health sectors; in the second section, mainstreaming gender in health within international organizations is illustrated.

Gender mainstreaming within national health sectors

South Africa's *Gender Policy Guidelines for the Health Sector* were developed in order to support the Department of Health and Public Health Institutions to systematically identify and address gender considerations in health, and within the organizations responsible for managing and delivering health care services (Government of South Africa 2002). The guidelines set a series of objectives for 'institutional' gender mainstreaming, i.e., promoting gender equity and equality within institutions of the health sector. These included: elimination of gender-based discrimination in human resource procedures, such as appointments and promotions; changing institutional rules and culture to create an environment supportive of gender equity and equality; and enhancing the capacity of staff and senior management for mainstreaming gender concerns within health policies, programmes, research, and training (Government of South Africa 2002).

In order to achieve these objectives, structures and mechanisms were created. Full-time gender focal points were appointed at the national and provincial levels, to provide technical support for implementing the gender policy. A Health Sector Co-ordinating Committee (HSCC) was constituted of representatives of health departments at different levels (national, provincial, and local) and civil society actors, to help with gender analysis, to develop a gender action plan and a framework for monitoring and evaluation, and to facilitate the development of a Management Information System (Government of South Africa 2002).

The Gender Equity Strategy of the Ministry of Health and Family Welfare (MOHFW) in Bangladesh was developed through a consultative process, and adopted in 2003. The overall objective of the Strategy was to enhance the capacity of the MOHFW to address gender inequities in health, which were detrimental to overall health development. Gender considerations were systematically identified, and strategies to address them were outlined, within each of five essential components of the Health and Population Sector Programme (HPSP). The Gender Equity Strategy included, enhancing women's participation in senior management, creating a supportive a safe and harassment-free work environment for female staff, and promoting skills and sensitivity among managers to identify and address gender issues in the workplace (Government of Bangladesh 2003).

Institutional mainstreaming in international organizations

The World Health Organization

The World Health Organization's (WHO) Gender Policy was formally adopted in 2002, although work towards formulating the policy had started several years earlier. The policy called for 'integrating gender considerations' into all research, policies, programmes, projects, and initiatives in which WHO is involved (WHO 2002). The lead agency for gender mainstreaming within WHO is the Gender, Women and Health Department at the WHO headquarters in Geneva. This department is responsible for providing technical support to all departments of WHO, for mainstreaming gender in their work through, among other things, the development of appropriate gender analysis tools and by building a substantial evidence base. A high-level Gender Task Force, consisting of senior managers within the organization, was appointed by the Director General to oversee the implementation of the Gender Policy. A WHO Gender Team was constituted, consisting of gender focal points from departments and initiatives at WHO headquarters, and core gender specialists in the Department of Gender, Women and Health.

During the years following the adoption of the Gender Policy, the lead agency, the Department of Gender, Women and Health, has produced an impressive array of publications contributing to building the evidence base on gender and health, and developing and refining tools and guidelines for gender mainstreaming in research. These tools and publications have been the result of successful collaboration with a number of technical departments at the headquarters. The gender units of the WHO Regional Offices have also been engaged in similar activities.

While these achievements are impressive, especially given the relatively understaffed and under-resourced character of the lead agency and regional gender units, they are a long way from 'mainstreaming' or integrating gender into the organization's way of doing business. Gender focal points in different departments carry out their gender-related tasks as an add-on to their regular tasks. Capacity building for integrating gender has not happened systematically, or anywhere near the scale it ought to be. Gender considerations are not routinely integrated into policies, programmes, strategies, or research; or within organizational structures created to implement new initiatives and programmes. A quick scan of the organization's website will bear testimony to these observations. The experience of institutional mainstreaming at the WHO is shared by many multilateral and bilateral organizations, as the discussion in the next section will illustrate.

Other international organizations[6]

A review of gender mainstreaming experiences of 14 international organizations by Moser and Moser (2005) provides comprehensive information on progress made with respect to institutional mainstreaming in international organizations. The review covers bilateral donors, international financial institutions (IFIs), United Nations (UN) agencies, and non-governmental organizations (NGOs). Although these are not institutions within the health sector, their experiences are relevant because the processes involved and the emerging challenges are likely to be similar across sectors. Table 2 presents information on the presence of various components of institutional gender mainstreaming across the 14 organizations (Moser and Moser 2005).

All of the reviewed institutions had adopted the terminology of gender equality and gender mainstreaming. Gender analysis, gender training, and development of tools and techniques for monitoring and evaluation were

Table 2 Components and associated activities of gender mainstreaming policies in 14 international organizations.

Components	Activities	DFID	CIDA	Sida	IDB	ADB	WB	UNIFEM	Habitat	UNICEF	UNDP	ActionAid	OXFAM	HIVOS	ACORD	%
Dual strategy of mainstreaming and targeting gender equality	Mainstreaming into policies, projects, and programmes (all stages of cycle)	X	X	X	X	X	X	X	X	X	X	X	X	X	X	100
	Actions targeting gender equality	X	X	X	X	X	X	X	X	X	X	X	X	X	X	100
Gender analysis	Sex disaggregated data and gender information	X	X		X			X	X		X					43
	Analysis of all programme cycle stages	X	X	X	X	X	X	X	X			X	X		X	79
	Gender sensitive budget analysis										X					7
Internal responsibility	Responsibilities shared between all staff and gender specialists/focal points	X	X	X			X		X	X	X	X	X	X	X	79
Gender training	Understanding and implementation of gender policy for staff and counterparts	X		X								X	X	X	X	43
	Staff/counterpart gender sensitization												X			7
	Staff/counterparts gender training skills	X	X	X	X	X	X		X	X	X	X	X	X	X	93
	Manuals/tool kits	X				X	X		X	X	X					43
Supporting women's decision making and empowerment	Strengthening women's organizations through capacity building and training			X				X				X	X	X		36
	Support women's participation in decision making/empowerment	X	X	X	X			X	X	X	X	X	X	X	X	86
	Working with men for gender equality		X	X						X			X	X	X	43

Table 2 (cont'd)

Components	Activities	DFID	CIDA	Sida	IDB	ADB	WB	UNIFEM	Habitat	UNICEF	UNDP	ActionAid	OXFAM	HIVOS	ACORD	%
Monitoring and evaluation	Effective systems and tools for M & E	X	X	X	X	X	X		X	X	X	X	X	X	X	93
	Gender sensitive indicators								X			X				
Work with other organizations	Strengthening gender capacity at work with government donors, private sectors			X	X	X	X	X		X	X	X	X	X	X	93
	Capacity building of civil society	X	X					X	X		X					14
	Support to national women's machineries		X	X				X								11
Budgets	Allocation of financial resources to staff to carry out gender policy	X			X	X		X			X	X		X		50
	Publication of knowledge base for best practice and effective strategies			X	X	X		X			X		X		X	50
Knowledge resources	Networks		X					X			X					21
	Online databases							X			X					14

Source: Moser and Moser 2005.
CIDA: Canadian International Development Agency; DFID: Department for International Development (UK); Sida: Swedish International Development Agency; IDB: Inter-American Development Bank; ADB: Asian Development Bank; WB: World Bank; UNIFEM: United Nations Development Fund for Women; Habitat: United Nations Human Settlements Programme; UNICEF: United Nations Children's Fund; UNDP: United Nations Development Programme; ACORD: Agency for Cooperation and Research in Development.

seen as important strategies for mainstreaming by most organizations. In a majority of the organizations, responsibility for gender mainstreaming was shared by a cross-section of staff, supported by gender specialists. However, half or more of the 14 organizations had not allocated financial resources to enable implementation of the gender policy; were not working with men for gender equality; and had not been involved in strengthening the capacity of women's organizations or working with civil society.

Proceedings of an informal consultation of Gender Focal Points from multilateral development organizations confirms these observations, and is much more critical of the limited progress made (MFA 2002). Many gender focal points reported that gender policies and strategies had been put in place as merely 'cosmetic' changes, without any attempt to allocate the necessary resources or personnel, to guide the processes, or monitor and evaluate what had been achieved.

According to one observer:

> ... gender has tended to be treated as a passing fad, and especially in between major conferences, been down-played, and resurrected for frantic activity, and dusted over and dry-cleaned like winter clothes in autumn, just before the institution would be called upon to account for past undertakings.
>
> (Chinery-Heisse 2002)

Challenges to mainstreaming gender in health

Major findings of this review

The present paper attempts to review progress made in mainstreaming gender in health policies and programmes, research, and training within health system institutions. We found that many tools and guidelines had been developed on how to implement gender mainstreaming, and that there were many descriptions of gender mainstreaming initiatives. However, few publications provided insights on the processes adopted, or on the outcomes of gender mainstreaming initiatives.

Descriptive accounts of gender mainstreaming initiatives indicate that more has been done in 'operational' mainstreaming, as compared to institutional mainstreaming, of gender equity concerns within the health sector. Attempts at institutional mainstreaming seem to be suffering from the apparent tendency to 'appear to do much' rather than making fundamental changes. Institutions seem to have superficially gone through the motions of adopting a gender policy and creating a few structures without investing any more into making these actually work. Most attempts have been top-down, without scope for democratic participation, both within international organizations and national government institutions. At the government level: '... gender mainstreaming has become a mechanical process to attract funding but does not change practices of discrimination embedded in government institutions' (Sandler 2002). These weaknesses in institutional mainstreaming of gender make it difficult, if not impossible, for operational mainstreaming to be large-scale or sustained over a long period.

Within operational mainstreaming, service-delivery and training interventions that have been implemented and evaluated are mainly community-based and carried out by non-governmental organizations with external funding. Many of these tend to focus on women's specific needs without challenging gender roles and norms. Attempts at integrating gender issues in the training of health personnel have remained, largely, small-scale attempts initiated in a few settings by committed individuals or advocacy groups. There are only a small number of examples of planned and system-wide initiatives for mainstreaming gender, guided by policy and implemented by the state. Even when successful in terms of improving health outcomes and promoting gender equity, micro-level, small-scale, or ad-hoc interventions, are not likely to make the health sector completely more gender-equitable. Where health policies are concerned, the task of mainstreaming gender in their content has barely begun. More has been done to identify 'gender-gaps' within existing policies, rather than address these gender gaps within policies and in their implementation. With the exception of Sweden's public health policy, these have not considered gender as part of human rights and social justice agendas.

Factors constraining mainstreaming gender in health

What are some reasons for the limited progress with respect to gender mainstreaming in health? The discussion below draws on the authors' own experiences, in addition to published literature reviewing gender mainstreaming (Chinery-Heisse 2002, Hannan 2002, Sandler 2002, Porter and Sweetman 2005). Our focus is more on the larger systemic challenges than on issues related to management and organizational structures within institutions. We deal first with the specific challenges in mainstreaming gender in the health sector, and then with factors common to gender mainstreaming efforts across sectors.

Challenges specific to the health sector

Gender mainstreaming is a difficult undertaking in any sector, but mainstreaming gender in health has to contend with some specific challenges:

- Because there are biological differences between women and men in both health needs and experiences, there is a tendency to attribute all male–female differences to biology. The consequence is that maternal health programmes are seen as an adequate response to addressing differences in health between sexes. The need for examining gender issues in all

- health problems, as well as in delivery of health care services, remains unrecognized.
- While the disadvantages experienced by women in sectors like education, employment, or political participation are evident from available data, the case of health is more complex. Women outlive men in most countries of the world, and, for many health conditions, male mortality exceeds female mortality. Many policy makers and programme managers, therefore, remain unconvinced of any gender-based inequalities in health, and of the need for gender mainstreaming. Other dimensions of gender inequality in health, such as in morbidity, access to health care, and social and economic consequences of ill health are seldom examined.
- Health sectors in many countries are informed by a bio-medical approach to health and disease under the leadership of health professionals who may not see the relevance of understanding the social dimensions and determinants of health. Health care providers tend to see themselves as technical persons who solve problems presented to them, and may believe themselves to be free from any gender (or other social) biases. Gender mainstreaming, in their view, may represent a diversion of valuable time and resources away from the far more important task of 'saving lives'.

Challenges faced across sectors

Confusion about concepts

The two complementary components of gender mainstreaming (viz. working on women-specific projects to bridge the gap between women and men, and mainstreaming gender across all areas of work) have often been interpreted as competing approaches from which one approach has to be chosen and adopted. This has sometimes led to drastically trimming, or even dismantling, of Women's Bureaus and Gender Units (Chinery-Heisse 2002). Some critiques believe that this may be a deliberate attempt to sabotage gender mainstreaming by doing away with a focus on women (Hannan 2002).

De-politicization of gender mainstreaming

Another reason for gender mainstreaming remaining at a superficial level is the reduction of gender equality work into a set of tools and activities, delinked from the women's movement and from a rights and social justice agenda (Sandler 2002). Gender mainstreaming is not just about identifying gender-gaps through gender analysis and 'including' women where they were previously excluded. It is also about asking why women were excluded in the first place, identifying the forces that perpetuated such exclusion, and challenging these forces. It is about taking on patriarchy, misogyny, and discrimination, and the structures that uphold them.

Adoption of an 'integrationist' agenda

Many gender mainstreaming efforts in health have been 'integrationist', politically conservative, merely trying to add women to the existing agendas, without challenging the validity of the agendas themselves (Jahan 1995, as quoted in Porter and Sweetman 2005). This is also true of the health sector, where attempts at gender mainstreaming have been made without questioning some of the fundamental problems in the sector, such as health sector reforms promoting commodification of health care services.

Changes in the global policy environment

The global policy environment is increasingly hostile to justice and equity concerns (Rao and Kelleher 2005). Conservative governments in many donor countries are less willing to commit to development aid overall. The Millennium Development Goals, which are guiding development priorities and funding, have failed to integrate gender issues in all the goals, narrowing the scope of funding for gender mainstreaming. The scant attention paid to gender in Poverty Reduction Strategy Papers of many low-income countries (Zuckerman and Garrett 2003) will further constrain development funding for gender.

Paradigm shifts in favour of privatization

Paradigm shifts within the social sectors, including health, in favour of privatization and retraction of the state's role, and in support of promoting the development of a market for health, education, and other social services, are developments that have the potential effect of widening the gender (and other social) gap(s). In addition, the focus is more on efficiency rather than on equity and, hence, policy support for gender mainstreaming as an equity issue will be limited. The bigger issue is what shape gender mainstreaming should take in a health sector that is increasingly privatized. How do we ensure gender-sensitive health facilities and services within the private sector? How can we enforce any policy in a weak-regulatory environment?

Where do we go from here?

We believe that rather than doing more of the same, hoping that sustained efforts will bear fruit, it is time to acknowledge that we were probably 'working hard on the wrong things' (Sandler 2002). We need to transform both our agenda and our way of doing business:

- It may be time to frame gender mainstreaming explicitly as an issue of equity, rights, and justice, health as a basic human right, and gender equality as a basic consideration in health.

- The focus should shift from 'integration' of gender issues into existing agendas to reframing the agenda in a way that promotes gender and social equity in health. For example, rather than make sure that women's interests do not get excluded from the health sector reform agenda, the attempt would be to transform the agenda to make it equity-oriented. This approach has been named as 'agenda-setting' gender mainstreaming by Jahan (see Porter and Sweetman 2005).
- The approach would emphasize setting agendas which consider gender inequity within the context of inequities by caste, class, ethnicity, and so on, as a cross-cutting issue; gender will be 'mainstreamed' within a health equity agenda.
- Investment will be made in institutional mainstreaming of gender equity concerns so that structures are in place to support and sustain operational gender mainstreaming.
- Alliances may be forged with those advocating for, and researching, attention to the social determinants of health inequity.
- Rather than being top-down initiatives, political mobilization to create demand for gender equity in health must be seen as necessary groundwork for mainstreaming gender in health.

Acknowledgements

This paper is an abridged version of a report submitted to the Gender and Women's Equity Knowledge Network of the WHO Commission on Social Determinants of Health in November 2006.

Notes

1 A wide range of terminologies are found in the literature on gender mainstreaming, such as 'integrating gender considerations', or 'adopting a gender-perspective'. In so far as they refer to the same processes, described above, we have treated these as synonymous to gender mainstreaming.
2 Information on progress of the project is available only in Spanish, and could not be included in this paper.
3 Figures do not add to 27 because more than one outcome was reported by some interventions.
4 As cited in Caron (2003).
5 The initiative was located at the Achutha Menon Centre for Health Science Studies, Sree Chitra Tirunal Institute for Medical Science and Technology, Kerala, India, and funded by the Ford Foundation.
6 These do not work specifically on health.

References

Caron, J. (2003) *Report on Governmental Health Research Policies Promoting Gender or Sex Differences Sensitivity* (Alberta, Canada: Institute of Gender and Health).

Chinery-Heisse, M. (2002) Experiences in promoting gender equality. In *MFA, Strategies for the Promotion of Gender Equality. Is Mainstreaming a Dead End?* Report from an informal consultation of gender focal points in multilateral development organisations, 6–9 November 2002 (Oslo: Norwegian Ministry of Foreign Affairs).

Commonwealth Secretariat (2002) Establishment of the gender management systems in the health sector. In *Gender Mainstreaming in the Health Sector: Experiences in Commonwealth Countries* (London: Commonwealth Secretariat, 52–65).

Gomez-Gomez, E. (2002) *Gender Equity and Health Policy Reform in Latin America and the Caribbean* (Washington, DC: Pan American Health Organization).

Government of Bangladesh (2003) *Gender Equity Strategy* (Dhaka: Ministry of Health and Family Welfare).

Government of South Africa (2002) *Gender Policy Guidelines for the Health Sector* (Pretoria: Department of Health, 39–40).

Gunnar, A. (2003) *Sweden's New Public Health Policy: National Public Health Objectives for Sweden* (Stockholm: Swedish National Institute of Public Health, 20–21).

Hannan, C. (2002) Promoting gender equality in multilateral development organisations. In MFA, *Strategies for the Promotion of Gender Equality. Is Mainstreaming a Dead End?* Report from an informal consultation of gender focal points in multilateral development organisations, 6–9 November 2002 (Oslo: Norwegian Ministry of Foreign Affairs).

Harris, D. J. & Douglas, P. S. (2000) Enrollment of Women in Cardiovascular Clinical Trials Funded by the National Heart, Lung, and Blood Institute. *The New England Journal of Medicine*, 343(7), 475–480.

Health, Welfare and Food Bureau (2006a) Provision of public toilets by food and environmental hygiene department. In *Gender Mainstreaming, The Hong Kong Experience: Implementing Gender Mainstreaming in the Government of the Hong Kong Special Administrative Region* (Hong Kong: Women's Commission Secretariat, 42–43).

Health, Welfare and Food Bureau (2006b) Publicity programme on electricity and gas safety by electrical and mechanical services department. In *Gender Mainstreaming, The Hong Kong Experience: Implementing Gender Mainstreaming in the Government of the Hong Kong Special Administrative Region* (Hong Kong: Women's Commission Secretariat, 47–48).

IGWG (2004) *The 'So What' Report: A Look at Whether Integrating a Gender Focus Into Programmes Makes a Difference to Outcomes* (Washington, DC: Interagency Gender Working Group Task Force Report).

Jahan, R. (1995) *The Elusive Agenda: Mainstreaming Women in Development* (London: Zed Books).

Khanna, R., Pongurlekar, S., Ubale, U. and de Koning, K. (2002) *Gender-Sensitisation of Health Care Providers: Experiences of the Women-Centred Health Project, Mumbai, India* (Mumbai, India: Women-Centred Health Project).

LACWHN (2002) *Gendered Health Research for Development: A Vital Contribution to Health Equity* (Santiago, Chile: Latin American and Caribbean Women's Health Network).

MFA (2002) *Strategies for the Promotion of Gender Equality. Is Mainstreaming a Dead End?* Report from an informal consultation of gender focal points in multilateral development organisations, 6–9 November 2002 (Oslo: Norwegian Ministry of Foreign Affairs).

Moser, C. and Moser, A. (2005) Gender Mainstreaming since Beijing: A Review of Success and Limitations in International Institutions. *Gender and Development*, 13, 12–13.

National AIDS Control Council (2002) *Mainstreaming Gender into the Kenya National HIV/AIDS Strategic Plan: 2000–2005* (Nairobi, Kenya: Gender and HIV/AIDS Technical Sub-Committee of the National AIDS Control Council).

Ostlin, P. and Diderichsen, F. (2003) *Equity-Oriented National Strategy for Public Health in Sweden: A Case Study* (Copenhagen: European Centre for Health Policy). Accessed 15 June 2007, available at http://www.un.org/womenwatch/daw/csw/GMS.PDF

PAHO (2007) Accessed 16 September 2007, available at http://www.paho.org/English/AD/GE/Policy.htm

Porter, F. and Sweetman, C. (2005) Mainstreaming: A Critical Review. *Gender and Development*, 13(2), 2–10.

Rao, A. and Kelleher, D. (2005) Is There Life After Gender Mainstreaming? *Gender and Development*, 13, 57–69.

Ravindran, T. K. S. (2005) *Report of the Small Grants Programme on Gender and Social Issues in Reproductive Health Research* (Trivandrum, India: Achutha Menon Centre for Health Science Studies).

Ravindran, T. K. S. (2006) Integrating gender into the curricula of health professionals: Experiences and lessons learned. Paper presented at the WHO Meeting on integrating gender in the curricula of health professionals (Geneva: World Health Organization).

Salmon, A., Poole, N., Morrow, M., Greaves, L., Ingram, R. and Pederson, A. (2006) *Improving Conditions: Integrating Sex and Gender into Federal Mental Health and Addictions Policy* (Vancouver: British Columbia Centre of Excellence for Women's Health, 37).

Sandler, J. (2002) Promoting gender equality in different international organisations (UNIFEM). In *Strategies for the Promotion of Gender Equality. Is Mainstreaming a Dead End?* Report from an informal consultation of gender focal points in multilateral development organisations, 6–9 November 2002 (Oslo: Norwegian Ministry of Foreign Affairs).

Theobald, S., Elsey, H. and Tolhurst, R. (2004) Gender, Health and Development I: Gender Equity in Sector-Wide Approaches. *Progress in Development Studies*, 4, 58–63.

UN (2000) Further actions and initiatives to implement the Beijing declaration and the Platform for action. Unedited final outcome document as adopted by the plenary of the twenty-third special session of the General Assembly on 10 June 2000 (New York: United Nations). Accessed 14 February 2008, available at http://wcd.nic.in/bej5plus.htm

UNECOSOC (1997) Gender Mainstreaming. Extract from the Report of the Economic and Social Council for 1997 (A/52/3, 18 September 1997) (Vienna: Division for Advancement of Women. UN Department of Economic and Social Affairs). Accessed 14 February 2008, available at http://www.un.org/documents/ga/docs/52/plenary/a52-3.htm

WHO (2002) *Integrating Gender Perspectives in the Work of WHO: WHO Gender Policy* (Geneva: World Health Organization, 2).

Women's Health Council and WHO/EURO (n.d.) *Integrating the Gender Perspective in Irish Health Policy: A Case Study* (Dublin: Women's Health Council and Copenhagen: World Health Organization, Regional Office for Europe).

Zuckerman, E. and Garrett, A. (2003) *Do Poverty Reduction Strategy Papers (PRSPs) Address Gender? A Gender Audit of PRSPs*. Accessed 15 June 2007, available at http://www.genderaction.org/images/2002PRSP&Gender.pdf

46

REFORMING GENDERED HEALTH CARE
An assessment of change

Mary K. Zimmerman and Shirley A. Hill

Source: *International Journal of Health Services*, 30:4 (2000), 771–95.

> Health policy in the United States has changed dramatically over the past three decades, with the main concern shifting from expanded health care coverage to containment of health care costs. The current focus on providing cost-effective health services, reflected in the growth of managed care initiatives, has elevated concern about the quality of health care. The authors contend that quality of health care has always been the key focus in the women's health movement, which evolved in the late 1960s as the first significant challenge to modern medicine. In this article, they apply the analytic lens of gender to develop a fresh perspective on U.S. health care organizations and policies, examining the six broad demands of the feminist consumer model of health care, all of which hinge on the issue of quality care for women, to determine whether women's health needs are now being better addressed. The authors conclude that, despite some notable gains in the roles of women as consumers and providers of health care, many of the new health reforms have replicated and solidified the historical inequities in the health care system.

The United States' health care policy during the latter decades of the 20th century can be viewed as an evolving, even dialectical, struggle between expanding health care access and containing health care costs that too frequently leaves quality of care hanging in the balance. In contrast, quality of care has long been a central goal of the women's health movement. Analyzed recently as a "megamovement" with numerous "waves" dating back to the popular health movement of the 1830s and 1840s (1), the women's health movement can be considered the first significant consumer voice since the rise of modern medicine. It pre-dates other prominent consumer voices in health care such as the patients' rights and disability rights movements (2) and arguably has advanced a broader, more extensive critique of mainstream health care. Especially since the mid-1960s, the women's health movement has established a precedent of questioning and actively confronting medical assumptions and practices while at the same time offering an alternative vision of health care (1, 3, 4).

In this article, we apply the analytic lens of gender in order to develop a fresh perspective on U.S. health care organization and policies, expanding our understanding of the nature of health care systems and elaborating the workings of gender as a major form of social differentiation and stratification. Our point of departure is the current debate over the consequences of managed care, especially the implications for health care quality. A fundamental issue in this debate is whether the rational efficiency and improvements promised since the 1980s by proponents of managed care have prevailed over the strong economic incentives in the U.S. market-based system that often pit patient well-being against corporate profits. Specifically, we are interested in the gendered nature of the health care system and the extent to which recent policy changes have improved the position of women as consumers and providers of health care.

To address this question, we revisit the women's health movement of the late 1960s and early 1970s to identify principles from its feminist critique, which we employ as quality indicators in an examination of the current status of women in the health care system. Women, of course, are not a monolithic group, and we endeavor, where possible, to address this issue in race and class context. We seek to clarify whether women's health needs are now better responded to or, on the other hand, the patriarchal practices of the past are simply being replicated in new forms. We begin by describing the broad parameters of the feminist critique of health care and presenting the original feminist model of health care. Hindsight reveals that the women's health movement anticipated many of the problems and issues that policy analysts and decision-makers are wrestling with today. We briefly examine the gendering of health care within the framework of capitalism and patriarchy, and then provide an analysis of the extent to which that gendered system of health care has been reformed.

The feminist consumer model of health care

During the late 1960s and 1970s, the women's health movement emerged with reforming health care as an explicit objective. The movement identified the basic causes of inadequate health care for women to be androcentrism and male dominance in medicine (1, 3, 4). Some groups focused on women's entry into medicine, their prevalence as physicians, and women's overall lack of access to health care. Other, more radical groups attempted to develop a vision and culture that would form an alternative to the paternalism and perceived insensitivity of the dominant biomedical model of health care (5–7). Quality of care was the fundamental objective in the early women's health movement (1, 8), with greater control over medical decisions and one's own body perceived as a solution (3). Gender bias was seen as a key barrier to quality health care for women in clinical decision-making and in treatment approaches (9–11). Inappropriate medical responses to women also reflected the lack of research on women and women's health problems (12–14), as well as financial arrangements and cultural ideas that encouraged the over-treatment of some persons and problems and the undertreatment of others (15). The women's health movement was at the forefront of advocating for personal autonomy in health decisions and in debating the limits of personal responsibility for health (16, 17). Further, women's health advocates of this period were well ahead of their peers in focusing on a number of other issues, including the need to shift emphasis from specialty medicine to primary care and prevention; to adopt a patient-centered or consumer approach in health care delivery with greater emphasis on communication, service, and satisfaction; and to implement and maintain an integrated sociomedical care model.

Six broad, overlapping principles of women's health care were promoted by the early women's health movement:

1. Increased control for women in decisions and actions affecting their bodies and health.
2. The de-medicalization of women's life events and problems, that is, defining health care issues so as to release women's experiences from needless medical ownership and excessive therapeutic control.
3. An emphasis on information, prevention, and less invasive treatment.
4. An atmosphere of interpersonal respect between physician and patients regardless of gender, race and class.
5. The centrality of a sociomedical as opposed to a biomedical model of health.
6. A commitment to health care as a right, including access to physicians and hospitals regardless of financial or insurance status (2–4, 6, 18, 19).

Before analyzing the extent to which these principles have been realized, we briefly explore the origins of gender inequities in the U.S. health care system.

Capitalism, patriarchy, and gendered health care

Theorists of the women's health movement argue that achievement of their objectives has been thwarted in part because of the context of capitalism and patriarchy within which U.S. medicine developed. The gendered nature of the health care division of labor (20) is perhaps the most obvious indicator of patriarchy in medicine. Allopathic physicians in the United States have always been predominantly white males, despite the fact that women in colonial America were integrally involved in the provision of health care through domestic medicine and midwifery (21). By the mid-1800s, a few women had entered medical apprenticeships and even applied to medical schools (22, 23), but for the most part women faced systematic opposition in their efforts to become physicians. The discovery of scientific medicine and the emergence of an industrial economy during the 19th century became key elements in keeping women out of medical practice. The germ theory of disease and new medical technologies were more readily accepted by allopathic physicians, who used them to develop new standards for medical education and to effectively lobby for legal statutes defining the parameters of medicine and medical licensure, which solidified their dominance and, as a result, the exclusion of women (22).

The doctrine of separate spheres, a gender ideology that coincided with industrialization's separation of home and economic production, further bolstered the patriarchal social order. Women were excluded from the rapidly developing scientific practice of medicine, relegated to the home and "cult of domesticity" where their major responsibilities in life were defined as domestic work (23–25). Working-class and race-ethnic women, however, typically were unable to meet this middle-upper-class ideal and, because of economic necessity, continued to labor outside their homes in agriculture, factories, and other sites of employment. Frequently, they encountered denigration for even striving to perform homemaker and mother roles. Women's health during this period was often informed by the unscientific and stereotypic theories that abounded in medical schools. Mental health professionals defined normal, healthy women in terms of female passivity and a desire for marriage and motherhood, and often penalized those who did not conform to that stereotype (26). Physicians commonly sought to treat middle- and upper-class women for neurasthenia or hysteria, as evidenced by symptoms of fatigue, depression, or anxiety (27), at the same time using indigent, lower-class white women and women of color as subjects for experimental surgeries (28). The health problems of women were rarely linked to social factors, such as the upheaval in gender roles that was occurring in relation to rapid industrialization. Instead, these problems were seized upon in order to expand the authority of male physicians, as justification for the exclusion of women, and to reinforce cultural norms such as women's dependency and subservient social positions.

These developments were clearly linked to the capitalist economy of U.S. health care. As a commodity, health care was initially available only to those who could pay for it. By the late 1930s, labor unions successfully negotiated with employers for health benefits and an employment-based health insurance system. This system was especially attractive to businesses, as state laws were passed making contributions to employee health insurance plans tax deductible for employers (29, 30). This, however, also intensified the gendering of health care because most women were not employed. The services covered by insurance plans reflected the needs and priorities of male workers; women were insured primarily as the dependents of their husbands, making their access to health care contingent on marriage. While the U.S. health care system was developing as an expression of market capitalism, it was also being built on the patriarchal assumption that women's unpaid labor as caregivers for friends and family would be freely available (31).

The feminist agenda of the late 1960s and early 1970s advocated a radical reorganization of standard health care attitudes, philosophies, and practices. Since then, the entry of women into medical school has increased substantially, from around 5 percent of entrants in the early 1960s to over 43 percent in the late 1990s (16). Health care organizations that focus specifically on women's health have emerged, often under the sponsorship of well-established hospitals and health systems. In addition, health care reform efforts, especially initiatives that fall under the rubric of "managed care," have promised access, cost improvements, and quality health care that are consistent with the goals of the feminist agenda, although the evidence that these goals are being met is, at best, inconsistent (32).

Our research objective is to examine to what extent these changes may have altered historical gender inequities in health and medicine—or, rather, to what extent they may have been coopted by the powerful forces of capitalism and patriarchy. In the remainder of this article, we consider these questions as we review the current circumstances of women's health care in terms of the six principles of the feminist consumer model of health care.

Increased control over health decisions and actions

Consumer choice, personal responsibility, and an emphasis on self-care are all concepts with important implications for women's decision-making and control in their health care. Managed care programs are explicitly designed to enhance the cost effectiveness of health care by shifting risk and accountability to the providers, using strategies such as prepaid financing, case management, and the use of medical practice guidelines. Health maintenance organizations (HMOs) often implement managed care principles by emphasizing primary care, sometimes from a pre-selected pool of physicians, and by limiting access to specialists.

Consumer choice of physician has become a central issue in health care because maintaining continuity of care by seeing the same physician or group of physicians is thought to promote positive health outcomes (33). The issue of consumer choice is especially important for women, as women need and use more health care services than men, receive more coverage in heavily managed plans, and have unique health care issues that require greater provider choice and flexibility. Women routinely need care from multiple physicians, from obstetrician-gynecologists for a variety of reproductive and contraceptive issues and from internists or family practitioners for general care (34). Multiple providers, however, are not consistent with the efficiency concepts of managed care. As of 1994, 70 percent of HMO plans in the United States allowed women to self-refer to an obstetrician-gynecologist other than their primary care provider, but half of these plans limited the visits to one per year (35). The overall picture is one of either no or limited access to obstetrician-gynecologists, which may increase the risk of inadequate prevention and monitoring for key women's health problems (36).

Taking personal responsibility for illness may seem to increase the control of women in health issues, but it also has immense potential for disproportionately harming women. The traditional (Parsonian) sociological view of sickness holds that sick individuals do not intentionally become incapacitated and so can be exempted from their normal social roles and responsibilities without blame, as long as they legitimately try to get well (37). For Parsons, the sick role allowed society to differentiate between the "sick" and the "bad," a distinction that is now being blurred as individuals are increasingly seen as causing their own illness by either engaging in risky behaviors or failing to engage in healthy ones. Parsons did not offer a gendered perspective on the sick role; however, Miles (38) argues that women are more easily placed in the sick role, and once there may find it more difficult to leave the sick role, than men. If the sick role is more readily occupied by women, then they may be more likely to be blamed for their illnesses than men, especially with increasing acceptance of the idea that persons are responsible for their own illnesses.

This is particularly ominous if punishment or negative sanctions follow the blame, for example, if health benefits are denied to women because they are perceived to have contributed to or "caused" their own illnesses (19). Violence against women, an obvious example of a health risk created by a patriarchal society, provides a dramatic example (39). Rape and battery affect women much more than men and are responsible for a much greater proportion of subsequent illness than is recognized. More than four million women are assaulted by their domestic partners each year, resulting in thousands of physician visits and hospital stays (40). In 1992 the American Medical Association's Council on Ethical and Judicial Affairs (41) reported that injury to women from battering and rape accounted for as much as 35 percent of all emergency room visits; however, more recent studies indicate that a much smaller percentage of women visiting the emergency room report current (2 to 3 percent) or past-year (14 percent) sexual abuse (42). African American women are even more likely to be victims of violence; one study found the rate of domestic violence to be 400 percent higher among blacks than among whites (43). Despite the absurdity of holding these women responsible for the acts perpetrated against them, a 1994 survey reported by Ezzard (44) found that half of 16 large insurers surveyed used domestic violence as a risk criterion for denying health, life, or homeowners' insurance to women.

Poverty and lack of adequate health coverage affect the ability of individuals to care for themselves and therefore undermine the health of women and their children. As Rothman (17) has noted, the recent spate of "behave yourself" campaigns encouraging expectant mothers not to smoke, drink alcohol, or use drugs and to get good prenatal care increasingly make women responsible for the health of their infants. But, as Rothman points out, few of these campaigns address issues such as women being battered during pregnancy, the growing rate of homelessness among women and their children, inadequate welfare benefits, or lack of access to health care.

Self-care is an appealing aspect of personal responsibility that on first glance seems consistent with the principles of the women's health movement in that it represents individuals taking more control over their bodies and lives. Both self-care and the underlying notion of personal responsibility offer only the illusion of control, however. There is no power or equity for women if they are held responsible for what they cannot alter or avoid, such as rape or domestic violence and exposures to health risks linked to conditions of poverty, one's workplace, or the environment of one's neighborhood. Many popular cultural norms of self-care, such as certain diet and exercise regimens, are embedded in middle-class life styles and are unrealistic for low-income individuals, especially women and minorities.

In one sense, women engage in self-care more readily than men. Researchers contend that men are more stoic in responding to symptoms and therefore less likely to take corrective actions, whereas women are thought to pay greater attention to their bodies and to monitoring health signs and symptoms (38, 45). To the extent that personal responsibility encourages this type of self-care, then women may do more and men may do less, with men depending instead on women. At the same time, it has been argued that the trend toward increased personal responsibility, including self-care, is a way to deflect attention away from the deficiencies of the U.S. health care system.

De-medicalization of women's life events and problems

Feminist sociologists have written extensively about the medicalization of women's lives, especially within the context of growing social control by physicians over the behaviors and experiences of women. Much of this work has centered on the medicalization of the reproductive activities of women, from the displacement of midwives by physicians in labor and delivery to the general medicalization of pregnancy, childbirth, menstruation, and menopause (46–49). In the 1970s, when insurance payments for complicated surgeries were generous and the use of technology unrestrained, medicalization of childbirth was manifest in escalating cesarean delivery rates, which rose from 5 percent of all births in 1970 to 25 percent in the late 1980s (50). By the 1990s, financial incentives had shifted under managed care, and some cesarean rates began to decline, from a low of 16 percent in Colorado to a high of 28 percent in Arkansas. Moreover, rates within health care systems varied to an even greater extent: for example, one study found cesarean rates ranged from 12.8 percent in a public system to 28.1 percent in a for-profit system (50).

Despite the overall drop in cesarean rates, childbirth practices continue to exemplify both medicalization and marketing. Although childbirth is typically a nonmedical event with an increasingly short length of hospital stay, hospitals now offer sophisticated technology and personal amenities in their efforts to "bond" with patients and establish ties that may bring future business. These characteristics in the United States stand in sharp contrast to childbirth experiences in developing countries, where the key issue is the survival of the mother and infant (51). The average rate of maternal deaths in developing nations is 420 per 100,000 live births; in the developed world, the rate is dramatically lower at 26 per 100,000 (11).

Midwifery was another casualty of the medicalization of childbirth in the United States. Midwives were largely eclipsed by physicians, who argued they should control labor and delivery (52). Offering a tradition in which the woman takes charge of her own childbirth, midwives serve as the main health care personnel for labor and delivery in many European countries (53). In Sweden and Finland, for example, the vast majority of prenatal care and all normal deliveries are presided over by nurse midwives, with physicians brought in by the midwife only when medical complications require it. In the Netherlands, childbirth is also less medicalized than in the United States, and approximately one-third of births take place at home.

The medicalization of premenstrual symptoms (PMS) as a mental illness, known since 1994 as premenstrual dysphoric disorder, reveals the controversy that still exists over the distinction between illness and normality (54, 55). Many women's groups saw this as stigmatizing a normal female characteristic, while others welcomed it as legitimating their symptoms as a "real illness" for which they could claim treatment and insurance benefits. This debate underscores the authority medicine wields in culturally constructing what is normal and abnormal, what is to be accepted or tolerated, and what is to be avoided or stigmatized. While not limited to women, medicalization is directed more to them because of the patriarchal nature of society and, specifically, the political economy of women.

Nowhere is this clearer than in the medicalization of appearance, the dramatic expansion of medicine into cosmetic surgery (56), eating problems, body shaping, fitness and exercise (57, 58), and fertility. Americans reportedly spend more than $30 billion annually in pursuit of weight loss, $43 billion on fitness, and millions more on plastic surgery and infertility (58). In these areas, women in particular are vulnerable to fraud and overtreatment by medicine. In 1990 the Federal Trade Commission settled out-of-court at least four times with infertility clinics that claimed their success rates were substantially higher than they in fact were (59). The life-threatening health problems to which women were exposed by their use of diet medications such as fenfluramine-phentermine (fen-phen) in the mid-1990s show how the health benefits of these procedures may prove minimal in the light of their possible adverse outcomes (60).

We conclude that the health care financing reforms in the United States over the past few decades have served to *increase* rather than decrease the medicalization of women's lives. There has been some de-medicalization in childbirth practices; however, this is outweighed by the medical takeover of weight control, fitness, cosmetic surgery, and infertility, all areas where women are the primary clients. While these gendered services have artificially inflated health care utilization and costs, cost-effective measures, such as the increased use of midwives for normal childbirth, have been kept marginal.

Emphasis on information, prevention, and less invasive treatment

Providing information to women was one of the earliest strategies of the women's health movement, which grew in part by educating women about their bodies and health care. The Boston Women's Health Book Collective, for example, began reviewing and critically analyzing existing research on women's health as early as the late 1960s (6). At the same time, it was recognized—and soon became a focal concern of the women's health movement—that much medical knowledge about women is, in fact, extrapolated from studies of men. Knowledge about special groups of women, such as American Indian women or African American women, is even more rare. Research on women finally became a public priority in the 1990s (1); however, it remains to be seen how soon or how well the significant gender gaps in evidence-based medicine will be remedied.

Receiving preventive services has been a central objective in reforming health care for women. Managed care, compared with other care arrangements, provides more prevention and early intervention services (61). Available data show that HMO members have lower hospital admission rates, shorter hospital lengths of stay, and less use of expensive procedures and tests (35). A 1993 survey found that women in HMOs received more screening tests for early detection of disease, such as clinical breast examinations, mammography, pelvic examinations, and Pap tests, than did insured women not in HMOs (62–64). Further, HMOs were substantially more likely to cover all types of reversible contraception than were other forms of health insurance (64). For example, 81 percent of HMOs covered diaphragm fittings whereas only 21 percent of conventional plans did so. The increased access provided to women, combined with the long-established finding that women are more likely to engage in preventive health practices than are men (38), seems to suggest that managed care will enhance preventive care among women. The effects for men are less clear. While research suggests that men are less oriented to prevention, much also depends on the extent to which HMOs and other managed care organizations emphasize screening and encourage prevention practices appropriate for men. Prevention in men may also reflect the health monitoring and family caregiving provided by female relatives and friends.

As discussed in the previous section on medicalization, recent health care reforms have increased incentives for responding to women's perceived problems with *invasive* health care procedures—that is, for example, addressing women's concerns about their aging bodies and changes in physical appearance and attractiveness with liposuction and other forms of reconstructive and cosmetic surgery, or addressing difficulty in becoming pregnant with technically and ethically complex surgical procedures. While mainstream U.S. medicine has continued to adhere to standard invasive medicine (and even extended its control through medicalization), the use of unconventional or alternative therapies has increased (65, 66), and there is some evidence that allopathic physicians are becoming increasingly open to complementary use of some previously unconventional treatments. There has been very little research into who uses alternative therapies. One recent study using a nationally representative sample found that 39 percent of men and 41 percent of women had used an alternative therapy within the past year (65); however, little is known about gender differences in the extent of use or the primary reliance on alternative therapy.

In conclusion, during the past several decades, women have received greater amounts of information about their health, although research specifically on women has lagged and remains severely deficient. Women are receiving increasing levels of preventive care as a result of managed care plans. Still, medical care in the United States remains highly invasive, although there seems to be greater acceptance and greater access to alternative therapies.

An atmosphere of respect

Reforming the historically patriarchal physician-patient relationship was another primary objective of the women's health movement of the 1960s. Among the objectionable features thought to be characteristic of the relationships of physicians (only a tiny fraction of whom were women) to women were: patronizing or "talking down" to them, dismissing or treating their symptoms lightly, making stereotypic assumptions and judgments about women, and a tendency to consider all problems first in relation to the reproductive system (38). Socio-cultural differences, including gender differences, create conditions for prejudice and the accompanying indignities and offenses; social inequality increases the likelihood that these will occur.

The physician-patient relationship involves multiple sources of social inequality, starting with the imbalance of expertise, the vulnerability of a sick patient, and the typically high social status of physicians. Class differences are further compounded by gender and race differences. These differences in social position between physicians and patients create differing expectations from and for doctors and patients, which, along with patients' anxiety and stress about prognosis and the significance of symptoms, escalate the chances for miscommunication and misunderstanding. Gendered behavior among physicians can mean that male and female patients are treated differently, and that male and female physicians behave differently. In recent years, considerable attention has been placed on studying these social aspects of physician-patient interaction; however, gender has received comparatively little attention in these studies.

We know that physicians do not treat all patients in a uniform way and that attitudes and values play a role in shaping physician behavior, including the way they relate to women (38). Although the majority of practicing physicians (more than 75 percent) are still men, there is evidence that female physicians differ from males in their attitudes toward and encounters with patients. Female medical students have a stronger sense of responsibility toward disadvantaged patients (67), provide more preventive care and spend more time with patients (68), and are less likely than male physicians to be deficient in breast examinations, PAP tests, and mammograms (69). Women may also be more likely to establish egalitarian relationships with patients (38). Overall, it is too early to conclude that women bring a more "humane" touch to medical encounters; studies have mixed results and patients' perceptions of care are shaped by gendered expectations (11, 38). What does seem clear is that as physicians, women do not receive the same respect and deference as do men. In communicating with patients, female physicians are interrupted more by male patients than are male physicians (70), and the vast majority (77 percent) report being sexually harassed at least once in their career (71).

The contention that women's presenting complaints and both subjective and measured symptoms are viewed less seriously than men's is difficult to confirm. There are, however, rapidly accumulating studies to indicate that similar conditions in men and women are treated less aggressively and less effectively in women. Corea (72) has documented the struggle over diagnostic criteria for AIDS, which for a number of years did not include common infections in women, such as gynecological infections, keeping thousands of women from qualifying for health care programs and assistance while men with equivalent disease status received these benefits. Studies of treatment for heart disease consistently show that women are undertreated even when their medical condition is similar to (or sometimes worse than) men's (73). Iezzoni and colleagues (74) found that women who suffered heart attacks were less likely than men to receive coronary angiography to diagnose the extent of heart damage or to undergo bypass surgery, and they were more likely to die in the hospital (74). Furthermore, these gender differences could not be explained by either age or severity of illness. Concern over physicians' inadequate response to women's subjective reports of symptoms are well demonstrated in the case of chronic fatigue syndrome, with a debate currently raging in the medical literature over the "psychosomatic" nature of women's experiences (75, 76).

Health reform policies have recently adopted a greater "consumer" focus, which includes both public and private health care entities placing greater emphasis on patient satisfaction. Except for this alteration, the reform efforts of the past several decades have paid little attention to the social and psychological dynamics of physicians and patients, focusing instead on health care financing arrangements. For a time, hospital-sponsored women's health centers attempted to attract female patients by offering improved physician-patient encounters; however, they were limited in the extent to which they could emphasize this because in so doing they criticized the routine practices of their other physician providers (77). One place where the nature of the doctor-patient relationship has received considerable attention, however, is within medical schools and residency programs. Here, there have been both explicit changes in terms of educational content and implicit changes in terms of the extent to which the educational institutions themselves are gendered.

Medical education creates precedents for gender bias by the extent to which there is an atmosphere of respect (or disrespect) toward women and minorities (78). In medical schools and teaching hospitals, the most visible indicator is the gender and race hierarchy evident in the composition of the health care workforce. Medical school admission, primarily restricted to white males prior to the 1960s, has since been extended to more women and racial minorities. During the 1996–1997 school year, 43 percent of students entering medical school were women, and one-third of those entering were either black, Asian, Hispanic/Latino, or American Indian. Most aspects of medical education, however, continue to be gendered, including specialization and residency choices. In 1997, female residents were concentrated in pediatrics and obstetrics-gynecology and were slightly overrepresented in family practice and psychiatry. Men, on the other hand, dominated in surgery (81 percent), especially orthopedic (93 percent) and thoracic (95 percent) surgery (79). There is a gender imbalance in residency programs and among faculty as they progress through the professorial ranks (80, 81). About one-fourth of U.S. medical school faculty members are women, and they are much more likely than men to be junior rather than senior faculty. Full professors and top administrators are overwhelmingly men; for example, in 1997, only seven of the 125 accredited U.S. medical schools were headed by women (79).

The medical curriculum is a significant way in which medicine functions as an institution of social control (82). We have already noted that medical research on women is grossly inadequate and that much of medical knowledge is built around a hypothetical white male patient. Within the medical curriculum's skewed view of what is normal, therefore, women and minorities quickly become "the other," the outliers, exceptional cases, deviations from the norm (83). The lack of an evidence base for women's health care makes it easier for cultural assumptions and attitudes that devalue and subordinate women to persist in medical knowledge (4). These biases also can serve to perpetuate medicine's historically outdated preoccupation with the reproductive system as the source of women's medical problems. In addition to the content of the curriculum, students learn a gendered form of respect for patients through the way in which gender issues are handled within their own medical institutions.

The climate of medical schools for women was often nonsupportive, even hostile, in the late 1960s and early 1970s (84). Even before admission to medical school, female applicants in the mid-1980s reported being questioned more intensely than men about their marriage and family plans (85). While much overt sexism seems to have disappeared, there is evidence that the climate remains less friendly to women than to men (80,86). In a recent national probability survey of medical residents, 63 percent of women reported experiencing at least one episode of sexual harassment or discrimination compared with just 15 percent of men (87). Subtle gender bias, though difficult to measure, includes gender preferences in faculty and guest lecturers and in the evaluation of student awards, research assistantships, and other opportunities; sex bias and inappropriate stereotypes in classroom material; and a lack of programs and resources to address women's issues, such as inadequate insurance coverage, maternity and parental leave opportunities, child care, and flextime work arrangements (88).

For decades, women activists have claimed that they were discriminated against in mainstream medicine and health care, leading to lower quality health care. Based on the accumulated evidence, the call for more respectful consideration of women is still relevant at the beginning of the 21st century. Reform in medical attitudes and demeanor is not contingent on financing reforms and cannot be either blamed on or promised by managed care, except in the sense that more rationality in health care should increase the evidence base in medicine and help eliminate practices based on culture or gender-biased attitudes. By most counts, sensitivity to gender issues in medicine has increased and overt hostility and sexism have diminished. On the other hand, medicine remains gendered. In 1995, the U.S. Council on Graduate Medical Education concluded that "Gender bias is the single greatest deterrent to women physicians achieving their full potential in every area and aspect of the medical profession and across all stages of medical careers" (89, p. 32). These problems are only compounded for women of color and ethnic minorities. We conclude that, despite some progress toward a less gendered climate, there is not yet a fully respectful environment in health care for women—as medical students, as physicians or other health care workers, or as patients.

Emphasis on a sociomedical model of health

The biomedical model has served as the modern basis for medical education and for the organization of health services in the United States (90). Reflecting a narrow view of disease and disease etiology, it focuses primarily on establishing patterns of normal and pathological biophysiology. The social context and the psychosocial parameters of illness are typically left out of this model, or at best given secondary consideration (91). For these reasons, a number of scholars have called for revisions to the biomedical model (90–92). Less commonly recognized is that the biomedical model has a gendered impact. There are two basic reasons: the model takes an androcentric view of patients and their bodies, and it ignores the social context of health and illness. Within the confines of the biomedical model, the persistent patriarchal nature of society is easily overlooked, as well as the social reality of unequal resource distribution on the basis of gender—in addition to inequalities of distribution on the basis of class and racial-ethnic group. The biomedical model misses the relationship between women's health and the immutable socioeconomic dependency that often accompanies women's lives. Variation in morbidity and mortality rates on the basis of race, class, and gender provides confirmation. For example, a recent study found that, although black and white women in the United States experience similar rates of heart disease morbidity, the 1997 rate of heart disease mortality for black women between the ages of 45 and 64 was more than twice that of white women of the same age (93). These findings revealed that poverty, female-headed families, and residential isolation were key factors accounting for the racial difference in mortality. Similarly, there is evidence that breast cancer mortality rates are significantly higher among black than among white women (94).

The dominance of the biomedical model has also resulted in the separation of mental health from the rest of health care, with a resulting lack of attention to mental health services, an arrangement that is being perpetuated by recent developments in managed care (95, 96). The availability of appropriate mental health services, meaning accurate diagnoses and effective therapies, is crucial for women, as they are more likely than men to be diagnosed with a mental disorder (97). Current data suggest that gender differences (which may in part be due to gender bias) in mental illness diagnoses are declining, although men are still most likely to be diagnosed with paranoid or antisocial personalty disorders and women with histrionic personality disorders, phobias, and depression (26). Depression is experienced by 24 percent of women over the course of their lifetime, compared with 15 percent of men, with only about one in ten persons receiving adequate treatment (98). A recent consensus statement from the National Depressive and Manic-Depressive Association charged managed care systems with failing to adequately provide specialized care for depressed patients, concluding that "too many patients with depression are treated for very brief periods of time and then lost to the health care system" (98, p. 337). At the same time that depressed patients, especially women, may not be receiving adequate psychotherapy services, 64 percent of doctor's visits at which psychotropic medications are prescribed are made by women (99). Under managed care, access to quality mental health services frequently is diminished when mental health services are removed ("carved out") from the primary care service package and designated to agencies that focus more on changing overt behaviors than on remedying the underlying causes of illness. Though managed care has meant that many Americans have gained access to mental health coverage, the depth of coverage—and possibly its quality—appears to have decreased (100).

For quality health care, women's social circumstances must be integrated with biophysiology. Social position is often reflected in health status, so gender itself must be considered in terms of its potential risks and as an important contextual variable in planning treatment (51). As Sobel (91) has pointed out, physical symptoms as a consequence of psychological distress account for as many as half of all medical visits. To be effective, diagnosis and treatment must recognize and address both body and mind, and how they are related to each other and to the social environment—in other words, a sociomedical model.

Commitment to health care as a right

The United States stands alone among industrial and post-industrial democratic nations in having failed to enact a national health insurance plan (101). This problem is compounded by declines in access to health insurance through employment. The percentage of the population with private health insurance dropped from 80 to 70 percent between 1980 and 1995 (102). Women are more likely than men to be covered in the public sector of the health care system, especially Hispanic (33 percent) and black (40 percent) women (103). Despite the implementation of Medicaid in the 1960s to extend health coverage to the poor, 30 percent (11 million) of the poor had no health insurance of any kind during 1995 (104). Even those with Medicaid face many barriers to access due to the difficulty in finding and getting to providers who accept Medicaid and have openings for appointments. Overall, the existing patchwork system of public and private services leaves over 17 percent of the population—40.3 million individuals—with no way to pay for health care except from their own pockets (105), and millions with coverage inadequate to protect them against financial ruin in the event of a major illness (106, 107).

Women have been especially disadvantaged by the historical linking of health insurance to employment. Until recently, most white women were not employed and were insured as their husband's dependents; in 1995, 40 percent of privately insured women were covered as dependents (108). White women are about twice as likely as women of color to have such coverage (103). This same legacy of disadvantage can be seen in Medicare. Although Medicare is viewed by most Americans as a program for *all* elderly persons age 65 and older, in reality, 5 percent of the population—predominantly women—is ineligible because they have not qualified for social security (109). As Meyer and Pavalko (110) have pointed out, employment-based health insurance assumes more stability in family life and employment than currently exists in the United States, especially given the growing number of people who are single, divorced, or widowed. Furthermore, although women's labor force participation has increased in recent years, women are much more likely than men to work in lower positions, receive a lower hourly pay, find employment in smaller firms with fewer benefits, be non-unionized, and hold part-time jobs—all factors that work against favorable insurance coverage. In 1996, only 42.7 percent of workers in jobs paying an hourly wage of $7.00 or less were offered health insurance, compared with 93.4 percent of workers making more than $15.00 per hour (111). Even among full-time employees, men are more likely than women to have employer-paid insurance (68.3 percent versus 60.5 percent). The same discrepancies are found for those working part-time (26 percent of men and 17 percent of women) (112).

Gender differences in insurance coverage are important to explore as yet another part of the gendered health care system. On the surface, gender statistics on private health insurance coverage in the United States suggest only small differences. For example, in 1993, 73 percent of women and 74 percent of men reportedly were covered by private insurance. Recent in-depth analyses, however, suggest that aggregate percentages mask significant discrepancies in how health care insurance serves the health care needs of men and women. Two forces help create this pattern. First, women may have fewer options and less adequate coverage simply because poorer coverage/less choice is associated with lower paying, lower status jobs. A double standard in health coverage often exists within the same company. A recent *New York Times* (113) article, for example, compared top executives with other employees at the Charles Schwab firm. Top executives, more likely to be white and male, had unlimited doctor and hospital choice; other employees were required to use a primary care physician for referrals. The executives had no deductibles and full coverage for office visits; other employees had a $500 deductible and a $15 cost for visits within the specified network.

Ideally, because of differences in health care requirements, insurance should work somewhat differently for women and men. Miles and Parker (112) have concluded that in all forms of insurance—in Medicare and Medicaid as well as in private coverage—men are served better than women in relation to their needs. Men and women have different life spans and illness patterns, making their health care needs substantially different and requiring accessibility to different types of health care services. Men tend to have more acute conditions that can result in hospitalization, whereas women more often suffer from chronic problems that require ambulatory or home health care. The Medicare reimbursement structure is geared to hospital care, so among older people women bear a greater financial burden, which may impede their access to care (8). Inadequacies also exist for younger women. For example, 9 percent of privately insured women have policies that exclude maternity coverage (114), and 27 to 36 percent of insurance plans do not cover induced abortion (115). All but 16 percent of HMOs cover oral contraceptives, but only 31 to 60 percent of other plans provide such coverage. Another study that included a range of health plans found that 85 percent covered medication and services related to impotency, whereas only 59 percent covered oral contraception and only 7 percent covered infertility (116). Managed care limitations on hospital stays for mental health diagnoses are making it increasingly difficult for individuals with anorexia nervosa, the vast majority of whom are women, to get appropriate treatment (117).

In the final analysis, gendered insurance coverage is also important to explore because these biases may lower the quality of health care for women (118). For example, women are more likely to move in and out of jobs owing to childbirth, making them vulnerable to loss of services or higher premiums to cover medical conditions that develop while they are between jobs. Women require preventive screening that is not always provided, such as mammograms and Pap tests, as well as birth control and abortion services. Because women live longer than men, they are more likely to require nursing home services. And associated with living longer, older women have chronic illnesses and disability and are therefore more likely than men to require adaptive aids, home health, community-based services, and outpatient prescriptions. As we have seen, Medicare covers hospital costs well, but it provides less adequate coverage for non-hospital care, including the very services women need most, such as home health care, outpatient medicines, and adaptive aids.

Conclusions

In this article we have examined the impact of recent U.S. health care policies, including managed care initiatives, on the quality of health care for women. We have discussed the historical gendering of the health care system in terms of patriarchy and capitalism, and outlined the feminist challenge to that health care system. We have argued that gender is a fundamental way of organizing social life, that health care has historically been gendered because men and women occupy different positions within it and because the system itself has been established with patriarchal assumptions and practices structurally embedded. Furthermore, health care has been driven by the profit motive and dominated by the viewpoint and interests of physicians who are predominantly white and male. Both patriarchy and capitalism have contributed to the social construction of a gendered institution, including norms that stereotype women, marginalize their roles in medicine as both patients and providers, and diminish their access to quality health care. Theorists disagree about the relative importance to assign to these two forces; however, it is clear that patriarchal practices work to the disadvantage of women in various types of economies throughout the world (51). The gendering of medical knowledge and of the doctor-patient relationship, and the extensive medicalization of female-related mental and biological phenomena, have lessened the respect accorded women and their control over their own bodies. Has the overall quality of health care available for women in the United States improved since the 1970s? We have used the demands of the feminist consumer model of health to address this issue and have concluded that, despite some notable gains, neither managed care nor other health policies have significantly altered the gendered nature of health care.

Since the feminist critique of the U.S. health care system took form, some things have definitely improved: health policies have adopted a greater "consumer focus" and now place more emphasis on patient satisfaction; HMOs have provided more preventive services; the medicalization of some female-related events has decreased; mental health diagnoses are less gender stereotyped; more women have entered medical school; and the emphasis on self-care and self-responsibility may have fostered health-promoting behaviors among some women. Yet these changes are meager when compared with the continuing and, in some cases, growing gender inequities in health care.

While managed care has increased the scope of preventive services available, there is little evidence that it has increased overall access to care for women. Moreover, managed care arrangements have seriously restricted the choices in providers for women to meet their health care needs, leading us to conclude that women have gained little ground in being able to take control over medical decisions and their own bodies. The growing emphasis on personal responsibility and self-care may have enhanced activism and vigilance by promoting healthy behaviors, yet it ignores social forces over which women, especially those who are poor, have very little control. To be more specific, women's health care must be understood in the context of male dominance and domestic abuse and violence. It must be understood in the context of harassment and discrimination, low-status, low-paying jobs with little authority, and poverty. Women's health must also be understood in the context of motherhood, where a woman's decisions are constantly being mediated by her responsibility for children. It must also be considered that women have the primary caregiving responsibilities for other family members, friends, and relatives, and this also restricts their choices for themselves. Rather than indicating greater autonomy for either men or women, personal responsibility and self-care may simply give the illusion of control over one's health.

Medicalization has been a central issue in the women's health care agenda. We have noted a slight decline in some areas of medicalization, such as the rate of cesarean sections, but we contend that new areas of medicalization—specifically, weight loss, infertility, fitness, and plastic surgery—have more than offset the decline. The growing medicalization of women's bodies and experiences is fed by the combination of capitalism and patriarchy. Additional impetus comes from the health care reforms of the 1980s and 1990s, especially the financial pressures on hospitals and medical practices to survive and profit in a competitive health care market. Rather than following health care needs, demand for many health care services has followed marketing strategies that play on the vulnerabilities of the insured middle classes, especially women.

Despite an increase in the number of women entering medical school in recent decades, the majority of practicing physicians are still men, and the doctor-patient relationship for women continues to be a gendered encounter. Research suggests that, compared with men, women may still face more barriers to medical school entry, experience the medical school setting as more hostile and unsupportive, and be more victimized by sexual harassment In addition, there is significant gender segregation in specialty areas, with men dominating the more financially lucrative areas of medicine. While it is certainly too early to conclude that female physicians are improving the quality of health services available, studies so far do show that women have more egalitarian relationships with patients, feel a stronger sense of responsibility toward disadvantaged patients, and provide more preventive health care services.

Women are as likely to have health care insurance coverage as are men; yet this ostensible equity masks gender differences in the services provided and the likelihood of receiving care in the public sector of the health care system. We have pointed out that 40 percent of privately insured women receive health insurance as dependents on their husbands' policies, and that the services offered by such policies are often organized around the potential health care needs of men. The quality of health care for women is diminished by insurance schemes that favor men and fail to cover basic services for women, such as access to obstetricians-gynecologists and contraceptive and abortion services. The health care coverage of employed women is also diminished by their greater likelihood of having jobs that are low-paying or part-time, or both. Managed care does not guarantee equitable coverage for consumers; rather, as Waitzkin (32) has noted, it often provides "bare-bone packages" for those in low-premium plans and expanded services for those in high-premium plans.

The evidence so far suggests that gender disparity is still firmly embedded in health care. If the goal for the future is continued quality improvement, then policymakers, health care personnel, and consumers must be vigilant in analyzing managed care and other initiatives. They must become aware of the effects of patriarchy and capitalism and must be willing to promote policies to correct those that are harmful, whether because of overuse, underuse, or misuse of health care resources. Such vigilance is crucial lest new health reforms replicate and further solidify the gendered inequities of the past.

References

1. Weisman, C. S. *Women's Health Care: Activist Traditions and Institutional Change*. Johns Hopkins University Press, Baltimore, 1998.
2. Rodwin, M. A. Patient accountability and quality of care: Lessons from medical consumerism and the patients' rights, women's health and disability rights movements. *Am. J. Law Med.* 20: 147–167, 1994.
3. Ruzek, S. B. *The Women's Health Movement: Feminist Alternatives to Medical Control*. Praeger, New York, 1978.
4. Zimmerman, M. The women's health movement: A critique of medical enterprise and the position of women. In *Analyzing Gender: A Handbook of Social Science Research*, edited by M. M. Ferree and B. Hess. Sage, Thousand Oaks, Calif., 1987.
5. Bart, P. Seizing the means of reproduction: An illegal feminist abortion collective and how it worked. In *Women, Health and Reproduction*, edited by H. Roberts. Routledge and Kegan Paul, London, 1981.
6. Boston Women's Health Book Collective. *The New Our Bodies, Ourselves*. Simon & Schuster, New York, 1992 [1973].
7. Federation of Feminist Women's Health Centers. *A New View of a Woman's Body*. Simon & Schuster, New York, 1981.
8. Sofaer, S., and Abel, E. Older women's health and financial vulnerability: Implications of the Medicare benefit structure. *Women and Health* 16(3/4): 47–67, 1990.
9. Scully, D., and Bart, P. A funny thing happened on the way to the orifice: Women in gynecology textbooks. *Am. J. Soc.* 78: 1045–1050, 1973.
10. Fisher, S. *In the Patient's Best Interest: Women and the Politics of Medical Decisions*. Rutgers University Press, New Brunswick, N.J., 1986.
11. Lorber, J. *Gender and the Social Construction of Illness*. Sage, Thousand Oaks, Calif., 1997.
12. Kirschstein, R. L. Research on women's health. *Am. J. Public Health* 81: 291–293, 1991.
13. Rosser, S. V. Gender bias in clinical research: The difference it makes. In *Reframing Women's Health*, edited by A. Dan. Sage, Thousand Oaks, Calif., 1994.
14. Narrigan, D., et al. Research to improve women's health: An agenda for equity. In *Women's Health: Complexities and Differences*, edited by S. B. Ruzek, V. L. Olesen, and A. E. Clarke. Ohio State University Press, Columbus, 1997.
15. Friedman, E. *An Unfinished Revolution: Women and Health Care in America*. United Hospital Fund of New York, New York, 1994.
16. Zimmerman, M. K., and Hill, S. A. Health care as a gendered system. In *The Handbook of Gender Sociology*, edited by J. S. Chafetz. Plenum, New York, 1999.
17. Rothman, B. K. *Recreating Motherhood: Ideology and Technology in a Patriarchal Society*. Norton, New York, 1989.
18. Weitz, R. *The Sociology of Health, Illness, and Health Care: A Critical Approach*. Wadsworth, Belmont, Calif., 1996.
19. Doyal, L. The politics of women's health: Setting a global agenda. *Int. J. Health Serv.* 26: 47–65, 1996.

20. Riska, E., and Wegar, K. (eds.). *Gender, Work and Medicine: Women and the Medical Division of Labour.* Sage, Newbury Park, Calif., 1993.
21. Cassady, J. H. *Medicine in America: A Short History.* Johns Hopkins University Press, Baltimore, 1991.
22. Walsh, M. R. *Doctors Wanted: No Women Need Apply.* Yale University Press, New Haven, Conn., 1977.
23. Morantz-Sanchez, R. M. *Sympathy and Science: Women Physicians in American Medicine.* Oxford University Press, New York, 1985.
24. Cott, N. F. *The Bonds of Womanhood: Women's Sphere in New England, 1780–1835.* Yale University Press, New Haven, Conn., 1977.
25. Weltner, B. The cult of true womanhood: 1820–1860. In *The American Family in Social Perspective*, Ed. 3, edited by M. Gordon. St. Martin's Press, New York, 1983.
26. Cooksey, E. C., and Brown, P. Spinning on its axes: DSM and the social construction of psychiatric diagnosis. *Int. J. Health Serv.* 28(3): 525–554, 1998.
27. Smith-Rosenberg, C., and Rosenberg, C. The female animal: Medical and biological views of women and her role in nineteenth-century America. *J. Am. History* 60: 332–356, 1973.
28. Ehrenreich, B., and English, D. *For Her Own Good.* Doubleday-Anchor Books, Garden City, N.Y., 1978.
29. Starr, P. *The Social Transformation of American Medicine.* Basic Books, New York, 1982.
30. Staples, C. L. The politics of employment-based insurance in the United States. *Int. J. Health Serv.* 19: 415–431, 1989.
31. Glazer, N. Overlooked, overworked: Women's unpaid and paid work in the health services "cost crisis." *Int. J. Health Serv.* 18(1): 119–137, 1988.
32. Waitzkin, H. Is our work dangerous? Should it be? *J. Health Soc. Behav.* 39: 7–17, 1998.
33. Bindman, A. B., et al. Primary care and receipt of preventive services. *J. Gen. Intern. Med.* 11: 269–276, 1996.
34. Bartman, B. A. Women's access to appropriate providers within managed care: Implications for the quality of primary care. *Women's Health Issues* 6: 45–50, 1996.
35. Bernstein, A. B. Women's health in HMOs: What we know and what we need to find out. *Women's Health Issues* 6: 51–59, 1996.
36. Johns, L. Obstetrics-gynecology as primary care: A market dilemma. *Health Aff.* 13: 194–200, 1994.
37. Parsons, T. *The Social System.* Free Press, Glencoe, Ill., 1951.
38. Miles, A. *Women, Health and Medicine.* Open University Press, Philadelphia, 1991.
39. Schafran, L. H. Topics for our times: Rape is a major public health issue. *Am. J. Public Health* 86: 15–17, 1996.
40. Gerbert, B., et al. Experiences of battered women in health care settings: A qualitative study. *Women and Health* 24: 1–17, 1996.
41. Council on Ethical and Judicial Affairs, American Medical Association. Physicians and domestic violence: Ethical considerations. *JAMA* 267: 3190–3193, 1992.

42. Dearwater, S. R., et al. Prevalence of intimate partner abuse in women treated at community hospital emergency departments. *JAMA* 280: 433–438, 1998.
43. Straus, M., Gelles, R., and Steinmetz, S. *Behind Closed Doors: Violence in the American Family*. Doubleday, Garden City, N.Y., 1980.
44. Ezzard, M. Insurance companies exhibit no respect for abused women. *Kansas City Star*, December 17, 1995.
45. Mechanic, D. *Medical Sociology*. Free Press, Glencoe, Ill., 1968.
46. Bell, S. E. Changing ideas: The medicalization of menopause. *Soc. Sci. Med.* 24: 535–542, 1987.
47. Riessman, C. K. Women and medicalization: A new perspective. *Social Policy*, Summer 1983, pp. 3–18.
48. Sullivan, D., and Weitz, R. *Labor Pains: Modern Midwives and Home Birth*. Yale University Press, New Haven, Conn., 1988.
49. McCrea, F. The politics of menopause: The discovery of a deficiency disease. *Soc. Prob.* 31: 111–123, 1983.
50. Public Citizen Health Research Group. Unnecessary cesarean sections: Curing a national epidemic. *Med. Benefits*, July 30, 1994.
51. Doyal, L. *What Makes Women Sick: Gender and the Political Economy of Health*. Rutgers University Press, New Brunswick, N.J., 1995.
52. Weitz, R., and Sullivan, D. The politics of childbirth: The re-emergence of midwifery in Arizona. *Soc. Prob.* 33: 163–175, 1986.
53. DeVries, R. A cross-national view of the status of midwives. In *Gender, Work, and Medicine: Women in the Medical Division of Labour*. Sage, London, 1993.
54. Figert, A. *Women and the Ownership of PMS: The Structuring of a Psychiatric Disorder*. Aldine de Gruyter, New York, 1996.
55. Gold, J. H. Premenstrual dysphoric disorder: What's that? *JAMA* 278: 1024–1025, 1997.
56. Sullivan, D. Cosmetic surgery: Market dynamics and medicalization. *Res. Sociol. Health Care* 10: 97–115, 1993.
57. Wolf, N. *The Beauty Myth: How Images of Beauty Are Used Against Women*. William Morrow, New York, 1991.
58. Hesse-Biber, S. *Am I Thin Enough Yet? The Cult of Thinness and the Commercialization of Identity*. Oxford University Press, New York, 1996.
59. 4th infertility clinic settles on charges of fraudulent claims. *Modern Healthcare*, November 4, 1991, p. 20.
60. Connolly, H. M., et al. Valvular heart disease associated with fenfluramine-phentermine. *N. Engl. J. Med.* 337: 581, 1997.
61. Miller, R. H., and Luft, H. Managed care plan performance since 1980. *JAMA* 271: 1512–1519, 1994.
62. Louis Harris and Assoc. Commonwealth Fund Survey of Women's Health. New York, 1993.
63. Makuc, D. V., Freid, M., and Parsons, P. E. *Health Insurance and Cancer Screening Among Women*. Advance Data No. 254. National Center for Health Statistics, Hyattsville, Md., August 3, 1994.
64. Alan Guttmacher Institute. *Uneven and Unequal: Insurance Coverage and Reproductive Health Services*. Alan Guttmacher Institute, New York, 1994.
65. Astin, J. A. Why patients use alternative medicine: Results of a national study. *JAMA* 279: 1548–1553, 1998.

66. Eisenberg, D., et al. Unconventional medicine in the United States. *N. Engl. J. Med.* 328: 246–252, 1993.
67. Crandall, S. J., Volk, R. J., and Loemker, V. Medical students' attitudes toward providing care for the underserved: Are we training socially responsible physicians? *JAMA* 269: 2519–2523, 1993.
68. Lurie, N., et al. Preventive care for women: Does the sex of the physician matter? *N. Engl. J. Med.* 329: 478–482, 1993.
69. Franks, P., and Clancy, C. M. Physician gender bias in clinical decisionmaking: Screening for cancer in primary care. *Med. Care* 31: 213–218, 1993.
70. West, C. *Routine Complications: Troubles with Talk Between Doctors and Patients.* Indiana University Press, Bloomington, 1984.
71. Phillips, S. P., and Schneider, M. S. Sexual harassment of female doctors by patients. *N. Engl. J. Med.* 329: 1936–1939, 1993.
72. Corea, G. *The Invisible Epidemic: The Story of Women and AIDS.* HarperCollins, New York, 1992.
73. Pearson, T. A., and Myerson, M. Treatment of hypercholesterolemia in women: Equality, effectiveness and extrapolation of evidence. *JAMA* 277: 1320–1321, 1997.
74. Iezzoni, L. I., et al. Differences in procedure use, in-hospital mortality, and illness severity gender for acute myocardial infarction patients. *Med. Care* 35: 158–171, 1997.
75. Ware, N. C. Suffering and the social construction of illness: The delegitimation of illness experience in chronic fatigue syndrome. *Med. Anthropol. Q.* 6: 347–361, 1992.
76. Abbey, S. E., and Garfinkel, P. E. Neurasthenia and chronic fatigue syndrome: The role of culture in the making of a diagnosis. *Am. J. Psychiatry* 148: 1638–1646, 1991.
77. Thomas, L. W. A critical feminist perspective of the health belief model: Implications for nursing theory, research, practice, and education. *J. Prof. Nursing* 11: 246–252, 1995.
78. Zimmerman, M. Status Report on Women's Health in Medical Education and Training. Paper prepared for the Canada–U.S. Forum on Women's Health. U.S. Department of Health and Human Services, Office on Women's Health, Washington, D.C., 1996.
79. Baransky, B., Jonas, H. S., and Etzel, S. I. Educational programs in U.S. medical schools, 1996–1997. *JAMA* 278: 744–784, 1997.
80. Bickel, J., and Ruffin, A. Gender-associated differences in matriculating and graduating medical students. *Acad. Med.* 70: 552–559, 1995.
81. Bickel, J. Scenarios for success—Enhancing women physicians' professional advancement. *West. J. Med.* 65: 165–169, 1995.
82. Zola, I. K. Medicine as an institution of social control. *Sociol. Rev.* 20: 487–503, 1972.
83. Harrison, M. The woman as other: The premise of medicine. *J. Am. Women's Med. Assoc.* 45: 225–226, 1990.
84. Campbell, M. *Why Would a Girl Go into Medicine?* Feminist Press, Old Westbury, N.Y., 1974.
85. Grant, L. The gender climate of medical school: Perspectives of women and men students. *J. Am. Women's Med. Assoc.* 43: 109–119, 1988.

86. Komaromy, M., et al. Sexual harassment in medical training. *N. Engl. J. Med.* 328: 322–326, 1993.
87. Daugherty, S. R., Baldwin, D. C., and Rowley, B. D. Learning, satisfaction, and mistreatment during medical internship. *JAMA* 279: 1194–1199, 1998.
88. Philibert, I., and Bickel, J. Maternity and parental leave policies at COTH hospitals: An update. *Acad. Med.* 70: 1056–1058, 1995.
89. Council on Graduate Medical Education, U.S. Department of Health and Human Services. *Fifth Report: Women and Medicine.* USDHHS Publication No. HRSA-P-DM-95-1. Washington, D.C., July 1995.
90. Mishler, E. *The Social Contexts of Health, Illness, and Patient Care.* Cambridge University Press, New York, 1981.
91. Sobel, D. S. Rethinking medicine: Improving health outcomes with cost-effective psychosocial interventions. *Psychosom. Med.* 57: 234–244, 1995.
92. Engel, G. L. The need for a new medical model: A challenge for biomedicine. *Science* 196: 129–136, 1977.
93. LeClere, F. B., Rogers, R. B., and Peters, K. Neighborhood social context and racial differences in women's heart disease mortality. *J. Health Soc. Behav.* 39: 91–107, 1998.
94. Kronenfeld, J. J. Gender and health status. In *The Handbook of Gender Sociology*, edited by J. S. Chafetz. Plenum, New York, 1999.
95. Mechanic, D. Mental health services in the context of health insurance reform. *Milbank Q.* 71: 349–364, 1993.
96. Mechanic, D. Integrating mental health into a general health care system. *Hosp. Community Psychiatry* 45: 893–897, 1994.
97. Linzer, M., et al. Gender, quality of life, and mental disorder in primary care: Results from the PRIME-MD 1000 study. *Am. J. Med.* 101: 526–533, 1996.
98. Hirschfeld, R. A. M., et al. The National Depressive and Manic-Depressive Association consensus statement on the undertreatment of depression. *JAMA* 277: 333–340, 1997.
99. Pincus, H. A., et al. Prescribing trends in psychotropic medication. *JAMA*, February 18, 1998.
100. Jensen, G., et al. Mental health insurance in the 1990s: Are employers offering less to more? *Health Aff.* 17(3): 201–208, 1998.
101. Evans, R. G. Going for the gold: The redistributive agenda behind market-based health care reform. *J. Health Polit. Policy Law* 22: 427–465, 1997.
102. U.S. General Accounting Office. *Private Health Insurance.* GAO/HEHS-97-122. Washington, D.C., July 1997.
103. Leigh, W. A., and Lindquist, M. A. *Women of Color Health Data Book: Adolescents to Seniors.* Office of Research on Women's Health, National Institutes of Health, Bethesda, Md., 1997.
104. Bennefild, R. L. *Health Insurance Coverage: 1995.* Bureau of the Census P60-195. Economics and Statistics Administration, U.S. Department of Commerce, Washington, D.C., 1996.
105. Fronstin, P. Employee Benefit Research Institute Brief No. 185: Trends in health insurance coverage. *Med. Benefits* 14: 2, 1997.
106. Himmelstein, D. U., and Woolhandler, S. *The National Health Program Book: A Source Guide for Advocates.* Common Courage, Monroe, Me., 1994.

107. Zimmerman, M. K. TLC or CFO? Conflicted Caregivers in the Health Care Market. Paper presented at the annual meetings of the Midwest Sociological Society, April 1999.
108. U.S. General Accounting Office. *Employment-Based Health Insurance.* GAO/HEHS-97-35. Washington, D.C., February 1997.
109. Doress, P. B., and Siegal, D. L. *Ourselves Growing Older.* Simon & Schuster, New York, 1987.
110. Meyer, M. H., and Pavalko, E. K. Family, work, and access to health insurance among mature women. *J. Health Soc. Behav.* 37: 311–325, 1996.
111. Cooper, P. F., and Schone, B. S. More offers, fewer takers for employment-based health insurance: 1987 and 1996. *Health Aff.* 16: 142–149, 1997.
112. Miles, S., and Parker, K. Men, women, and health insurance. *N. Engl. J. Med.* 336: 218–221, 1997.
113. A double standard in health coverage. *New York Times*, March 17, 1997.
114. Braverman, P. *West. J. Med.* December 1988.
115. Horton, J. A. (ed.). *The Women's Health Data Book: A Profile of Women's Health in the United States*, Ed. 2. Jacobs Institute of Women's Health/Elsevier, Washington, D.C., 1995.
116. Health plan exclusions for medication and services: Reproduction and sexual dysfunction. *Med. Benefits* 15(18): 1–2, 1998.
117. Chase, M. Insurers are obstacle for anorexics. *Kansas City Star*, March 28, 1999.
118. Burstin, H. R., Lipsitz, S. R., and Brennan, T. A. Socioeconomic status and risk for substandard medical care. *JAMA* 268: 2383–2387, 1992.

Part 11

THE IMPACT OF GENDERED ASSUMPTIONS ON HEALTH AND HEALTHCARE

47
A FUNNY THING HAPPENED ON THE WAY TO THE ORIFICE
Women in gynecology textbooks[1]

Diana Scully and Pauline Bart

Source: *American Journal of Sociology*, 78:4 (1970), 1045–51.

The gynecologist is our society's official specialist on women, legitimately commenting on their psyches as well as on the illnesses of their reproductive tracts (Novak, Jones, and Jones 1970; Green 1971). Nevertheless, gynecologists are overwhelmingly male (93.4% [*Time* 1972, p. 89]); and the tools of the sociology of knowledge suggest that one's perspectives are constrained by one's place in the social structure and thus gynecologists may not adequately represent the worldview and the interests of the group they are supposed to attend and advocate. Indeed, examination of gynecology textbooks, one of the primary professional socialization agents for practitioners in the field, revealed a persistent bias toward greater concern with the patient's husband than with the patient herself. Women are consistently described as anatomically destined to reproduce, nurture, and keep their husbands happy. So gynecology appears to be another of the forces committed to maintaining traditional sex-role stereotypes, in the interest of men and from a male perspective.[2]

The contents of 27 general gynecology texts published in the United States since 1943 were analyzed. Complete lists of texts and authors were obtained from the Index Catalog of the Library of the Surgeon General's Office, National Library of Medicine. We attempted to read all the texts available, rather than to sample (27 books out of 32). To allow for emergent trends based on new information about female sexuality, the books were divided into three periods; pre-Kinsey, 1943–52 (six of nine were used); post-Kinsey, pre-Masters and Johnson, 1953–62 (nine of 10 were used); post-Masters and Johnson, 1963–72 (12 of 14 were used). Only the latest edition of each text was read. The numbers represent authors active in the field rather than total volumes published.

1943–53[3]

In this period, prior to the work of Kinsey and Masters and Johnson, there was little empirical data about female sexuality. Of the four books in this group, two did not index female sexuality. One of the four (Janney 1950) presented a strikingly egalitarian approach to sexuality. Two others are characterized by a double standard. Thus Cooke stated: "The fundamental biologic factor in women is the urge of motherhood balanced by the fact that sexual pleasure is entirely secondary or even absent" (Cooke 1943, pp. 59–60). Since women were assumed to be "almost universally generally frigid," while the male "is created to fertilize as many females as possible and has an infinite appetite and capacity for intercourse" (Cooke 1943, p. 60), two texts instruct gynecologists to teach their patients to fake orgasm. "It is good advice to recommend to the women the advantage of *innocent simulation* [italics added] of sex responsiveness, and as a matter of fact many women in their desire to please their husbands learned the advantage of such innocent deception" (Novak and Novak 1952, p. 572; Lowrie 1952, p. 671).

The Kinsey era, 1953–62

Once Kinsey et al. published *Sexual Behavior in the Human Female* (1953), the medical field had an authoritative and definitive (albeit from a nonrandom sample) source of information on the female. For the most part, these texts used Kinsey's report selectively; findings which reinforced old stereotypes were repeated, but the revolutionary findings significant for women were ignored. For example, one often finds in the textbooks that the male sets the sexual pace in marital coitus, but nowhere is it mentioned that women are multiorgasmic, a Kinsey finding which raises questions concerning the gynecologist's belief in the stronger male sex drive.

Though Kinsey is not usually credited with the discovery, he debunked the myth of the vaginal orgasm. "The literature usually implies that the vagina itself should be the center of sensory stimulation but this as we have seen is a physical and physiologic impossibility for nearly all females" (Kinsey 1953, p. 582)

Gynecologists, however, have tenaciously clung to the idea of the vaginal orgasm as the appropriate response and labeled "frigid" and immature those patients who could not experience it. The content analysis (see table 1) showed that no text read in any of the three decades said that portions of the vagina had no nerve endings and lacked sensation (a Kinsey finding); only one, in the 1963–72 decade, said that the clitoris was the seat of sensation; three in the second decade and two in the most current decade said that the vaginal response was the "mature response"; and two, one in the current decade and one in the 1952–63 period, stated the vagina and clitoris were equally

Table 1 Female sexuality and orgasm in three decades of gynecology texts.

	1943–52		1953–62		1963–72	
	N	% of Indexed Item (N)	N	% of Indexed Item (N)	N	% of Indexed Item (N)
Texts which indexed female sexuality	(4)	...	(8)	...	(9)	...
Sex primarily for reproduction*	...	25 (1)	...	62 (5)	...	67 (6)
Male sex drive stronger	...	50 (2)	...	62 (5)	...	89 (8)
Women characterized as frigid	...	25 (1)	...	37 (3)	...	33 (3)
Female sexuality not indexed	(2)	...	(1)	...	(3)	...
Total texts	(6)	...	(9)	...	(12)	...
Texts which indexed orgasm (clitoral-vaginal)	(4)	...	(4)	...	(4)	...
Vaginal mature response	...	0	...	75 (3)	...	50 (2)†
Not discussed in these terms	...	75 (3)†	...	25 (1)	...	0
Orgasm not indexed	(2)	...	(5)	...	(8)	...
Total texts	(6)	...	(9)	...	(12)	...

* Of those books in which female sexuality was indexed, some had more than one reference area. Therefore the total number of references is greater than the number of books.
† One text in the 1963–72 period indicated the clitoris to be the seat of sensation, and two texts, one in the 1963–72 and one in the 1943–52 period, indicated no difference in clitoral and vaginal orgasm.

sensitive. For example: "Investigators of sexual behavior distinguished between clitoral and vaginal orgasm, the first playing a dominant role in childhood sexuality and in masturbation and the latter in the normal mature and sexually active women.... The limitation of sexual satisfaction to one part of the external genitalia is apparently due to habit and aversion to normal cohabitation" (Ruben 1956, p. 77). Indeed as late as 1965, gynecology texts were reporting the vagina as the main erogenous zone (Greenhill 1965, p. 496). In 1962: "The transference of sensations from the clitoris to the vagina is completed only in part and frequently not at all.... If there has been much manual stimulation of the clitoris *it* [italics added] may be reluctant to abandon control, or the vagina may be unwilling to accept the combined role of arbiter of sensation and vehicle for reproduction" (Parsons and Sommers 1962, pp. 501–2). But, even if she is "truly frigid ... the marital relations may proceed without *disturbing* [italics added] either partner" (Parsons and Sommers 1962, p. 494).

1963–72

In the early 1960s reports began to flow from the laboratories of Masters and Johnson, and, though their findings are not generally quoted, there has been some indirect influence. Two-thirds (eight) of the books of that decade failed to discuss the issue of the clitoral versus vaginal orgasm. Eight continued to state, contrary to Masters and Johnson's findings, that the male sex drive was stronger; and half (six) still maintained that procreation was the major function of sex for the female. Two said that most women were "frigid," and another stated that one-third were sexually unresponsive. Two repeated that the vaginal orgasm was the only mature response (Greenhill 1965; Jeffcoate 1967).

Although sex roles are never indexed, we learn from reading the texts that when they deal with the subject, the traditional female sex role is preferred (nine out of 12 in the recent decade). Thus Jeffcoate states: "An important feature of sex desire in the man is the urge to dominate the women and subjugate her to his will; in the women acquiescence to the masterful takes a high place" (Jeffcoate 1967, p. 726). In 1971 we read: "The traits that compose the core of the female personality are feminine narcissism, masochism and passivity" (Willson 1971, p. 43).

So it appears that in gynecology texts the basic underlying image of woman and her "normal adult female role in the marital relationship" (Green 1971, p. 436) has changed little even though new data contradicting such views have been available. A 1970 text states: "The frequency of intercourse depends entirely upon the male sex drive. . . . The bride should be advised to allow her husband's sex drive to set their pace and she should attempt to gear hers satisfactorily to his. If she finds after several months or years that this is not possible, she is advised to consult her physician as soon as she realizes there is a real problem" (Novak, Jones, and Jones 1970, pp. 662–63).

The gynecologist's self-image as helpful to women combined with unbelievable condescension is epitomized in this remark: "If like all human beings, he [the gynecologist] is made in the image of the Almighty, and if he is kind, then his kindness and concern for his patient may provide her with a glimpse of God's image" (Scott 1968, p. 25).

Summary

A review of 27 gynecology texts written from 1943 to 1972 shows that they are written, as a sociology-of-knowledge framework would lead us to expect, from a male viewpoint. Traditional views of female sexuality and personality are presented generally unsullied by the findings of Kinsey and Masters and Johnson, though the latter resulted in some changes in rhetoric.

In the last two decades at least one-half of the texts that indexed the topics stated that the male sex drive was stronger than the female's; she was interested in sex for procreation more than for recreation. In addition, they said most women were "frigid" and that the vaginal orgasm was the "mature" response. Gynecologists, our society's official experts on women, think of themselves as the woman's friend. With friends like that, who needs enemies?

Notes

1. We thank Marlyn Grossman for a careful reading of this paper and valuable criticism. Another version of this paper was presented at the American Sociological Association meetings in 1972. A longer version is available from the authors. This paper is on file at the Women's History Research Center in Berkeley, Calif.
2. There is a growing literature detailing the emphasis on traditional sex roles in works ranging from children's story and school books through college history and sociology texts and academic disciplines (e.g., Ehrlich 1971; Weitzman et al. 1972).
3. Our analysis is based not only on indexed items but on a general reading of the texts.

References

*Behrman, Samuel J., and John R. C. Gosling. 1959. *Fundamentals of Gynecology*. New York: Oxford University Press.
*Benson, Ralph C. 1971. *Handbook of Obstetrics and Gynecology*. Los Altos, Calif.: Lange Medical Publishers.
*Brewer, John I., and Edwin J. DeCosts. 1967. *Textbook of Gynecology*. Baltimore: Williams & Wilkens.
*Cooke, Willard R. 19543. *Essentials of Gynecology*. Philadelphia: Lippincott.
*Crossen, Robert James. 1953. *Diseases of Women*. Saint Louis: Mosby.
*Curtis, A. H. 1946. *A Textbook of Gynecology*. Philadelphia: Saunders.
*Danforth, David. 1971. *Textbook of Obstetrics and Gynecology*. New York: Hoeber.
*Davis, Henry Carl, ed. 1964. *Gynecology and Obstetrics*. 3 vols. Hagarstown, Md.: Prior.
Ehrlich, Carol. 1971. "The Male Sociologist's Burden: The Place of Women in Marriage and Family Texts." *Journal of Marriage and the Family* 33:421–30.
*Gray, Laman. 1960. *A Textbook of Gynecology*. Springfield, Ill.: Thomas.
*Green, Thomas H. 1971. *Gynecology: Essentials of Clinical Practice*. Boston: Little, Brown.
*Greenhill, J. P. 1965. *Office Gynecology*. Chicago: Yearbook Medical Publishers.
*Huffman, John Williams. 1962. *Gynecology and Obstetrics*. Philadelphia: Saunders.
*Janney, James C. 1950. *Medical Gynecology*. Philadelphia: Saunders.
*Jeffcoate, Thomas. 1967. *Principles of Gynecology*. London: Butterworth.
*Kimbrough, Robert A., ed. 1965. *Gynecology*. Philadelphia: Lippincott.
Kinsey, Alfred C., et al. 1953. *Sexual Behavior in the Human Female*. New York: Simon & Schuster.
*Kistner, R. W. 1964. *Gynecology*. Chicago: Yearbook Medical Publishers.
*Lowrie, Robert J. 1952. *Gynecology, Diseases and Minor Surgery*. Springfield, Ill.: Thomas.

*Meigs, J. V., and S. H. Sturgis. 1963. *Progress in Gynecology*. New York: Grune & Stratton.

*Novak, Edmund R., Georgeanna Seegar Jones, and Howard W. Jones. 1970. *Novak's Textbook of Gynecology*. Baltimore: Williams & Wilkens.

Novak, Emil, and Edmund R. Novak. 1952. *Textbook of Gynecology*. Baltimore: Williams & Wilkens.

*Parsons, Langdon, and Sheldon C. Sommers. 1962. *Gynecology*. Philadelphia: Saunders.

*Pettit, Mary DeWitt. 1962. *Gynecologic Diagnosis and Treatment*. New York: McGraw-Hill.

*Reich, Walter, and M. Nechtow. 1957. *Practical Gynecology*. Philadelphia: Lippincott.

*Rubin, I. C., and Josef Novak. 1956. *Integrated Gynecology: Principles and Practice*. New York: McGraw-Hill.

Scott C. Russell. 1968. *The World of a Gynecologist*. London: Oliver & Boyd.

*Scott, William A., and H. Brookfield Van Wyck. 1946. *The Essentials of Obstetrics and Gynecology*. Philadelphia: Lea & Febiger.

*Taylor, Edward Stewart. 1962. *Essentials of Gynecology*. Philadelphia: Lea & Febiger.

Time, March 20, 1972, p. 89.

Weitzman, Lenore J., Deborah Eifler, Elizabeth Hokada, and Catherine Ross. 1972. "Sex-Role Socialization in Picture Books for Preschool Children." *American Journal of Sociology* 77 (May): 1125–50.

*Wharton, L. R. 1943. *Gynecology*. Philadelphia: Saunders.

*Willson, James Robert. 1971. *Obstetrics and Gynecology*. Saint Louis: Mosby.

*One of the 27 gynecology textbooks used in this study.

48
DOCTOR–PATIENT NEGOTIATION OF CULTURAL ASSUMPTIONS

Sue Fisher and Stephen B. Groce

Source: *Sociology of Health and Illness*, 7:3 (1985), 342–74.

Abstract

This paper simultaneously examines the relationship between norms as features of the social structure and norms as interactional accomplishments. Doctors as cultural members share a set of social facts about women as part of their common stock of knowledge. By posing these facts in a reflexive relationship with the interactional work participants do in specific settings we are able to display how doctors acting as 'secret apprentices' ferret cultural assumptions from medical interactions. A detailed comparison of two cases with the same doctor provide the data to examine the ways norms about patients *qua* women emerged and were negotiated against a background of cultural expectations or assumptions about women. This comparison reveals how divergent assumptions about women emerge, structure the discourse and influence the delivery of health care.

Introduction

Social action is a basic concept in sociology. Through time questions have been asked about how individuals come to behave appropriately and explanations have been generated which link norms or rules for behaviour with action. Parsons (1951) accounted for this phenomenon by positing that individuals internalize a shared set of norms. For Durkheim (1938), it was a collective consciousness that was shared in an external and constraining social world. And for Marx (1964), economic conditions provided the primary basis of the explanation.

These theorists lead us to believe that norms govern action – a position that has a long history of revision and criticism (see for example Gurwitsch, 1964; Winch, 1958; Wittgenstein, 1952; among others). In this tradition Garfinkel and Cicourel have redefined and extended the concept of normative action. Garfinkel (1967) contends that individuals actively construct their behaviour. Rather than being 'judgmental dopes' who internalize deterministic norms into their cognitive systems, individuals are 'secret apprentices', ferreting from their daily interactions the information needed to act appropriately. While Garfinkel alludes to the context of action, he does not specify the relationship between norms and actual situations in the construction of behaviour. Mehan and Wood (1975) call this neglect of the social situation in which behaviour is constructed a 'constitutive bias'. It is this bias which Cicourel (1973) addresses when discussing the relationship between structure and process. Cicourel asks how individuals decide which norms are operating or relevant for the negotiation of social situations and concludes that general rules or policies (norms) must be interpreted within emergent, constructed action scenes. Meaning is constructed in this process of interpretation.

In this paper we simultaneously examine the relationship between norms as features of the social structure and norms as interactional accomplishments. We do so by analyzing medical conversations in a specific setting – a model family practice resident training programme in the southeastern part of the United States. In this setting, resident doctors diagnose illness and treat patients under the supervision of attending staff physicians. The patients are women who are using the clinic for the first time. Although the patients come from varied socioeconomic backgrounds, the residents and staff physicians in this hospital, as in most medical settings in the United States, are predominantly white, middle-class men (Navarro, 1976).

We explore how cultural assumptions about patients as women emerge, develop and are negotiated and displayed as doctor and patient communicate over the course of an initial medical interview. Although at one level the argument can be taken as self-evident – the literature on the delivery of health care to women documents the pervasive use of medical domination in the form of sexism (cf. Scully, 1980; Ruzek, 1978) – our point here is more subtle. We first examine *how* medical domination in the form of sexism is enacted and then we quantify our description. By posing cultural definitions of patients as women in a reflexive relationship with the interactional work participants do in a specific setting to construct action we can shed light on how doctors act as secret apprentices, ferreting from their medical interactions with new women patients cultural assumptions (or norms) about these patients as 'good' or 'bad' women. Once assumptions about women develop interactionally, they are evident in the discourse, structure the remaining exchange of information between doctor and patient and have consequences for the delivery of health care.

A growing body of literature suggests that doctors typify their clientele as either 'good' or 'problem' patients. Lorber (1975) finds that doctors evaluate those patients as 'good' who do not make trouble for the hospital staff and who do not interrupt established medical routines. Those who violate these norms of the medical relationship are considered 'problem' patients. Biener (1983) adds that factors such as the social distance between doctors and patients, the seriousness of presenting complaint and perceived patient cooperation influence doctors' perceptions and evaluations of their patients. Finally, Barr (1983) suggests that the perceived seriousness of presenting complaint is the strongest predictor of doctors' responses to patients.

The afore-mentioned studies (and many others like them) locate doctors' evaluations of patients within the normative framework of the doctor–patient relationship and the medical encounter itself. These studies suggest that 'patient' is the master status operating when a person visits the doctor. Macintyre (1977) has also discussed doctors' categorizations of patients, but has located the source of doctors' categorizations *outside* the framework of the doctor–patient relationship. She argues that during the course of consultations concerning unwanted pregnancies, doctors typify their clients as 'good' or 'bad' *women* rather than 'good' or 'bad' *patients*. Doctors ferret from the culturally produced collage of norms governing gender–role behaviour, sexuality and family interactions information which allows them to categorize their patients as 'good' or 'bad' women.

Following Macintyre, we suggest that *woman* emerges as the master status and overrides the status of *patient* in the interactional production of doctors' categorizations and evaluations of their clients. However, whether the master status is patient or woman, extant studies all take the negotiation of categorizations as unproblematic. Not only do we focus on woman as the master status, but we also analyze the *process* through which patients are identified as good or bad women and discuss how this identity, once formed, structures the discourse and influences the delivery of health care.

Cultural assumptions and medical dominance

Cultural assumptions about women take on increased significance when considered in the context of the structure of the medical relationship. Navarro (1976) argues that the social and political factors woven into the fabric of society are mirrored in the shape of the health care system. In this system, class and gender interplay to give predominantly white, male physicians top position in the medical hierarchy. Physicians, as the top 6% in this hierarchy, are the highest earners in the United States (see Conrad and Kern, 1981, for a more complete discussion of these points). While 85% of all physicians are men, 75% of all medical workers are women, and there is almost no movement from one category of medical jobs to another, because each has its own education and requires its own set of skills (Caress, 1975, 1977).

The issue of control by a predominantly white, middle-class, male professional group carries over to the doctor–patient relationship. Sociological examinations of the medical relationship describe it as asymmetrical. Early discussions point out the imbalance between the role of doctor and that of patient (Szasz and Hollender, 1956). Patients are described as passive dependent; doctors as active and dominant (Parsons, 1951). This asymmetry is ascribed to doctors' specialized medical knowledge, their technical skill, the professional prestige of their role (Parsons, 1951), and the organization of the profession and the practice of medicine (Freidson, 1970), as well as other demographic and interactional variables (Zola, 1972; Mechanic, 1968; Davis, 1963; Roth, 1963).

Waitzkin and Waterman (1974) claim that most patients lack the medical knowledge to be equal partners in the medical situations. Furthermore, they describe this gap as widening at the lower end of the socioeconomic spectrum. Patients at the lower end of the spectrum not only share different life experiences, have less medical knowledge, and have fewer choices over the medical setting in which they receive care, but they are also perceived as irresponsible and forgetful (Ehrenreich and Ehrenreich, 1970). Patients who seek help in relative ignorance assume a subordinate position, while doctors assume a superordinate one (Waitzkin and Waterman, 1974). The woman's role also contributes to being powerless. Ehrenreich and Ehrenreich (1970) report that doctors assume women are difficult, neurotic, emotional, and unable to understand complex explanations.

The asymmetry in the doctor–patient relationship, whether criticized or accepted, is widely acknowledged by social scientists, medical providers, and patients alike. Less well documented is whether doctor–patient interaction in this asymmetrical relationship influences medical discourse and shapes the delivery of health care. Recently a few researchers have taken the doctor–patient relationship as a topic in its own right and begun to investigate how doctor and patient transmit information during medical interviews. For example, Strong (1979) suggests that the medical relationship is responsive to a variety of medical factors: the nature of the medical problem, the perceived social class of the patient, and the organization of the setting. Frankel (forthcoming) examines the details of doctor–patient communications and points out a 'dispreference' for patient-initiated questions during medical interviews. Others (Todd, 1983, 1982; Fisher, 1982; West, 1982; Silverman, 1981) argue that the lack of reciprocity in the practitioner–patient relationship creates gaps and misunderstandings in medical communication. They explore why the medical relationship is characterized by this lack of reciprocity and how the asymmetry in the medical relationship and the institutional authority of the physician's role influence medical decision-making in ways which have the potential to negatively influence the delivery of health care. In each of these analyses, the assumption, whether explicated or not, is that the asymmetry or paternalism which characterizes physician–patient discourse creates problems in the delivery of health care.

Medical interactions are social and micro political (Henley, 1977; Waitzkin and Stoeckle, 1976). They reflect and sustain cultural, structural and institutional factors and, in turn, are shaped by them. While medical encounters are interactions between individuals, the interactants – doctor and patient – are not equal interactional partners. Doctors have knowledge and skills that patients lack. By virtue of the authority vested in their professional role, doctors act as gatekeepers dominating the medical process. Since patients live in the same social world and frequently share a reciprocal view of the appropriate roles for doctors and patients, it is not too surprising that they often accept the subordinate role without question.

The issue here is *not* that the patient never has any power or that the doctor always has all of the power. Patients can and do ask questions, interrupt, change topics and claim and/or maintain the floor. Doctors' styles of communication can and do vary – some being more dominant and others more equalitarian. It is the institutional authority of the medical role and the control it provides for medical practitioners that does not change.

When doctors are men and patients are women, this imbalance is heightened.[1] In our society, the man–woman and the doctor–patient relationships recapitulate and reinforce each other, locking male physician and female patient in an asymmetrical relationship – a relationship in which female patients are dependent on their male physicians' judgments about them as women.[2] These judgments are often abstracted from the daily lives of women and frequently coloured by traditional assumptions about the appropriate roles for women in today's society.

The negotiations of cultural assumptions about women

Our data were gathered during the summer of 1981 in a model family practice clinic of a teaching hospital. Forty-three medical interviews of residents' initial visits with new women patients were audio and video taped and transcribed for later analysis. As we reviewed the transcripts we noticed a recurrent pattern: doctors were relying on cultural assumptions to categorize and evaluate their patients. In some cases the actual assumptions were directed toward the women *qua* patient and in other cases they are directed toward the woman *qua* women. The following examples, while showing the different forms cultural assumptions may take, all indicate this 'sizing-up' procedure:

Initiation	*Response*	*Comment*
P: I did put iodine on it. A lady told me it was good for ringworm so I thought it was ringworm	D: don't think this is ringworm	P: I don't think it is either
Later		
P: I read up on it and I thought I had ringworm	D: well it didn't quite fit with ringworm	P: no I didn't think so

Initiation	Response	Comment
And later		
D: what I would do is just keep an eye on this if it starts to spread a lot more if it's not getting better starts itching something like that let us see you again otherwise it should start fading over the next few weeks or it might take a month or more but it ought to go away//okay you want me to write that down for you	P: no I its all in that medical book at home I//	P: //uhhuh
D: //I'll write it down for you so you can remember what it is uh you have any other questions	P: nuhuh not that I know of	
D: alright otherwise we'll just see you back as we need to uh if a problem comes up		

This example illustrates cultural assumptions of woman *qua* patient. The patient says, 'I put iodine on it. A lady told me it was good for ringworm.' And later she continues, 'I read up on it and I thought I had ringworm.' In each case the doctor signals the inappropriateness of her behaviour by discounting her 'diagnosis' of ringworm. Finally, near the end of the interview, the patient tells the doctor that he need not write anything down for her because it's all in her medical book at home. The doctor interrupts her to say: 'I'll write it down for you so you can remember' (cf. Groce and Fisher, 1984 for a discussion of doctors' reactions to patient deviance as manifestations of social control). In each instance the woman displays behaviour inconsistent with the norms for 'good' patients, i.e. that patients allow the doctor to make diagnoses and treatment decisions and in each instance the doctor let the patient know that her behaviour is in some way inappropriate. In the end, the patient is cut off rather abruptly.

These transcripts also highlight assumptions or norms concerning woman *qua* women:

Initiation	Response	Comment
D: are you and your husband still having relations?	P: no no	
D: how long has that been	P: oh honey it's been I don't know I don't even know it's not a problem for either one of us	
D: oh so neither one of you care about that anymore	P: no no no	
D: he doesn't say if you'd like to	P: no no//he's sick too he's sick people you just	D: //okay
D: so that's not a problem	P: no nuhhuh	
D: so that's not a part of what's making you sad	P: lord no honey lord no	

In this example, despite the patient's assurance that the absence of sexual relations in her marriage is *not* a problem to either her or her husband, the doctor repeatedly asks a variation of the same question; namely, is the absence of sex a problem. The patient's 'Lord no, honey, Lord no', provides an emphatic denial. In this case the doctor seems to be operating on the normative expectation (cultural assumption) that married women *should* engage in sexual relations with their husbands and if they do not, problems *should* result.

We found that the negotiation of cultural assumptions was a pervasive pattern that occurred in the majority of transcripts in our data set. There were instances, particularly in briefer medical interviews, where these negotiations were less evident. Overall twenty-eight (67.4%) interviews contained evidence of the negotiation of norms. In twelve (27.8%) norms about women *qua* patient emerged and were negotiated against a background of cultural expectations about patients. These occurred somewhat less frequently and were not for us the most interesting. While doctors interrupted women who were not acting like good patients and even evidenced some mild disapproval, we could find little evidence of how this behaviour influenced medical outcomes. In sixteen (36.0%) norms about woman *qua* women emerged and were negotiated against a background of cultural expectations about women. In these instances doctors' behaviour seemed to indicate that they 'liked' or 'did not like' patients as women and these evaluations, once triggered, emerged more clearly as the medical interview unfolded to influence the delivery of care. To illustrate this relationship we chose two archetypal cases with the same doctor as examples – one in which the picture of woman *qua* women that emerged was not consistent with cultural norms about good women and another in which there was consistency. Since it was our purpose to shed light on the intricacies of the reflexive relationship between cultural assumptions or norms about women and the communicational work doctors and patients do to produce and sustain them, we analyze these two interviews in depth. A detailed comparison of them not only reveals divergent sets of cultural assumptions, but how these assumptions emerge, structure and are expressed in the discourse, and influence the delivery of health care.

In each case, we explore how cultural assumptions are negotiated over the course of the medical interview and comment on the relationship between these assumptions and the delivery of health care. Then we examine the ways in which these assumptions structure the discourse. The analysis extends beyond the linguistic boundaries of the transcripts to blend linguistic data with more impressionistic ethnographic data. It seems reasonable that neither residents nor patients say aloud all that contributes to the medical interview process. For example, patients rarely say aloud that they do not trust their medical practitioners or that they feel unheard, manipulated, and dissatisfied with the medical care they have received. Similarly, residents do not say aloud that patients look like poor women or talk like uneducated women. They do not say that the way patients talk, act, or dress leads them to believe that they are 'good' or 'bad' women and influences the medical interview and ultimately the delivery of health care. Yet while they are not said in so many words, our observations suggest that these factors and a host of similar ones are expressed in the discourse and contribute to the diagnostic-treatment process.

The first patient is Maria, a 24-year-old, unmarried, overweight Mexican-American woman. She moved to this region from the far west, accompanying the boyfriend she currently lives with. Maria arrives for the interview dressed in a pair of jeans and a loose-fitting shirt. Her presenting complaint is a leg injury sustained during a motorcycle accident. While discussing the circumstances surrounding the accident, the resident's questions and his comments begin to display the unfolding of his cultural assumptions about Maria's 'character', i.e., what kind of woman she is:

Initiation	*Response*	*Comment*
D: All right now let's see you were on your motorcycle and what happened	P: well I was . . .	
D: were you on the back	P: no I was driving	D: you were driving
D: what kind do you drive	P: a 450 . . . it's too big	D: //a 450

DOCTOR-PATIENT NEGOTIATION

Initiation	Response	Comment
D: that's a big hod ain't it	P: yeah it's too big//it's an older model and it's too heavy//so it took off and left me behind	D://uhhuh D://uhhuh
D: so you fell off	P: yeah, I fell off	D: hhmmff

The negotiation of cultural assumptions has begun. In the second exchange the resident asks, 'Were you on the back?' Maria responds that she was driving the motorcycle and the resident recycles this information repeating, 'You were driving'. And continues by asking, 'What kind do you drive?' Maria tells him that she drives a big motorcycle – 'a 450' and again the resident recycles the information repeating, 'a 450'. While these exchanges might indicate the resident's awe, Maria has not successfully managed the bike. She is at the clinic because of a leg injury. We suggest instead that the structure of the discourse provides time for the resident to regroup and displays a disjuncture between the norms or cultural assumption about the appropriate roles for women and the behaviour of this woman as it has emerged in the medical interview. This disjuncture is highlighted in the next exchange. The resident 'code switches' (Bernstein, 1973). His 'ain't it' combines with the way he has recycled information and his emphatic 'hhmmff' to display the disjuncture further. As cultural members we would agree that it is more common for women to ride on the back of a motorcycle, not to drive one – especially such a big one. Maria displays her shared understanding that her behaviour was somehow inappropriate. The issue for her is the size of the motorcycle. Twice she acknowledges that the motorcycle is 'too big'.

During an exchange later in the interview, the picture of Maria is developed further:

Initiation	Response	Comment
	P: ... when I put the alcohol on it ((her leg)) I thought I was going to pass out from the pain//and I can take pain too	D: //oh
D: so you needed to take the alcohol internally and not ...	P: yeah, I tried that and that didn't work either no not a bit	

And later:

D: how much alcohol do you drink	P: uhm ...	
D: do you drink every day	P: uhm no no//about a few times a month	D: //no

Maria explains that when she washed her injured leg with alcohol the pain was so severe that she thought she was going to pass out. She makes her point more emphatic by boasting that she can tolerate high levels of pain. The resident takes alcohol used externally – to wash a wound – and switches to alcohol used internally – to ease pain. Later in the medical history phase of the interview the resident returns to the topic of alcohol use – drinking.

In a conservative Bible belt area where many people do not drink and some would be offended if asked about drinking, it is most unusual to hear questions phrased in such ways that seem to presume alcohol consumption – '*How much* alcohol do you drink?' – and even more unusual to suggest that this behaviour occurs daily – 'Do you drink every day?' Nowhere else in our data do we see questions about alcohol use phrased in this way. The more typical question is, 'Do you drink alcohol?' If answered affirmatively, this question is on some occasions followed by another more specific one – 'How much alcohol do you drink?' Why the switch from a medicinal to a more social concept of use, why the change in the form of the questions asked about alcohol consumption and why the suggestion that the patient needs to drink alcohol for her leg pain?

This resident is a fundamentalist Christian raised in a 'Bible Belt' area.[3] His conservative attitudes toward drinking are well known in the clinic. We speculate that jostling Maria about drinking displays his religious beliefs as well as his developing picture of her as a woman. The structure of the discourse developed thus far suggests that he is coming to see her as an unfeminine, hard-drinking, motorcycle-riding woman who can take pain. The emerging picture of Maria is increasingly discrepant with traditional assumptions about women.

As the medical interview unfolds, Maria contributes further to the assumptions building about her:

Initiation	*Response*	*Comment*
D: have you ever been in the hospital	P: yeah	
D: what for	P: abortion	D: abortion
D: okay, how many times have you been pregnant	P: four	D: four times
D: what happened to all the pregnancies	P: three abortions and one miscarriage	D: one miscarriage
P: and I have a question too	D: uhhuh	
P: I feel that I might be again do you perform that kind of thing here	D: abortions, no no we don't	

DOCTOR–PATIENT NEGOTIATION

Initiation	Response	Comment
And later:		
D: what kind of birth control are you on	P: well I was on the pill for the longest time and I quit//and I just been going without for a few months	D: //uhhuh
P: I was spotting on that ((the birth control pills))	D: spotting on that okay well that's another subject//but I'll be glad to work with you on that//anyway I'll want to talk to you about all the different forms of birth control and explain all the different side effects of the pill//and some of the good effects and then go from there	P: //yeah P: //okay P: //okay P: okay
D: when was the last time you were at Planned Parenthood	P: uhm about 16 months ago	
D: well you need another Pap smear//*as many times as you've been pregnant*//has your foot been hurting		P: //yeah definitely P: //definitely

In answer to a standard question usually asked while taking a medical history, 'Have you ever been in hospital?' Maria tells the doctor that she has had three abortions and one miscarriage. The doctor recycles each piece of information, 'abortion', 'four times', and 'one miscarriage'. Each recycle provides time for him to reformulate and continue and each expresses a disjuncture between commonly held norms or cultural assumptions about women and the picture of herself this woman presents.

Once again Maria illustrates her shared understanding. She says, 'I feel I *might be again* do you perform *that kind of thing here.*' The elliptical way she refers to her suspicion that she might be pregnant and need another abortion further supports our suggestion that both doctor and patient recognize her pregnancies and abortions as somehow at odds with generally accepted cultural norms. Maria then goes on to justify her lack of birth control by saying that she spotted (bled) on the birth control pill so she stopped taking them and has '. . . been going without for a few months'.

The medical attitude toward abortion is common knowledge at the hospital. Doctors who perform them are talked about disparagingly and patients are often told that abortions can be obtained more inexpensively from an outpatient abortion clinic in the community. When placed in this conservative Bible belt context, the data are easier to understand. When asked about abortions, the resident claims that he cannot provide them. And the grounds stated by the resident to establish the need for Pap smear are, . . . 'as many times as you've been pregnant'. Again common medical assumption is displayed in the discourse: the increased sexual activities of today's population of young women plus the added strain of multiple abortions place women at a greater risk from cervical cancer (see Spletter, 1983; Fisher, 1982a for a more complete discussion of the social assumptions associated with cervical cancer).

In the next sequence, medication for Maria's leg is discussed and we begin to see how the resident's picture of her as a woman influences the delivery of health care:

Initiation	*Response*	*Comment*
D: well I'm really hesitant about medication//you're not, sure even though you know you might say have an abortion ((while he reads the label on some medicine))	P: definitely	P: //yeah
D: you may uh well the medication I want to use it's not recommended during pregnancy for treating nursing mothers or during pregnancy, tell you what to do what kind of if you just don't do anything you're alright	P: oh alright	

In this sequence, there is more concern with protecting an unborn foetus than there is with treating the pain from Maria's leg injury. The resident says, 'the medication I want to use, it's not recommended during pregnancy', and decides against *any* medication. He reaches the decision in spite of the fact that Maria has indicated that she had intense pain. Although an unwillingness to prescribe medicine that is unsafe for pregnant women is laudable, we question why the resident neither looks further for safer medication, nor takes Maria's statement that she 'definitely' wants an abortion into consideration.

Over the course of the medical interview, personal information about Maria has been gathered piece by piece. She not only rides motorcycles, she *drives* them – and rather large ones at that; she is a strong woman with an ability to withstand pain; she drinks; she has a history of abortions – not one, but three plus the possibility of another one in the near future; she lives, unmarried, with her boyfriend; and, while sexually active, she is not using birth control. This view of Maria, obtained over the course of the medical interview, influences the delivery of health care. Maria left the clinic without the Pap smear that both she and the resident agreed she needed, without the birth control information which the resident told her he would provide, without the abortion information that she requested, and without *any* medication to treat her leg pain. Finally, in closing the interview, Maria is not encouraged to return to the clinic:

Initiation	*Response*	*Comment*
D: it was nice meeting you	P: same to you I'll come back whenever I need to see a doctor . . .	
D: hopefully 24 year old ladies don't need many doctors	P: yeah okay thanks a lot bye bye	

Before discussing further the relationship between cultural assumption and the delivery of health care, we examine a case which contrasts with Maria's. The patient, Sarah, is a shy, 23-year-old. She is well-dressed in conservative, middle-class attire. As the medical interview unfolds, Sarah displays herself very differently than Maria did.

Initiation	*Response*	*Comment*
D: . . . we'll do a Pap smear and a pelvic today . . . well//		
P: //what's a pelvic	D: . . . the big thing is feeling your uterus and your ovaries and uh Pap smear is the scraping uh//	P: //of the uterus?
D: you had that before	P: no I never have	
D: never had it before	P: nuh uh ((no))	D: well how did//
P: //well I just never had it I heard that it wasn't necessary actually	D: nah I don't think anybody would tell you that it's not necessary	
P: well someone told me that as long as you weren't sexually active it isn't necessary	D: uhm//there may be a little in that//but it's not really true	P: //but then
P: //but

Early in the interview, as the resident reviews the upcoming procedures, Sarah interrupts him to ask, 'What's a pelvic?' After explaining a pelvic examination and Pap smear, the resident says, 'You had that before'. Sarah indicates her sexual inexperience by saying that she has never had a Pap smear. Again the resident signals a disjunctive. He recycles this information and repeats his question. Sarah explains that she had heard that it was not necessary if a woman was not sexually active.

As the interview unfolds, both the doctor's assumptions about women and Sarah become more evident:

Initiation	*Response*	*Comment*
D: you ever been on birth control	P: no I haven't	
P: but that's something else I want to talk to you about	D: okay	
D: let's see are you married	P: no I'm not	
D: okay what do you do	P: what do I . . . I've just been using over-the-counter suppositories	

Sarah has never used prescription birth control, but wants to talk about it during this visit. Birth control may, in fact, be the reason for her visit – her hidden agenda. This request signals her emerging status as a sexually active woman and elicits the next question. The resident asks, 'Are you married?' and Sarah replies that she is not.

The resident's next question, 'Okay, what do you do?' is ambiguous. He could be asking for her occupational status, or asking how she manages sexual relationships outside of marriage so as not to get pregnant. He could be checking his cultural assumptions about women and constructing a view of Sarah in the process. If she is unmarried and sexually active, is she responsible? Even if she is without the social acceptability that sexual relationships within marriage provide, if she used some birth control measure to prevent unwanted pregnancy, her behaviour may still be consistent with commonly held cultural assumptions – although sexual behaviour is changing, responsible people use some form of birth control. He could, in addition, be making a more subtle assumption about the relationship between responsibility and social class. The resident's question, 'Okay, what do you do', could signal his conclusion that Sarah is an intelligent and responsible middle-class woman who would be using birth control. The phrasing of the question leaves Sarah momentarily confused. She responds, 'What do I . . . ?' After a brief hesitation, she validates the resident's conclusion: 'I've just been using over-the-counter suppositories'.

Later in the interview, more evidence is presented that Sarah has a good background. She comes from a 'normal', middle-class family:

DOCTOR–PATIENT NEGOTIATION

Initiation	Response	Comment
D: you just had your normal sore throats	P: uhhuh	
D: and all that and your childhood shots	P: uhhuh	
D: how about your *daddy* is he healthy	P: he's healthy, he's taking medication for high blood pressure	D: uhm
D: how about your *mama*	P: she's healthy	

Underlying the phrasing of questions in this exchange are assumptions about Sarah's background. She comes from an intact nuclear family and she received the necessary childhood immunizations: Sarah's answers validate these assumptions. It is particularly interesting to us that questions of this sort were not included in Maria's interview. The resident asks no questions about childhood diseases or immunizations and did not inquire as to the existence or the condition of Maria's parents.[4]

At this point, there is a picture of Sarah as a shy, newly sexually active, middle-class woman using over-the-counter contraceptives and inquiring about a more effective form of birth control. The resident summarizes the advantages and disadvantages of the available methods of contraception – birth control pills, diaphragms, IUDs, condoms, and spermicides. Throughout this discussion, an assumption is displayed: Sarah, although unmarried, cannot risk an unwanted pregnancy – she is a 'good' woman. To protect her a case for the birth control pill as the preferred contraceptive method is developed (see Fisher and Todd, forthcoming for a more complete discussion of this point):

Initiation	Response	Comment
D: you plan to get married sometime soon	P: uhhuh//it wouldn't be until I get out of school which should be next summer	D: //okay
D: well what would be perfectly acceptable for me if I was in your shoes is to be on the birth control pills until next summer for sure and uh that time you see how you did on them		

Once again, assumptions are reflected in the communication. If Sarah is sexually active, she will marry soon. As an intelligent and responsible woman, until she marries she will use an effective contraceptive. The resident declares that it is acceptable to him for her to use the birth control pill until she marries. Notice the use of authority. The doctor relies on the institutional authority of his role to control the flow of information and to 'help' the patient reach her decision about which method of contraception to use.[5] This institutionally based authority allows him to act as a gatekeeper, providing options to Sarah which were not provided to Maria.

Summary

The medical interviews just discussed produce two very different pictures of Maria and Sarah. In so doing, they illustrate commonly held cultural assumptions (norms) about women as well as how these norms are interactional accomplishments negotiated and displayed over the course of the medical interview. Assumptions about these patients emerged and were developed as doctor and patient discussed medical and social topics. In the first case, as the interview unfolded a negative picture of Maria developed. In the second case a positive picture of Sarah developed.

In each case, the delivery of health care was shaped by norms about the patients that were negotiated as the medical interviews unfolded. Maria came to the clinic with a painful leg injury. While this was her presenting complaint, several other medical problems emerged over the course of the medical interview. She left the clinic without having either her presenting complaint or the other problems which emerged during the medical interview dealt with. She received no prescription for pain and was encouraged not to return.

By comparison, Sarah came to the clinic requesting a Pap smear and a pelvic examination. Over the course of the medical interview, her need for information about menstrual pain and her interest in birth control information emerged. She left the clinic after both her presenting complaint and her emergent problems had been dealt with. She received a Pap smear and a pelvic examination as well as information about and prescriptions for menstrual pain and birth control. Again, the institutional authority of the medical role gave the resident control. He could provide medical services to Sarah (information and prescriptions) while denying them to Maria.

While the negotiation of norms about women and medical outcomes were interactional accomplishments, the institutional authority of the doctor's role gave the resident an interactional edge, which was expressed in the communication. Patients came to the clinic with what they perceived as medical problems. When the resident asked questions and they responded, presenting a social as well as a medical picture of themselves, patients may not have been aware of either the picture of themselves that was being developed or the consequences for them of that picture. Yet the data suggest that this information influenced the resident's conception of them as women as well as the health care he delivered.

We suspected that as a medical provider and a middle-class man the resident would hold certain culturally shared assumptions about women learned in society and reinforced in medical school (Scully, 1980; Ruzek, 1978; Scully and Bart, 1973). This suspicion has been taken as the topic under study. The data suggest that as the medical interview unfolded the resident matched his cultural assumptions about women with the information the patient presented about herself – he acted like a secret apprentice ferreting out and interpreting information and developing a picture of the kind of woman the patient was. When there was a disjuncture between the norms about the appropriate ways for women to behave and the ways the patient described her behaviour, the discrepancy was marked in the discourse: the resident recycled information. Information was recycled with both Maria and Sarah. In each case the resident expressed disapproval and incredulity: Maria drove such a big motorcycle and had repeated abortions; Sarah did not know that women, even if they were not sexually active, needed Pap smears.

The negotiation of cultural assumptions was marked in the discourse in another way as well: the resident switched codes to a less formal, less medically appropriate way of talking. Code switching was only done with Maria. The resident's 'ain't it' spoke down to Maria and, we claim, displayed his developing redefinition of her.

As norms about women patients were negotiated they structured the remaining exchange of information and the delivery of health care. Although Sarah received the care for which she came to the clinic, Maria did not. Not only did Maria not have her presenting complaint cared for, but, perhaps even more importantly, none of the medical problems which emerged as the medical interview unfolded were dealt with. This raises a question about the adequacy of the care she received. The resident's authority allowed him to control medical outcomes, at least in part, by controlling the structure of the discourse. The finding is clearer when the structure of the discourse is examined more closely.

Cultural assumptions, medical authority, and the structure of discourse

Fisher (1984) identifies four phases of medical interviews – opening, medical history, physical examination, and closing phases.[6] Each phase has a characteristic form and specific task function. She suggests that during the opening phase the task is to get the patient's story – why she initiated the medical visit. It is during this phase that patients have the most input into the medical interview. The task of the medical history and physical examination phases is to gather the medical and social information necessary to treat the presenting complaint, gaining sufficient background information to provide quality medical care. During the closing phase, the task is for the doctor to sum up his/her findings, make treatment recommendations, prescribe medications, and, in general, to present the information the patient needs to reach a medical decision.

She finds that the asymmetry in the doctor–patient relationship is reflected in the phase structure of medical interviews. Doctors initiate topics and control access to the floor (who speaks when) as well as the flow of medical information. Although patients initiate less and ask fewer questions, they do ask questions and initiate exchanges of information which call for responses from physicians. While it could be argued that the doctor's word output over the course of the medical interview is influenced by both personality and context variables, we make a different argument. To validate our quantification of doctor–patient communication we point to research which demonstrates a positive correlation between doctors' raw word output and outcome variables such as patient compliance and satisfaction (cf. Pfefferbaum et al. 1982; Slavin et al. 1982; Freemon et al. 1971). These and other studies show repeatedly that the more a doctor talks with/to a patient, the more satisfied the patient is with the medical encounter and the more likely s/he will be to comply with the prescribed regimen. Table 1 presents a numerical view of how information is exchanged across the phases of the interview and suggests that the ways the resident came to see Maria and Sarah affected the structure of the discourse.

Table 1 indicates a quantitative difference in the way information is both offered and responded to in the two interviews. The resident communicates more with Sarah than he does with Maria. In the opening phase, he responds to Sarah with an average of 14.0 words per response, while he responds to Maria with an average of only 5.0 words per response. In Maria's interview, the resident initiates at an average of only 6.4 words per initiation; in Sarah's interview, he initiates at 17.7 words per initiation. The resident's initiations are roughly two and one-half times longer in Sarah's interview. During the opening phase, the doctor both gathers and provides more information with Sarah than with Maria. This finding is consistent with and reinforces an earlier one: the way the resident came to see the two women is reflected in the structure of the discourse as well as the delivery of care.

This pattern continues through the medical history phase. In a phase typically characterized by short resident initiations, the table indicates a significant difference in the doctor's words per initiation. With Maria, he is short and

Table 1 Doctor's word output across medical interview phases.

Phase	Maria		Sarah	
	Words/initiation	*Words/response*	*Words/initiation*	*Words/response*
Opening	6.4	5.0	17.7	14.0
History	6.7	16.4	47.4	111.8
Closing	13.9	16.7	31.5	–*

The patient made no initiations during this phase.

to the point – only 6.7 words per initiation; with Sarah, though, his average words per initiation increases to 47.4. In terms of resident responses, we see a similar pattern. While he responds to Maria with only 16.4 words per response, he responds to Sarah with an average of 111.8 words per response. We once again argue that the doctor's typifications of Sarah and Maria influence the discourse, limiting the exchange of information.[7]

Since Sarah made no initiations during the closing phase of the interview, the only category with comparable figures is the resident's words per initiation. Here again, the developing pattern persists. Typically, the closing phase is characterized by a high incidence of doctor initiations as he sums up his findings and provides the patient with the information she needs to reach a medical decision. However, even here we see a discrepancy between the two interviews. The resident initiates exchanges with Sarah at an average of 31.5 words per initiation, a figure that suggests that he is providing information to her. His words per initiation average with Maria is only 13.9, which suggests that he provides her with less information. The lack of information provided to Maria is consistent with the limited health care which was delivered.

Our data indicate that cultural assumptions about these patients as women have an impact on how the resident manages both the patient's presenting complaint and the medically relevant topics that emerge during the course of the interview. Table 2 displays the patient's word outputs for topics that arise during the interview.

These tables indicate that both Maria and Sarah have preferences for certain topics. Maria clearly would rather discuss the availability of abortions than her motorcycle injury – her stated reason for coming to the clinic. Her words

Table 2 Patients' word output by topic.

Topic	Maria		
	Words per initiation	Words per response	Words per utterance
Presenting complaint	9.0	12.9	10.9
Birth control	5.8	10.5	8.2
Abortion	18.5	26.5	22.5
Topic	Sarah		
	Words per initiation	Words per response	Words per utterance
Presenting complaint	10.7	2.5	6.6
Birth control	17.7	5.8	11.8
Menstrual cycle	7.5	11.3	9.4

per utterance averages of 22.5 and 10.9 reflect her interest in the topics of abortion and the presenting complaint, respectively. Similarly, Sarah is least interested in discussing her presenting complaint (6.6 words per utterance). She is an unmarried, newly sexually active woman interested in contraceptive information and in obtaining a prescription for birth control pills. Her words per utterance average for this topic – 11.8 reflects such an interest.

Now that we have an idea of what topics the patients wish to pursue, how do they compare with the topics discussed by the resident? Table 3 shows the resident's word output for the topics discussed with Maria and Sarah.

Table 3 indicates a significant difference in the resident's approach to the two interviews. He exhibits the highest words per utterance average while attending to Maria's presenting complaint (25.2 words per utterance). His output for the remaining two topics is roughly similar – 17.6 words per utterance for the abortion topic and 15.9 words per utterance for the birth control topic. This pattern displays the asymmetry in the resident–patient relationship. The resident, not the patient, controls the flow of information and the topics under discussion. In addition, it reinforces the suggestion that the resident has adopted a narrow health care orientation, i.e., he primarily focuses his attention on Maria's presenting complaint.

When the typification of the woman is negative, as in Maria's case, the authority of the resident's role is reflected in the structure of the discourse. In turn, the structure of the discourse organizes the delivery of health care. When the typification of the woman is more positive, as in Sarah's case, both discourse and delivery of health care are organized differently. In Sarah's case, the resident not only generates a higher words per utterance average

Table 3 Doctor's word output by topic.

Topic	Maria		
	Words per initiation	Words per response	Words per utterance
Presenting complaint	11.4	39.0	25.2
Birth control	14.2	17.5	15.9
Abortion	13.0	22.5	17.6
Topic	Sarah		
	Words per initiation	Words per response	Words per utterance
Presenting complaint	36.8	18.3	27.6
Birth control	90.1	141.6	115.9
Menstrual cycle	43.2	3.0	23.1

for Sarah's presenting complaint than he does for *any* topic of discussion with Maria (27.6 words per utterance), but he also demonstrates a willingness to generate the most substantial amount of discourse toward Sarah's hidden agenda, her desire for birth control (115.9 words per utterance). This pattern suggests that, although the asymmetry in the resident–patient relationship has not lessened, the resident has adopted a broad health care orientation, i.e., he treats her present complaint as well as focuses on emergent topics so as to provide the most comprehensive care.

We observe this phenomenon once more when we examine how the resident responds to initiations by both patients. We have created a statistic, the RIR, to highlight such a comparison. This response–intitiation ratio is computed by dividing the resident's words per response by the patient's words per initiation. This demonstrates the resident's willingness to provide information in response to patients' questions – a willingness which we argue influences the adequacy of the health care he is able to deliver. The interpretation of the RIR provides a view of how many words the resident utters in response to every 1.0 words of patient initiation. Table 4 presents the resident's RIR for the topics discussed during the medical interviews.

Table 4 indicates the resident's preference for discussing Maria's presenting complaint. His RIR for her presenting complaint was 4.3 compared to an RIR of 1.2 for the abortion topic, the very topic that Maria wanted to discuss. Perhaps this reflects his abhorrence of abortion, his typification of Maria or, in this case, his narrow orientation toward her health care needs.

Sarah's case is just the opposite. The resident generates 8.0 words of response for every word of initiation by Sarah during the discussion of birth

Table 4 Comparison of patients' initiations and doctor's responses by topic.

	Maria		
Topic	Words per initiation	Words per response	RIR
Presenting complaint	9.0	39.0	4.3
Birth control	5.8	17.5	3.0
Abortion	18.5	22.5	1.2
	Sarah		
Topic	Words per initiation	Words per response	RIR
Presenting complaint	10.7	18.3	1.7
Birth control	17.7	141.6	8.0
Menstrual cycle	7.5	3.0	0.4

control. He is apparently quite willing to pursue topics important to Sarah other than the presenting complaint. Perhaps birth control is more consistent with his belief system, more congruent with his typification of Sarah or more compatible with his broader health care orientation.

Summary

We have argued that norms about women as features of the social system are in a reflexive relationship with the communicational work participants do in specific settings to construct them. Cultural assumptions and communication function as context and ground in the social production of both medical discourse and medical outcomes. Although discourse and outcomes are interactional accomplishments, doctors dominate in these interactions. Doctors have the institutional authority to orchestrate the medical interview and the delivery of health care. In the cases just discussed, norms about woman *qua* women and communicational processes between resident and patient produced two very different pictures of Maria and Sarah. These pictures, once developed, structured the discourse, organized the flow of information, and influenced the delivery of health care.

As the medical interview unfolded, the resident talked more with Sarah than with Maria. Not only did he talk more and provide more information for Sarah, but he evidenced more willingness to discuss with her the topics that emerged over the course of the medical interview. While both Maria and Sarah came to the clinic with presenting complaints – an injured leg and request for a Pap smear and pelvic examination, respectively – both also had hidden agendas which emerged as the interview progressed. These agendas were reflected in the talk. For Maria, the primary agenda, aside from her presenting complaint, was her need for information about abortions and for Sarah it was her desire for information about birth control.

The patients' presenting complaints and hidden agendas were treated differently by the resident. With Maria his behaviour indicated that he was more interested in talking about her presenting complaint than he was in talking about her preferred topic – abortion. Although he talked extensively with Sarah about her presenting complaint, he talked even more with her about birth control – her preferred topic. These differences in the structure of the discourse and the flow of information influenced medical outcomes. Even with a narrow definition of her medical problem, Maria left the clinic with less than she bargained for. Her leg injury was not treated, her hidden agendas were not dealt with, and it was questionable whether she received adequate medical care. In contrast, Sarah received all she bargained for and more. Her presenting complaint was dealt with as were her hidden agendas. Even if we were to take issue with how they were dealt with, for example, the persuasion used in the decision to use birth control pills (see Fisher and Todd, forthcoming), the medical knowledge, and technical skill at the resident's disposal were used to address all the issues raised during the medical interview.

Social and political production of cultural assumptions

An analysis of the reflexive relationship between cultural assumptions and the communicational work which produces them creates a link between what are traditionally characterized as two disparate viewpoints. Often in the history of sociology, the analysis of social structure and social interaction has been characterized as incompatible (Knorr-Cetina & Cicourel, 1981). By placing discourse between physicians and patients in its broader social and political contexts, these seemingly incompatible macro and micro approaches are recast so that social structure and social interaction are each seen to flow from and be part of the other (Mehan & Wood, 1975). On the one hand, the social and political milieu of the culture we live in informs the discussion of the social production of medical discourse and medical outcomes. On the other hand, an understanding of the social production of medical discourse and outcomes illuminates how these are shaped by larger structural and institutional forces which in turn reproduce them. The analysis of discourse during medical interviews is strengthened by posing social structure and social interaction, context and ground, in a reflexive relationship with one another.

From the structural perspective there is work that describes the medical relationship as a *product* of particular features of the social structure. The assumption here is that the asymmetry in the doctor–patient relationship is *caused* by structural or institutional factors. Similarly, for some researchers, medical communication is a mechanism for reinforcing and maintaining the power differentials produced in a society dominated by class and gender and a medical profession which mirrors this domination (Wallen et al., 1979; Navarro, 1976). Medical communication too is seen as a *product caused* by the structural and institutional arrangements of society.

Moving from a structural to an interactional approach, the doctor–patient relationship, and medical communication are presented as social productions. In each case, the focus is on process. In specific contexts, actors use language to produce meaning (cf. Bosk, 1979; Millman, 1976; Davis, 1963). The interrelationships of roles, values and attitudes are described as creating social realities (cf. Scully, 1980; Luker, 1975). In addition, there is work in medical settings which addresses the social organization of doctor–patient communication – how physician and patient, in concert, produce medical discourse (cf. Frankel, 1983).

In this paper, we have recast the problem. Rather than posing social structure and social interaction as separate analyses, we suggest that each flows from and is part of the other – a reflexive analysis. At the structural level, we accept the premise that society is male dominated – a domination reflected in the organization and practice of medicine – and characterized by sexist assumptions about women. As cultural members these social facts are part of our common stock of knowledge. We are also committed to the belief that both male domination and sexist assumptions are socially produced realities constructed by participants as they communicate over the course of events such as medical interviews. Participants engage in an ongoing process of negotiation and interpretation.

Revealed in an examination of the communication between resident and patient over the course of the medical event are the means by which language is used to actualize the resident's power. The analysis illuminates how the structure of the medical relationship and cultural assumptions about women are, at one and the same time, social facts and socially produced, emergent realities. In the medical interviews just discussed, the resident evidenced a knowledge of the cultural assumptions (norms) about patients as 'good' or 'bad' women – knowledge of social facts. Over the course of the medical event the communicational work participants did to negotiate these norms is also displayed. The medical interview provides the context in which norms emerge, are displayed, interpreted and acted upon – a socially organized production accomplished through the situated activities of the participants.

The medical interviews also revealed how the asymmetrical structure of the medical relationship is, at one and the same time, a social fact and a socially accomplished reality. As Freidson (1970) points out, the medical profession is autonomous. As a profession physicians monitor the education, licensure and conduct of their fellow practitioners. Physicians also have a state-supported monopoly over the right to practise medicine and thus are guaranteed top position among health care providers. With autonomy and monopoly comes social control. When combined with their financial resources, the medical profession and the medical corporate enterprises that market health-related services – the pharmaceutical companies, health insurance companies, and medical supply industries as well as proprietary hospitals and nursing homes – have powerful political lobbies with tremendous legislative clout. Those who are reaping the benefits from the system as it is currently organized have a vested interest in preserving it and have been successful in resisting and limiting change. These are the social facts of the medical relationship; however, they do not tell the whole story.

Doctors not only have medical knowledge and technical expertise, but during medical interviews they have the ability to control patients' access to information and to health care services. Their power is enacted as the medical interview unfolds. This upper hand was evidenced in the ways the resident defined the patients, structured the discourse, controlled the flow of information and influenced the medical outcomes. This is the socially accomplished reality of the medical interviews just discussed.

There are social and political factors woven into the definition of health and illness as well as into the fabric of the health care delivery system. While providing health care, physicians also engage in an activity that is both social and political in nature. Since medical work occurs during face-to-face interaction and is an infinitely practical activity, it is social in that sense. Medical work also reflects, helps to sustain, and reproduces the status quo, and as such is micro-political. In the process of doing their work, doctors, who are predominantly men, control access to medical knowledge and technical skill, legitimate illness and help to maintain the existing social order.

Acknowledgments

Acknowledgments and thanks for providing helpful comments in the preparation of this manuscript go to Hugh Mehan, Alexandra Todd and Donna Eder. An earlier version of the paper was presented at the annual meeting of the Southern Sociological Society, Atlanta (April 1983).

Notes

1 At present we are aware of *no* studies which examine interactions between doctors and men patients. In hopes of remedying this situation, the junior author is currently engaged in research which examines how doctors and men patients communicate to reach medical treatment decisions.
2 While there is new research on the differential influence of a patient's gender and social class, the present study focuses solely on gender. This is due primarily to restraints of the research setting. First, since the setting is a resident training facility, we can assume that very few of the community's affluent members come for treatment. Second, since it is a *model* family practice clinic established to mirror the practice of medicine, the patient population is limited much as it is in a private fee-for-service practice. Most of the patients have private insurance. Only about 25% of the patients are on Medicare or Medicaid and patients who cannot pay are rarely seen. The result is that the patient social class range is limited at both extremes and is concentrated on the middle.
3 This information surfaced during the gathering of background data at the model family practice clinic. As residents, staff doctors, and support personnel sat around discussing everyday topics, they often displayed attitudes and values which supported this analysis. For example, it was common knowledge that this doctor did not drink and would not perform abortions. The reasons stated were his religious beliefs.
4 Although it might be argued that the absence of history-taking in Maria's interview is justified on the basis of the presenting complaint (why take a full medical history for someone with a leg injury from a motorcycle accident?) a brief look at the organization of the family practice clinic suggests otherwise. As part of their training, residents are continually encouraged to obtain a full medical history from each patient on his/her initial visit. The logic of this practice is inescapable. Since the majority of the patients do return to the clinic at some future time and since classes of residents continue to enter and leave the programme, the patient's medical history, if taken during the initial visit, and duly recorded provides a needed foundation for future care. Furthermore, although a patient's medical history may have no immediate bearing on the presenting complaint, it is common practice for issues to emerge during the medical interview for which a more detailed history would

be helpful, if not essential. We could speculate that perhaps a less detailed history was required with a presenting complaint of leg injury than with a presenting complaint of a pelvic examination. However, as the interviews unfolded, both women displayed medical issues that make a detailed history seem appropriate. One was done with Sarah and not with Maria, suggesting that the doctor's assumptions structured the discourse as well as the delivery of health care.

5 Sarah is not such a responsible woman that she does not need to be protected. In the discussion of birth control, the resident makes it clear that diaphragms, which may be left in the drawer, and condoms, which may not be intact, are too risky to keep her safe until she is married. He recommends the birth control pill (see Fisher & Todd, forthcoming).

6 In these two cases, we have no data on the physical examination. For Maria's leg injury, none was performed. With Sarah, the doctor asked us not to tape, assuming that since she was shy and this was her first pelvic examination, she would be distressed.

7 A claim made stronger when the topic is considered. When responding to Sarah during the medical history phase, the doctor is primarily providing information about birth control – a topic he does not discuss with Maria.

References

Barr, Judith K. (1983), 'Physicians' Views of Patients in Prepaid Group Practice: Reasons for Visits to HMOs', *Journal of Health and Social Behavior*, 24: 244–55.

Bernstein, Basil (1973), 'Class, Codes and Control', In Gerald Berreman (ed.), *Toward a Theory of Educational Transmission*, London: Routledge & Kegan Paul.

Biener, Lois (1983), 'Perceptions of Patients by Emergency Room Staff: Substance Abusers Versus Non-Substance Abusers', *Journal of Health and Social Behavior*, 24: 264–75.

Bosk, Charles L. (1979), *Forgive and Remember: Managing Medical Failure*, Chicago: University of Chicago Press.

Caress, Barbara (1975), 'Sterilization', *Health-Pac Bulletin* 62, January/February, 1–13.

Caress, Barbara (1977), 'Womb-boom', *Health-Pac Bulletin*, July/August.

Cicourel, Aaron (1973), *Cognitive Sociology, Language and Meaning in Social Interaction*, London: Macmillan.

Conrad, Peter and **Rochelk Kern** (eds) (1981), *The Sociology of Health and Illness*, New York: St Martin's Press.

Davis, Fred (1963), *Passage Through Crisis*, Indianapolis: Bobbs-Merrill.

Durkheim, Emile (1938), *The Rules of Sociological Method*, Chicago: University of Chicago Press.

Ehrenreich, Barbara and **John Ehrenreich** (1970), *The American Health Empire*, Health-Pac Book, New York: Vintage.

Fisher, Sue (1982), 'The decision-making context: how doctors and patients communicate', in Robert J. Di Pietro (ed.), *Linguistics and the Professions*, Norwood, NJ: Ablex, pp. 51–81.

Fisher, Sue (1984), 'Doctor–patient communication: a social and micro-political performance', *Journal of Health and Illness*, 6(3): (March).

Fisher, Sue and Alexandra Dundas Todd (forthcoming), 'Friendly persuasion: the negotiation of the decisions to use oral contraception'. In *Discourse and Institutional Authority*, Sue Fisher and Alexandra Dundas Todd (eds), Norwood, NJ: Ablex.

Frankel, Richard M. (forthcoming), 'Talking in interviews: A dispreference for patient initiated questions in coming physician–patient encounters', in George Psathas and Richard Frankel (eds) *Interactional Competence*, Norwood, NJ: Ablex.

Frankel, Richard M. (1983), 'The laying on of hands: aspects of the organization of gaze, touch and talk in a medical encounter', in Sue Fisher and Alexandra Tood (eds) *The Social Organization of Doctor–Patient Communication*, Washington D.C.: Center for Applied Linguistics, pp. 19–54.

Freemon, B., V. F. Negrette, M. Davis, et al. (1971), 'Gaps in doctor–patient communication: Doctor–patient interaction analysis', *Pediatric Research*, 5: 298–311.

Freidson, Eliot (1970), *Profession of Medicine*, New York: Dodd, Mead.

Garfinkel, Harold (1967), *Studies in Ethnomethodology*, Englewood Cliffs, NJ: Prentice-Hall.

Groce, Stephen B. and Sue Fisher (1984), 'Doctor-Talk/Patient-Talk: Patients' Accounting Practices and Doctors' Social Control Strategies as Interactional Accomplishments', Paper presented at the Annual Meeting of the Southern Sociological Society, Knoxville, TN (April).

Gurwitsch, Aaron (1964), *The Field of Consciousness*, Pittsburg: Duquesne University Press.

Henley, Nancy (1977), *Body Politics: Power, Sex and Nonverbal Communication*, Englewood Cliffs, NJ: Prentice-Hall.

Knorr-Cetina, K. and A. V. Cicourel (eds) (1981), *Advances in Social Theory and Methodology: Toward an Integration of Micro- and Macro-Sociologies*, London and Boston: Routledge & Kegan Paul.

Lorher, Judith (1975), 'Good Patients and Problem Patients: Conformity and Deviance in a General Hospital', *Journal of Health and Social Behavior*, 16: 213–25.

Luker, Kristin (1975), *Taking Chances: Abortion and the Decision Not To Contracept*, Berkeley: University of California Press.

Macintyre, Sally (1977), *Single and Pregnant*, New York: Prodist.

Marx, Karl (1964), *The Economic and Philosophic Manuscripts of 1844*, Trans. Martin Milligan, Ed. with an introduction by Dirk Streuch, New York: International Publishers.

Mechanic, David (1968), *Medical Sociology*, New York: Free Press.

Mehan, High and Houston Wood (1975), *The Reality of Ethnomethodology*, New York: Wiley.

Millman, Marcia (1976), *The Unkindest Cut: Life In the Backrooms of Medicine*, New York: William Morrow.

Navarro, Vincente (1976), *Medicine Under Capitalism*, New York: Prodist.

Parsons, Talcott (1951), *The Social System*, New York: Free Press.

Pfefferbaum, B., P. M. Levenson and J. Van Eys (1982), 'Comparison of physician and patient perceptions of communications issues', *Southern Medical Journal*, 75: 1080–3.

Roth, J. A. (1963), *Timetables*, Indianapolis: Bobbs-Merrill.

Ruzek, Sheryl Burt (1978), *The Women's Health Movement*, New York: Praeger.

Scully, Diana (1980), *Men who Control Women's Health*, Boston: Houghton-Mifflin.

Scully, Diana and Pauline Bart (1973), 'A funny thing happened on the way to the orifice: women in gynecological textbook', *American Journal of Sociology*, 78: 1045-0.

Silverman, David (1981), 'The child as a social object: Down's Syndrome children in a paediatric cardiology clinic', *Sociology of Health and Illness*, 3(3) 254-74.

Slavin, L. A., J. E. O'Malley, G. P. Foocher and D. J. Foster (1982), 'Communication of the cancer diagnosis to pediatric patients: Impact on long-term adjustment', *American Journal of Psychiatry* 139: 179-83.

Spletter, Mary (1983), 'How important is a Pap test?' *Parade Magazine* (September 4): 10.

Strong, P. M. (1979), *The Ceremonial Order of the Clinic: Parents, Doctors and Medical Bureaucracies*, London: Routledge & Kegan Paul.

Szasz, T. S. and M. H. Hollender (1956), 'A contribution to the philosophy of medicine: the basic models of doctor–patient relationship', *A.M.A. Archives of Internal Medicine*, 97: (May): 585.

Todd, Alexandra Dundas (1983), 'A diagnosis of doctor–patient discourse in the prescription of contraception' in Sue Fisher and Alexandra Dundas Todd (eds) *The Social Organization of Doctor–Patient Communication*, Washington, D.C.: The Center for Applied Linguistics.

Todd, Alexandra Dundas (1982), 'The Medicalization of Reproduction: Scientific Medicine and the Diseasing of Healthy Women', Unpublished doctoral dissertation, University of California, San Diego.

Waitzkin, Howard, B. and John D. Stoeckle (1976), 'Information Control and the micropolitics of health care: summary of an ongoing research project, *Social Science & Medicine* 10: 263-76.

Waitzkin, Howard and Barbara Waterman (1974), *The Exploitation of Illness in Capitalist Society*, Indianapolis: Bobbs-Merrill.

Wallen, Jacqueline, Howard Waitzkin and John D. Stoeckle (1979), 'Physician stereotypes about female health and illness', *Women & Health* 4: 135-46.

West, Candace (1982), 'When the doctor is a lady: power, status and gender in physician–patient conversations', in Ann Stromberg (ed.), *Women, Health and Medicine*, Palo Alto, CA: Mayfield.

Winch, Peter (1958), *The Idea of a Social Science and its Relation to Philosophy*, London: Routledge & Kegan Paul.

Wittgenstein, Ludwig (1953), *Philosophical Investigations*, London: Basil Blackwell & Mott.

Zola, Irving (1972), 'Medicine as an institution of social control', *Sociological Review* 20, 487.

49

WOMEN AS PATIENTS
A problem for sex differences research

Kathy Davis

Source: *Women's Studies International Forum*, 7:4 (1984), 211–17.

Synopsis

Using the feminist critique of the health care system as a starting point, this article indicates some of the relevant issues facing women as patients in general practice: lack of control over our bodies and reproductive functions, 'psychologizing' of women's complaints, the medicalization of social problems experienced by women as a group. Current research on women as patients is primarily of the sex-differences tradition, i.e. the differences between men and women patients are investigated. The results of this research are critically discussed. My contention is that such research, aside from being methodologically impoverished, is—from a feminist point of view—counterproductive. Some directions for alternative research in this area are given.

Introduction

I have written this paper in the context of a research project concerning women as patients in General Practice. The project focuses on how women's complaints are diagnosed and treated in the context of a consultation. I am primarily interested in how the social fact of women's oppression is manifested in the interaction occurring between women patients and their physicians, my assumption being—fortunately, this is a project under the auspices of Women's Studies—that sexism does, in fact, 'rear its ugly head' in the doctor's office, just as it does in most other areas of daily life.

Furthermore, I shall be dealing with the kind of information presently available, concerning the situation of women patients, both from the feminist movement as well as from the research being done on the subject. It is to this research especially that I have addressed myself here. By taking a critical look at what is currently being done, I hope to offer some guidelines for myself and others concerning directions future research on women as patients might (more) profitably take.

The feminist critique

Since the advent of the feminist movement in the late '60s, considerable attention has been devoted to women's health issues as well as the kind of medical treatment we receive. In The Netherlands alone, there are already five women's health centers and numerous self-help groups, applying themselves to such varied concerns as menopause, breast cancer, vaginal self-examination, problems with overeating, etc. There is scarcely a community center or a women's organization which does not include a program on women and health on its agenda. Scientific conferences have been organized and women's studies has made her entrance in medical school programs. Literature abounds, not only at the level of personal testimony (de Bonte Was, 1978; *Gynaecologische praktijken*, 1980), but also more theoretical or empirical investigations (Manschot *et al.*, 1977; Baart and Dercks, 1981).

What I have repeatedly encountered, is that women seem be anything but satisfied with the treatment they receive at the hands of the male medical establishment. Feminist critique falls roughly, into three categories:

(1) *Medical monopolization of the control of women's reproductive functions.* Physically normal women are, by definition, viewed as sick and are required to seek the services of physicians upon entering puberty. Functions like menstruation, childbirth and menopause, formerly part of what it meant to be female, are now considered matters warranting almost constant medical surveillance (Ehrenreich and English, 1973a,b; 1979; Oakley, 1979; Roberts, 1981; Laws, 1983). Women, without the control over their own bodies and fertility, will also lack power over their lives.
(2) *Medical views that women's complaints are psychogenic in origin.* Women's complaints are frequently considered to be caused or aggravated by psychological factors. Thus, dysmenorrhea or pain in labor may be attributed to a 'faulty outlook' and infantile colic to the mother's insecurity and anxiety (Lennane and Lennane, 1973). Accompanying the notion that 'it's all in her head', is the negative stereotype of the woman patient taking up the busy doctor's time with a host of vague symptoms and endless complaining (Scully and Bart, 1973; Lorbeer, 1976; Cooperstock, 1978; Fidell, 1980; Lipsitt, 1982). This means that women's complaints are not taken seriously and often receive inadequate treatment.
(3) *General practice as institution of social control over women.* When under pressure, women may look to their family doctor for support and help. In consultation with him, however, her difficulties in her living and working situation are transformed into examples of individual pathology. Thus, boredom or anxiety may be smoothed away with a chat, a prescription

for valium, and the promise of another appointment. GPs use their authority to lull women into accepting and/or adapting to problems stemming from the oppressive contingencies of their lives (Barrett and Roberts, 1978; Standing, 1980).

Sex differences and the woman patient

It is not surprising that, in view of such an extensive critique of health care for women, particularly as patients in general practice, empirical investigations on the subject make their entrance. Social scientists, ever alert to signs of commotion, have always made it their business to find out what's going on 'out there', and supply empirical evidence. Consequently, several years after the emergence of the feminist movement, we have started to see studies on women as patients.

Obviously, there are various forms such research might have taken. What I found, however, upon examining the literature to-date is that the research deals almost exclusively with sex-differences, i.e. male and female patients are compared in terms of their respective complaints, illness behavior and utilization of the various health services. Women, I am told, distinguish themselves from their male counterparts in two main areas:

They tend to use all health services more frequently than men.
Women are more subject to 'vague' illnesses than men.

Despite an occasional critical note, I have encountered these notions with such regularity in research on sex differences that they threaten to become a self-fulfilling prophecy. For this reason, I feel that a closer look is warranted.

Frequency of visits

In all surveys to my knowledge, women as a group are shown to pay more visits to their GPs than men. This is estimated to be about one and a half times more (Nathanson, 1977). This appears to be true even when visits in conjunction with children and reproductive functions, i.e. pill controls, are taken into account. Whereas everyone is in agreement *that* women see their GP more often, the theories explaining *why* this is so tend to vary. Roughly, these theoretical explanations fall into three categories:

(1) *Women are sicker than men.* This, it is suggested, may be a reflection of biological differences. The higher incidence of genito-urinary infections among women may be accounted for in this way, for example. Futhermore, women may be exposed to stress induced by their role obligations which has a negative influence on their health. Gove and Hughes' (1979) 'nurturant role hypothesis' is a representative of such an explanation. They assert, for example, that women have role obligations which require

constant ongoing activities vis-à-vis their husband and children and that these obligations tend to interfere with self-care as well as having a negative effect on women's health.

(2) *Women demonstrate more sick role behavior than men.* This is the social psychological perspective. It is not so much concerned with organic dysfunction, but rather with differences in perceiving and reporting illness. Women are supposedly more inclined to define themselves as ill since they do not have as many 'fixed role obligations' (outside employment). In addition, the sick role is more compatible with traditional female roles, i.e. women are accustomed to being dependent and asking for help. Finally, women are assumed to be more sensitive to bodily changes and also more knowledgeable on health issues, making them more likely to seek the services of a physician.

The main proponents here are Nathanson (1975; 1977), Verbrugge (1976; 1977) and Mechanic (1976; 1978).

(3) *Women receive more treatment than men.* Physicians are more inclined to 'treat' their female patients. They tend to prescribe psychotropic drugs at the drop of a hat—women receiving 2.2 times as many tranquillizers and sedatives as men (Cooperstock, 1978)—as well as perform unnecessary surgery like hysterectomies (Scully, 1980). Physicians are also more likely to make appointments for follow-up consultations with their female patients (Fidell, 1980). Thus, physician behavior could also be influencing the frequency with which women utilize the health services.

'Vague complaints'

The other frequently-cited sex difference concerns the kind of symptoms presented by patients. Women not only visit the GP more often than men do, but they are apparently doing so without anything very much being wrong with them. Women, it is said, have a tendency to present 'vague' symptoms.

To begin with, I am inclined to ask what makes a complaint 'vague'. In viewing the actual symptoms: dizziness, insomnia, headaches (typical examples), it is not immediately clear what is so vague about them. They all have to do with physical distress. It seems, however, upon closer examination, that it is not so much the symptom itself which is vague, but rather the unfortunate fact that the physician is unable to locate a clear-cut somatic casual agent. In other words, the headache, prototype of the 'vague complaint', when accompanied by a brain tumor, does not fall into the category 'vague'. Without this appendage, however, it may very well.

Taking the physician's inability to discover a somatic etiology as the defining characteristic of a 'vague complaint', then both men and women exhibit symptoms which might safely be called 'vague'. In view of the prevalence of the stereotype concerning the nature of women's complaints, something else must be involved here.

According to various studies, women tend to report more symptoms at one time than men do (Copperstock, 1978). They also report more symptoms of emotional distress—symptoms which lend themselves (subsequently) to psychiatric labels (Phillips and Segal, 1969; Dohrenwend and Dohrenwend, 1976). Thus, there may be differences in the way women and men perceive and talk about bodily discomfort, as well as differences in the way physicians 'hear' and later describe the complaints presented to them by their male and female patients. It is to these differences I suggest turning to, then, in order to account for the designation 'vague' to women's symptoms.[1]

A critical look at sex difference research

Having briefly discussed some of the findings on sex differences in patient populations as encountered by the GP, a few critical remarks are in order.

The first is methodological. The picture presented is one of static, poorly conceptualized research. There are few cross-national comparisons. Explanations are used in an ad-hoc way to account for isolated findings. None of the studies presents a coherent framework for explaining sex differences in morbidity (Lorbeer, 1976; Mechanic, 1978). I am rather inclined to view them in the light of the frantic race for tenure (certainly understandable in the US today): a decade later the same, uninspired investigations are being ground out, adding nothing to our understanding of sex differences, i.e. what the above-mentioned differences mean, what they can tell us about the social fact of being male or female or a patient in general practice.

More important than these methodological questions, however, is the entire focus of the research on sex differences. This focus itself leads to serious and—it is my contention—insurmountable problems in finding out about the situation faced by women patients in general practice. Presumably, those scientists busily engaged in gathering their data on sex differences are motivated by some sort of emancipatory intention. Bernhard (1975), in tracing the historical development of the research tradition, points out that the original investigators were interested in finding scientific evidence for equality between the sexes. Later, scientists addressed themselves to understanding and helping women in their (different) emotional needs. The present wave of sex differences research is based on the idea that men and women occupy different roles and that women occupy an inferior position (*ibid*: 9). Thus, it is not the sex difference *per se* which is of interest, but rather how it is used to the disadvantage of women—in this case, women patients. In actual practice, however, this works just the other way around. The role structure and women's inferior position within it are confirmed and, thanks to the helping hand of science, legitimated. I shall attempt to show how this undesirable outcome, despite all good intentions, can occur and, finally, offer some suggestions concerning how it might be circumvented.

To begin with, *when the scientist looks for sex differences, sex differences are what she will find.*[2] By focusing on the ways that men and women differ, she will miss all of the ways that they are, in fact, similar (for example, as patients in general practice). She will also run the risk of distorting those differences, i.e. by using sex as an explanatory variable for behaviors or events which cannot be accounted for solely on the basis sex.

In her excellent critique of feminist research, Eichler (1980) suggests that sex difference research succumbs to what she calls the 'biological fallacy'. Sex is not only the biological fact of being male or female; it is also a social fact, i.e. being a woman or man in a particular culture at a specific point in history. The danger in using biological sex to explain various social phenomena, is that these differences may be reinforced. They become attributed irrevocably to sex, ignoring, at the same time, other important aspects of the social context.

This often happens in research concerning the woman patient. By measuring the number of times she visits her GP and comparing this with the male patient, a difference is 'discovered'. This opens the floor to the search for reasons which can account for the difference: women are sicker, or are pretending to be sicker, or don't mind acting sick or whatever. In any case, they are taking up a lot of the doctor's time. That the issue might be more complicated is obscured by this approach.[3]

Sex differences research, then, is essentially limited to studying differences in (illness) behavior and, subsequently, attributing those found to sex. The issue for women as patient is, however, infinitely more complex.

When a woman enters the doctor's office, a wide variety of contingencies are going to be making themselves felt: age, marital status, socio-economic background, cultural context, the medical setting, the GP's training, preferences and attitudes, the weather, their respective moods, etc. Moreover, they will be actively negotiating their various roles, as they perceive them to be, for themselves and each other, in a flexible and ongoing way. It is impossible to explain what happens in a consultation as a result of sex roles or sex differences (although participants may well be oriented towards them). To do so is to deny the complexity which is part and parcel of being a female in this society.[4]

A final critical note is in order concerning the presumed objective of sex differences research. As previously mentioned, I assume that the intention is to show that there are differences in order to eliminate some of the difficulties faced by women as patients. In many cases, the aim is to raise the public's attention that there are, in fact, problems. That these good intentions backfire is beautifully illustrated by an experience I had recently at a conference on social science research and women.[5]

The results of an investigation concerning the differences in verbal therapeutic behavior between male and female therapists with their male and female clients were presented by two women researchers.[6] They had 'discovered' all sorts of differences. For example, female therapists were more sympathetic, interrupted their clients less, talked about themselves more, were more encouraging, etc. Male therapists, on the other hand, tended to interrupt more, try to persuade their clients to change, and gave more directives and criticism. Both investigators were notably excited about the findings. The audience, predominately female, was smiling and nodding as well. Finally we all seemed to be thinking, some 'hard proof' for what we all had known, or had been suspecting, all along. Women are better therapists than men, and certainly for female clients.

This general glow of satisfaction was rudely interrupted, however, when one sharp methodologist pointed out that these findings—attractive as they were to the feminists among us—were in fact based on a very small sample. They could hardly be considered representative and, consequently, we were advised to use caution in our interpretations. The best we could do is say that these few therapists did seem to exhibit differential behavior based on their sex. We, all schooled in quantitative research, were properly chastened and stopped smiling.

This experience is informative in several ways. First, the reactions of the two investigators as well as the reaction of the audience indicates that we all seemed to hold a common sense notion[7] concerning women's experiences in psychotherapy as well as how women deal with one another, men with women, etc. The inquiry itself was a typical example of quantitative research, i.e. categories for therapeutic behavior were conceptualized and applied to data across various groups of therapists and clients. Behavior fitting into these categories was counted and reported in the form of statistics. These findings were received by us, however, using the information of our own experiences, ideas and attitudes as members of our particular culture, as social scientists, as women, as feminists, and so on. It was exactly these common sense notions which enabled us to give the findings meaning, allowed us to interpret them and, ultimately, led to all the smiling and nodding going on in the room. These notions remained unexplicated, and of course, as is the case in quantitative research in general (and sex differences research in particular). Everyone seems to be pretending that we are examining virgin territory with an open mind, but just can't quite suppress the smile.

The second point concerns the criticism which was made. The inquiry was based on such a small sample of therapists and clients that it could not be considered representative. This was, of course, true. Theoretically, the investigators might have included more subjects in their research in order to avoid this particular pitfall. The end result, however, would have been the same; namely, that caution is in order. This is an ironic by-product of research on sex differences, which the investigator cannot eliminate by means of more-of-the-same, no matter how carefully she sets up her design nor how generously she chooses her sample.

The 'problem'—finding evidence to support the contention that women as a group differ from other (male) patients in a way which might account for their oppression both within as well as outside the medical context—insoluble within the *mode*[8] on which such research is based. My everyday experiences and belief in the factual nature of social structures were what convinced me that the above-mentioned problem existed. What I wanted was to see this common sense understanding bolstered by some scientific support. What happened, however, was that I was left with a warning to be more careful about what I think I 'know' and more uncertain about whether it is 'really' so. This seems, in fact, to be moving in the opposite direction of my—and presumably the other women's—original intention which was to convince the public that there *is* a problem.

To sum up, many of these remarks apply to quantitative research methods in general and not just sex differences research. I have chosen to deal with this particular area in some detail because it so often the focus of women's studies. I realize, of course, that social scientists, including those affiliated with Women's Studies, will continue to investigate sex differences. For many, it would appear to be the only way to say anything about women. I would, however, like to suggest that there are other ways of tackling the issue of women as patients in general practice and the problems they face there. It might be worth our while to examine some of these avenues of approach.

Conclusion and some directions for further research

An attempt has been made to indicate some of the issues concerning women as patients. The feminist critique deals with three main areas: control over our bodies and reproductive functions, women's complaints not being taken seriously ('psychologizing' women's health problems, treating women patients in a patronizing fashion, negative medical views about the woman patient as a 'complainer' having nothing very much wrong with her, etc.), and the medicalization of social problems experienced by women as a group (general practice as an institution of social control).

Current research on women as patients has been discussed. I have paid particular attention to sex differences research as it comprises far and away the bulk of research on women as patients in medical settings. Having taken a critical look at this style of research, my conclusion is that, although it has its advantages in some cases, one and a half decades later it is beginning to show signs of wear, particularly for those with emancipatory intentions interested in discovering more about possible problems faced by women in medical settings.

It goes beyond the scope of the present paper to provide a detailed treatment of other research orientations. However, I would like to make some suggestions based on the above discussion for directions such research might profitably take, both for myself and for others engaged in similar research endeavors:

(1) In order to say something about the experience of women as patients in general practice, it is necessary—and here I agree with Eichler (1980)—to examine this particular context without using sex as a variable. Thus, I would like to treat the consultation as a routine example of a daily encounter within the highly organized structure of general practice. As such, I consider it to be reflecting the contingencies of this context. The members—GP and (female) patient—will, in fact, be sustaining and creating this context as they go along. In other words, 'general practice' or 'GPs and female patients' are simply aggregates for hundred of micro-events which are the consultations.[9]

This means that I might take an in-depth look at the actual interaction occurring in a consultation between a male GP and a female patient. This is, in fact, the 'normal' situation anyway, 95 per cent of the GP's being men and 66 per cent of their patients being women.[10] By describing their interaction in detail, I can get an idea of how the structure of general practice is maintained, its routine practices and procedures, as well as how members are oriented to their own and each others' cultural, professional, personal and gender identities. Having done this, I might then return to my original concern of women's oppression as patients and see whether or not my findings can shed some light on the problem. I have not limited myself to differences between male and female patients. Nor, incidentally, am I assuming in advance that the problems described apply solely to women patients.

(2) Members in any conversational context will be oriented to gender as a social 'fact' and engaged in constructing it on various levels in the course of their talk. Thus, for example, the GP will have his medical view of women and their (specific) ailments, perhaps tempered by the more modern medical ideologies. He will have his own cultural background; the everyday notions about women prevalent in his own society as well as the relative position women occupy in it; his own experiences with women in general and his women patients in particular; his idiosyncratic response to the individual woman in his office, etc. These sources of knowledge will be demonstrated and, at the same time, constructed in the ongoing talk. Not as neatly defined sex-role stereotypes, but in a flexible way, part of the integration process in which other sources of information (concerning patient behavior, complaints, etiology, duties and responsibilities of the physician, etc.) are also being tapped and utilized as resources for the conversation at hand.[11] Thus, stereotypes, as idealized notions, so familiar to those involved in the social sciences, may be revealed in actual interaction, not in the form that the responses to a sex-role stereotype questionnaire on physicians' attitudes towards female patients

might take, but in a creative and flexible way. In order to capture the complexity of this process, it may be best to examine how patients and doctors are talking to one another within the context of the medical consultation.

(3) Just as the GP and the female patient use common sense notions in creating and making sense of their conversation, so do I, as investigator. In the above example of the conference, I demonstrated how I employed my own notions about men and about therapists to interpret the research findings. In fact, investigators rely on our being able to fit the findings back into everyday contexts to give them meaning (Cicourel, 1982). These notions, however, remain implicit in most research. According to Cicourel, it is the task of the investigator to explicate these sources of knowledge. In other words, she must show *how* she knows what she knows. What this means in the context of my present research, where I am engaged in analysing transcripts of medical consultations, is that I shall be using my own resources in order to make sense of my data. My experiences as a patient and as a—in my case—therapist, my general knowledge of the medical setting and training programs for GPs, as well as my—admittedly—partisan stance as feminist, will effect what I 'hear' in the conversations being investigated. It is this 'tacit knowledge' which will, hopefully, enable me to recognize instances of, for example, patronizing behavior or 'psychologizing' of women's health problems, when I encounter them. Explicating what I know—Cicourel's term is my 'interpretative competence'—will be part and parcel of my inquiry. The rest will entail showing how what I 'know' to be happening happens.

(4) Last but not least, it is my contention that by demonstrating *how* women's complaints are dealt with in a medical setting in a way which is plausible and easy to reconstruct for the reader, the question of whether or not the problem exists will become redundant. If I, for example, 'see' a woman patient's problems reduced to something that's 'all in her head' or can follow how she is being belittled by the doctor, I have, at the same time, offered some convincing support for at least one of the much-cited problems faced by women in the doctor's office.[12] More important, however, additional information has been provided on how oppression works at a micro-level—something I believe we presently know relatively little about, despite its everyday, routine occurrence.

Acknowledgements

This paper is part of a research project on women as patients in general practice being conducted at the Faculty of Medicine of the Vrije Universiteit in Amsterdam. I should like to thank Mary Fahrenfort, Hanne van Herwerden, Marianne Dercks, Wientje Meeuwesen, and Marlies Terstegge for their helpful comments on an earlier draft of this paper.

Notes

1 I am by no means suggesting that women's complaints are in any sense 'vague'. I merely wish to clarify what is meant by the term, which one so frequently encounters in the literature.
2 For want of a neutral pronoun and for reasons of style, I have used 'she', 'her', etc. throughout this paper. Any appearance of excluding men from the groups in question, be it scientists, physicians or whatever, is strictly unintentional.
3 For example, if I took the line that general practice is an institution through which social control over deviant individuals may be exercized, then it would make more sense to compare deviance among men and women rather than comparing male and female patients. In that case, I might find myself examining various social institutions, or different ways men and women express discontent or deviance from norms and how this is treated respectively. This is, by no means, an original idea and it goes beyond the scope of the present paper to discuss it in any detail. Let it suffice at this point to say that a comparison between male and female patients may have little to say about what the frequent visits women pay to the GP actually mean.
4 In this context, Eichler makes an interesting point that no one uses the concept 'race role', although race and sex are direct parallels in that they are based on an immutable criterion which remains stable over the individual's lifetime. This is because we do not explain different behavior patterns on the basis of a power differential which coincides with racial distinctions (Eichler, 1980). In this respect, women have not been so lucky.
5 'Wijzer worden over Marie', Amsterdam, March 11, 1983.
6 Ineke Catsburg and Maria Osterholt of the Universeteit van Amsterdam.
7 'Common sense notion' is a term coined by ethnomethodologists to describe an attitude which people have towards social structure. It refers to a stock of knowledge and reasoning procedures gained from viewing social reality as factual, or 'actually out there' (Schutz, 1962).
8 For a critical discussion of the 'analogue model' (correlations between gender and other variables like occupation, sympomatology, etc.) as applied to men and women clients in psychotherapy, the reader is referred to Davidson and Abramowitz (1980).
9 The notion 'micro-event' is taken from Cicourel (1982) and refers to routine and observable practices of everyday life.
10 I am referring to the situation in The Netherlands, but I have found no indication that it is not representative of other Western European countries as well.
11 This is in line with Cicourel's conception of 'role', namely, not a social structure which *causes* the individual to behave in a particular way, as though she were nothing more than a puppet controlled by outside forces. On the contrary, her role is ongoingly created in interaction with others within a particular context (Cicourel, 1974).
12 For an example of this approach, the reader is referred to an earlier inquiry (Davis, 1983) in which I demonstrated how a woman's difficulties with her situation as full-time housewife and mother were transformed and individualized in the context of psychotherapy. Whereas my inquiry was based on one therapy conversation, it was plausible enough that even the die-hard behaviorists described it as a 'model of a therapy conversation'. There was no question of the process *not* occurring in most therapy conversations, although it was not my initial intention to gather evidence to indicate *that* it takes place, but rather *how* it can occur.

References

Baart, Ingrid and Marianne Dercks. 1981. En de cirkel is weer rond. . . . Een ander licht op het huisartsenbezoek van vrouwen. *Tijdschr. vrouwenstudies* **8** (2): 532–548.

Barrett, Michèle and Helen Roberts. 1978. Doctors and their patients. The social control of women in general practice. In: Smart, Carol and Barry Smart, eds, *Women, Sexuality and Social Control*. Routledge and Kegan Paul, London.

Bernhard, Jessie. 1975. *Women, Wives, Mothers. Values and Options*. Aldine, Chicago.

Cicourel, Aaron V. 1974. *Cognitive Sociology. Language and Meaning in Social Interaction*. Free Press, New York.

Cicourel, Aaron V. 1982. Notes on the integration of micro- and macro-levels of analysis. In: Knorr-Cetina, Karin D. and Aaron V. Cicourel, eds, *Advances in Social Theory and Methodology. Toward an Integration of Micro- and Macro-Sociologies*. Routledge and Kegan Paul, Boston.

Cooperstock, Ruth. 1978. Sex differences in psychotropic drug use. *Soc. Sci. Med.* **12B**: 179–186.

Davidson, Christine V. and Stephen I. Abramowitz. 1980. Sex bias in clinical judgement: later empirical returns. *Psychol. Women Q.* **4** (3): 377–395.

Davis, Kathy. 1983. Probleem (her) formulering in psychotherapie. Het proces van individualisering op gespreksnivo bekeken. *Psychologie en Maatschappij* **22** (1): 59–79.

Dohrenwend, Bruce P. and Barbara Snell Dohrenwend. 1976. Sex differences and psychiatric disorders. *Am. J. Sociol.* **81**: 1447–1454.

Ehrenreich, Barbara and Deirdre English. 1973a. *Complaints and Disorders. The Sexual Politics of Sickness*. Feminist Press, Old Westbury, New York.

Ehrenreich, Barbara and Deirdre English. 1973b. *Witches, Midwives and Nurses*. Feminist Press, Old Westbury, New York.

Ehrenreich, Barbara and Deirdre English. 1979. *For Her Own Good. 150 Years of the Experts' Advice to Women*. Pluto Press, London.

Eichler, Margrit. 1980. *The Double Standard. A Feminist Critique of Feminist Social Science*. Croom Helm, London.

Fidell, Linda S. 1980. Sex Role Stereotypes and the American Physician. *Psychol. Women Q.* **4** (3): 313–330.

Gove, Walter R. and Michael Hughes. 1979. Possible causes of the apparent sex differences in physical health: an empirical investigation. *Am sociol. Rev.* **44**: 126–146.

Gynaecologische praktijken. Zwartboek over het gynaecologische handelen van huisartsen en gynaecologen. 1980. Vrouwendrukkerij Virgina, Amsterdam.

Laws, Sophie. 1983. The sexual politics of pre-menstrual tension. *Women's Studies Int. Forum* **6** (1): 19–31.

Lenanne, K. Jean and John R. Lenanne. 1973. Alleged psychogenic disorders in women—A possible manifestation of sexual prejudice. *New Eng. J. Med.* **288** (6): 288–292.

Lipsitt, Don R. 1982. The painful woman: complaints, symptoms, and illness. In: Norman, Malkah T. and Carol C. Nadelson, eds, *The Woman Patient*, Vol. 3. Plenum Press, New York.

Lorbeer, Judith. 1976. Women and medical sociology: invisible professional and ubiquitous patients. In: Millman, Marcia and Rosabeth Moss Kanter, eds, *Another Voice. Feminist Perspectives on Social Life and Social Science*. Octagon Books, New York.

Manschot, Anke Andre Cuppen and Jos Dijkmans. 1977. *Huisvrouwen: een vergeten groep in de -mediese-hulpverlening*. Paradogma, Nijmegen.

Mechanic, David. 1976. Sex, illness behavior, and the use of health services. *J. Human Stress* **2** (4): 29–40.

Mechanic, David. 1978. Sex, illness, illness behavior, and the use of the health services. *Soc. Sci. Med.* **12B**: 207–214.

Nathanson. Constance A. 1975. Illness and the feminine role: a theoretical review. *Soc. Sci. Med.* **9**: 57–62.

Nathanson. Constance A. 1977. Sex, illness, and medical care. A review of data, theory, and method. *Soc. Sci. Med.* **11**: 13–25.

Oakley, Ann. 1979. A case of maternity: paradigms of women as maternity cases. *Signs* **4** (4): 607–631.

Phillips, Derek L. and Bernard E. Segal. 1969. Sexual status and psychiatric symptoms. *Am. sociol. Rev.* **34**: 58–72.

Roberts, Helen, ed. 1981. *Women, Health and Reproduction*. Routledge and Kegan Paul, London.

Scully Diana. 1980. *Men Who Control Women's Health. The Miseducation of Obstetricians—Gynecologists*. Houghton Mifflin, Boston.

Scully Diana. 1980. *Men Who Control Women's Health. The Miseducation of Obstetricians–Gynaecologists*. Houghton Mifflin, Boston.

Schutz, Alfred. 1962. *Collected Papers I: The Problem of Social Reality*. Martinus Nijhoff, The Hague.

Standing, Hilary. 1980. 'Sickness is a woman's business?': reflections on the attribution of illness. In: The Brighton Women & Science Group, ed., *Alice Through the Microscope. The Power of Science over Women's Lives*. Virago, London.

Verbrugge, Lois M. 1976. Females and illness: recent trends in sex differences in the United States. *J. Hlth. Soc. Beh.* **17**: 387–403.

Verbrugge, Lois M. 1977. Sex differences in morbidity and mortality in the United States. *Soc. Biol.* **23**: 275–296.

Vrouwen over hulp bij ziekte en problemen. 1978 De Bonte Was, Amsterdam.

50

SEX DIFFERENCES AND THE NEW POLITICS OF WOMEN'S HEALTH

Steven Epstein

Source: S. Epstein, *Inclusion: The Politics of Difference in Medical Research*, Chicago: Chicago University Press, 2008, pp. 233–57.

The prescription drug terfenadine (sold as Seldane) was a modest breakthrough of recent pharmaceutical science: the first antihistamine not to cause drowsiness. In 1989, as pharmacology expert Raymond Woosley recalled, Seldane was selling briskly by prescription and was soon to be made available over the counter, when a woman in Bethesda, Maryland, who was taking the drug blacked out and ended up at Bethesda Naval Hospital. Physicians there detected a cardiac arrhythmia and wondered if it might be caused by an interaction between Seldane and another of her medications. The physicians reported the potential "drug-drug interaction" to FDA officials, who then uncovered other such cases involving Seldane. FDA officials contacted Woosley, who had been studying a life-threatening drug toxicity called *torsades de pointes*, a form of arrhythmia associated with prolongation of the "QT interval" (the time period needed for the heart to recharge between beats). Thus, the stage was set for Seldane's eventual demise—it was formally taken off the market in 1998—but also for a spate of research by Woosley and others on the various medications associated with *torsades de pointes*.

In 1993 Woosley noticed something that had escaped his attention previously: about two-thirds of the cases of arrhythmia from Seldane and several other drugs were in female patients. "It was a bit embarrassing" not to have recognized the gender disparity earlier, said Woosley, "but we then started studying it." Soon the NIH's Office of Research on Women's Health and the FDA's Office on Women's Health had taken an interest and were supporting Woosley's efforts. It turned out that, after puberty, the QT interval becomes fractionally longer in women than in men—by about 20 milliseconds—perhaps because of effects of sex hormones on heart functioning. As a result, women are more vulnerable to medications that prolong the QT interval than are men, and therefore are more likely to experience, and sometimes die from, *torsades de pointes*.[1]

The sex difference in this case is not absolute: men are also vulnerable to drug-related arrhythmia. However, the link between women's elevated statistical risk and an observable physiological difference between the sexes (the length of the QT interval), along with the presence of a reasonable hypothesis about a sex-linked cause of that physiological difference (hormones), confers a powerful plausibility on the claim of a medically relevant sex difference. Nor are QT-prolonging drugs the only such example. In June 2005 *Science* magazine ran a special issue on women's health, featuring a series of articles, news reports, and commentaries on research into the health differences between females and males. A news report in the issue, entitled "Gender in the Pharmacy: Does It Matter?" suggested that the answer to that question more than occasionally was yes. For a variety of reasons, or for reasons unknown, the same medication might affect women and men differently—moreover, women might be more inclined to suffer the consequences in the form of increased risk of adverse drug reactions.[2]

Medically relevant biological difference findings by sex, like the corresponding difference findings by race, are both cause and consequence of the inclusion-and-difference paradigm. On one hand, advocates of change used early reports of such differences as one rationale for their proposed inclusionary reforms; and on the other hand, the establishment of new inclusionary policies and procedures for subgroup comparisons has resulted in the proliferation of difference findings. Thus, when Viviana Simon, Director of Scientific Programs at the Society for Women's Health Research, wrote an editorial for the special issue of *Science* about the "increasing awareness of significant biological and physiological differences between the sexes, beyond the reproductive ones," she attributed that awareness to the new "federal mandates" and the abandonment of "the old paradigm of the '70-kg white male'" as the normative patient.[3]

However, while new policies and regulations have resulted in findings about both sex differences and race differences, there is a noteworthy distinction to be drawn between the two cases: reports of biological difference by race have sparked a heated medical and public controversy about "racial profiling," but no corresponding debate seems to have arisen as yet with regard to biological differences by sex. A few commentators have suggested that "gender in the pharmacy" is not the problem it is made out to be, because most drugs have a relatively wide "therapeutic index"—that is, a substantial margin of safety between the effective dose and the toxic dose in each individual.[4] And Sally Satel, the inveterate critic of "political correctness" in medicine, has responded with a "not so fast" to what she calls the medical slogan of "Vive la Différence."[5] But for the most part, there has been little public discussion of the merits or risks of "sex profiling" in medicine—indeed, the phrase does not even exist.[6]

To what extent, if any, is the case of biological differences by sex or gender analogous to that of biological differences by race and ethnicity? What does it mean that racial profiling in medicine has become an intellectual battleground while sex profiling has not? These questions have received little direct discussion.[7] To the limited extent that analysts (in academia and elsewhere) have addressed the comparison, it has been to contrast the "tricky" case of race with the "easy" case of sex: obviously men and women are biologically different, while racial difference at the biological level—and even the determination of which racial categories to work with or whether "race" exists at all—is contested terrain. Thus (the argument goes), while choosing a medication on the basis of the patient's sex may be sensible and commendable, making such determinations according to race is deeply problematic. Even those who differ on the merits of racial profiling, such as the philosophers of science Ian Hacking and Michael Root, are in agreement when it comes to this point. Hacking has observed that "many medical differences between males and females are uniform, but medical differences between races are almost always only statistical."[8] Root has warned that some seek to endow racial profiling with legitimacy via the suggestion that racial differences in medicine have the same status as sex differences. In opposition to this appeal for legitimation, Root makes a careful argument about "the differences between the categories of race and sex":

> A gene X that regulates drug metabolism can vary with a gene Y on a sex chromosome, but there is no race chromosome or race gene Y for X to vary with. As a result, doctors have a reason to study sex differences but not racial differences in drug response and a reason to use sex but not race as a proxy for response when deciding how best to treat an individual patient. Sex has more explanatory and predictive power in the clinic because there are genes for sex and good reasons to believe that the genes for sex and some genes for drug metabolism are concordant.[9]

As the views of Root and others suggest, many critics of racial profiling in medicine have engaged in "boundary work," erecting a wall between sex and race in order to designate the study of sex differences as good science and the study of race differences as bad science.[10] Is this boundary work a problem, or is it commendable?

Certainly, the biological significance of sex and race are quite different cases. It is true that females as a class are biologically different from males as a class in easily identifiable respects. It also appears true that men and women *on average* are biologically different in a number of well-known as well as less obvious respects. To the degree that Hacking, Root, and others are correct about the differences across types of difference, then the tendency of the policies of the inclusion-and-difference paradigm to treat all forms of difference in a standardized way—to "flatten" or commensurate differences, as I described in chapter 7—deserves critical scrutiny.

However, it immediately bears saying that biological sex is *not* an either/or—not at the anatomic, the hormonal, or the chromosomal levels. There are no truly dichotomous variables in nature, and, as many scholars have shown, there is no precise or fully satisfactory biological means of demarcating all males from all females.[11] And if so, then the problems associated with profiling—such as the risk of treating individuals improperly on the basis of their group affiliations—may apply to medical research on sex differences, too, and not just to research on differences by race.

The new meanings of sex differences

In this chapter, my expository strategy is to follow the general logic of the previous chapter on race. After considering the plethora of reports of biological sex differences in medicine in recent years, I will describe the emergence and development of a movement calling for "sex-based biology" (or "gender-specific medicine"), and I will locate it in relation to other recent research on the biology and genetics of sex difference. While sex-based biology has not provoked a debate analogous to that over racial profiling, it is implicated within the tensions that have emerged between sectors of the broader women's health movement, and I will analyze what is at stake in those strategic disagreements. Then, I will proceed one-by-one through the various critiques that I launched at racial profiling in the previous chapter. In each case, I will ask whether and to what degree the critique might also apply to the case of sex profiling.

The explosion of difference findings

Emphasis on sex differences in medicine is part of a larger trend toward claiming or assuming the overriding significance of biology and genetics in understanding the behavior of males and females, in domains ranging from brain functioning to mating behavior.[12] As with race, arguments about sex differences drawn from genetics can cut both ways, and occasionally reports of fundamental genetic similarities make their way into public view. For example, in 2001 *The Scientist* magazine reported: "Genetic studies are revealing that men and women are more similar than distinct. So far, of the approximately 31,000 genes in the human genome, men and women differ only in the two sex chromosomes, X and Y, and only a few dozen genes seem to be involved." However, the notion that our usual distinction between "pink and blue" might be replaced with "a blurred rainbow of confusion"—as the article's author put it—runs up against the vast wave of commentary that assumes or reports on stark differences between the sexes.[13]

Nowhere is the attention to biological sex differences more pronounced at present than in biomedicine, and the concern with the effects of pharmaceutical drugs is an especially important example. An interesting aspect of the case of Seldane is that it concerns a group-specific difference related not to the more typical issue of the *pharmacokinetics* of a medication (how it is metabolized, absorbed, and ultimately cleared from the body) but rather to *pharmacodynamics* (the actual effects of a medication on bodily organs and processes). Over the course of the 1990s, a range of reports in the medical literature described differences in drug effects of both sorts, building on earlier research dating back to the early 1970s. A review in 2001 by pharmacologist Mary Berg noted a wide variety of sex- or gender-related differences, significantly including the effect of oral contraceptives in increasing or decreasing the speed of clearance of drugs such as aspirin, caffeine, and morphine. Berg also described research in "chronopharmacology"—the effect of bodily rhythms, such as the menstrual cycle, on how drugs are processed.[14] Another review essay—by Monica Gandhi and coauthors, published in 2004—attributed pharmacokinetic differences by sex not only to variation in the cytochrome P450 enzymes but also to a number of other factors, including body weight and gastric emptying time.[15] Gandhi and coauthors also discussed the burgeoning literature on sex differences in response to pain medications (believed to reflect differences in how men and women actually experience pain), as well as the evidence on differences in the effects and side effects of antipsychotic and antidepressant medications.[16] Antiviral drugs targeting HIV have provided yet another important example: women appear to have more frequent and more severe side effects with several classes of anti-HIV medications, though some research also indicates that such drugs may also be more efficacious for women in terms of keeping the virus in check.[17]

"We now know that gender is one of the most important factors that influences and predicts response to all kinds of treatments," FDA Commissioner Mark McClellan said in 2003 in a speech at a Society for Women's Health Research event. "The FDA is working to better define the genetic differences between men and women that influence how they are going to respond to a particular medication."[18] Indeed, research on these various differences in the effects of medications has been a priority at the various women's health offices, which have organized conferences and developed research agendas.[19] A particular concern has been the issue of adverse drug reactions, estimated by the FDA to affect women at least one and a half times as often as men.[20] In April 2004 the Agency for Healthcare Research and Quality (a DHHS agency) held a two-day meeting of experts to consider the problem of adverse drug reactions and to focus on the goal of "Improving the Use and Safety of Medications in Women through Sex/Gender and Race/Ethnicity Analysis."[21]

The growing literature on biological sex differences in medicine extends beyond the important issue of pharmacology to include attention to many other kinds of differences in biological processes with health implications. According to the "statement of editorial purpose" of an electronic journal devoted to women's health research, "It is increasingly evident that sex-based differences exist in a range of conditions, including heart disease, cancer, stroke, depression, HIV/AIDS, autoimmune disorders, neurologic diseases, bone and joint disorders, as well as in reactions to drugs."[22] Heart function and cardiovascular disease provide an excellent example, as the case of Seldane already has suggested. According to an editorial published in *Cardiovascular Research* in 2004 (entitled "A Radical Idea: Men and Women Are Different"), "gender has a pronounced influence on the type and severity of cardiovascular disease that will likely ensue during one's lifetime. Sex differences have been noted in most major cardiovascular diseases including coronary heart disease, stroke, and hypertension."[23] Women also tend to develop heart disease at a later age than do men, and women and men are reported to have different symptoms prior to heart attacks—indeed, the canonical symptom of chest pain "was notably absent or was described differently by the women," according to research reported in 2004.[24] Women are more likely than men to have a hidden form of coronary disease;[25] and women with coronary artery disease and implantable cardioverter-defibrillators also have been reported to develop a form of arrhythmia more often than do men with the device.[26] As described in a recent article in *Science* on the "Molecular and Cellular Basis of Cardiovascular Gender Differences," many of these differences may be linked to hormones, and some may be traced to developmental pathways laid down *in utero*.[27]

Given the story told in this book, perhaps the most interesting of the recent cardiovascular difference findings concerns the protective effects of aspirin. In chapters 4 and 5, I described how the Physicians' Health Study, a randomized trial of low-dose aspirin to prevent heart attacks, tested in male doctors over 40, became a *cause célèbre* in the congressional debate over women's health research and a prime example in the General Accounting Office's damning report in 1990 on the underrepresentation of women in clinical trials. While the Physicians' Health Study demonstrated the efficacy of aspirin for men, it left open the question of whether the finding could be extrapolated to women. However, the investigators were by no means unaware of this issue, and they launched a separate study with 40,000 female participants, called the Women's Health Study. In March 2005 the verdict finally was in: although aspirin protected women from a major form of stroke—something that had not been demonstrated in the trials in men—it failed to prevent the occurrence of first heart attacks in women younger than 65.[28] As an editorialist commented in the issue of the *New England Journal of Medicine* that reported the study's findings, this "difference between the sexes in the cardiovascular response to aspirin . . . is at once a puzzle and a coda to the recent crescendo of demands that clinical research must always be organized to account for the biologic differences between women and men."[29] Newspapers around the country ran the story on the front page. The Associated Press called it a "stunning example" of "polar opposite" medical findings by sex, while the *Washington Post* concluded that the study added "powerful new evidence to the growing body of data showing that men and women differ in fundamental ways on various aspects of health, and that research on men does not necessarily translate directly to women."[30]

The philosophy of sex-based biology

On April 25, 2001, the Institute of Medicine (IOM) of the National Academy of Sciences announced the forthcoming publication of a book-length report entitled *Exploring the Biological Contributions to Human Health: Does Sex Matter?* This 288-page volume was the product of a lengthy review by a sixteen-member panel of experts, and it was sponsored by a range of government agencies, advocacy groups, and pharmaceutical companies. The report answered the rhetorical question—"Does sex matter?"—emphatically in the affirmative: "Sex does matter. It matters in ways that we did not expect. Undoubtedly, it also matters in ways that we have not begun to imagine."[31] Calling for medical researchers to study sex differences "from womb to tomb," the panel reviewed the literature on sex differences in the efficacy of pharmaceutical drugs, sex differences in the etiology and pathogenesis of autoimmune conditions, sex differences in the experiencing of pain, sex differences in coronary heart disease, and so on. The panel also offered a raft of recommendations, including the quite radical one that researchers should "determine and disclose the sex of origin of biological research materials" and that "journals editors should encourage researchers . . . to specify the extent to which analyses of the data by sex were included in the study."[32]

By coincidence, the announcement of the IOM report preceded by only about a week the publication in the *New England Journal* of Robert Schwartz's editorial on racial profiling.[33] But where reports of medically relevant biological differences by race provoked controversy, the IOM report seemed almost universally to be praised. For example, in a 15-minute segment on the *NewsHour with Jim Lehrer*, the story was presented straightforwardly as an episode in the forward march of medical knowledge.[34] Particularly keen to promote the IOM's conclusions was the Society for Women's Health Research (SWHR), one of the groups that had sponsored the report. In the early 1990s, the SWHR had coalesced around the goal of inclusion of women in research and had campaigned for the NIH Revitalization Act. By the late 1990s, the Society's raison d'être was the furtherance of research on differences between men and women that bore medical significance. "This report substantiates everything we've been saying for six years," Phyllis Greenberger, the president of SWHR, told the press. "Many scientists see the emphasis on sex and gender differences as a passing fad, reflecting some kind of political agenda. But the Institute of Medicine has validated this as an important field of research."[35] Sometime later, at a conference sponsored by the NIH's Office of Research on Women's Health, Sherry Marts, the SWHR's scientific director, repeated the rhetorical question in the report's subtitle and suggested that the most pithy executive summary to the report might be the single word *yes*.[36]

The SWHR has been a key proponent of a social movement within biomedicine on which the IOM report conferred crucial legitimacy.[37] Along with academic medical researchers, NIH scientists, and scientists at pharmaceutical companies invested in women's health, the SWHR has sought to establish a new field of study known as "gender-based biology" or (more recently, in an attempt to clarify their interest in what they understand to be biological and not social processes) "sex-based biology." Others, such as the cardiologist Marianne Legato at Columbia University, have used the term "gender-specific medicine." As distinct from more generic proposals for the development of a women's health specialty in medicine, advocates of sex-based biology emphasize fundamental, thoroughgoing, biological differences between men's and women's bodies, from the heart to the brain to the immune system. Those who subscribe to this movement believe that women—and men—deserve separate medical scrutiny because they are biologically different at the level of the cell, the organ, the system, and the organism.[38] Indeed, one of the chief rhetorical strategies of its proponents is to insist on physiological sites of difference that seem far removed from parts of the body traditionally coded as "female" or "male." As Florence Haseltine, the NIH scientist who was central to the founding of SWHR and who claims credit for the invention of the term "gender-based biology," told me, "I always say the liver is the sexiest organ." She meant by this that men's and women's livers metabolize medications at different rates because of differences that affect the presence and function of metabolizing enzymes.[39] Marianne Legato's organ of choice is the heart, though she also has written on gender dimorphism in the brain and a variety of other sites of bodily difference.[40]

On its Web site, the SWHR defines *sex-based biology* as "the study of biological and physiological differences between men and women." The organization notes: "Sex differences have been found everywhere from the composition of bone matter and the experience of pain to the metabolism of certain drugs and the rate of neurotransmitter synthesis in the brain. Sex-based biology has revolutionized the way that the scientific community views the sexes."[41] Sex-based biology first became the topic of a national meeting in 1995, when this society made it the theme of its Scientific Advisory Meeting.[42] The journal published by the Society, the *Journal of Women's Health*, also has served as an important forum for the dissemination of this agenda.[43] Since the mid-1990s, the term *sex-based biology* and its variants have surfaced in a wide range of settings, and diverse collection of actors have gathered beneath its banner. This includes not only researchers who convene at conferences organized by SWHR, but also researchers and other representatives from many of the leading pharmaceutical companies. According to Sherry Marts, an irony of the term's growing ubiquity is the erasure of its origins: "This phrase keeps coming up and Phyllis [Greenberger] gets a little frustrated; she says, 'They aren't giving us any credit. Don't they know we invented that?' And I say, 'Phyllis, this is what we want. We want it to be a household word.' ... In effect, you want people to forget who invented it, because by then you know it's out there."[44] To be sure, the SWHR's goals extend well beyond the simple diffusion of the concept. "In another 10 years," Marts told a reporter for *The Scientist*, sex-based biology "is going to be like neuroscience, [which] started out as a few physiologists and a few biochemists, and pretty soon you've got a core group that's really moving the field forward. Then folks start to realize that this is actually something you can build a career on."[45]

In 1997 Marianne Legato opened up what a reporter described as a "second front in the movement,"[46] founding the Partnership for Women's Health at Columbia University (renamed the Partnership for Gender-Specific Medicine in 2002). The Partnership also puts out an academic journal, the *Journal of Gender-Specific Medicine* (renamed *Gender Medicine* in 2004), and has published a medical textbook on the principles of gender-specific medicine.[47] Legato also has founded an Association for Gender-Specific Medicine,[48] which helped organize the First World Congress on Gender-Specific Medicine in Berlin in 2006.[49] Meanwhile, across the country at Stanford, the university's medical school has revamped its women's health program to include attention to research on sex-based biology. The Web site of "Women's Health @ Stanford" asserts: "When it comes to the way our bodies fight off and process disease, sex truly does matter."[50]

The ORWH also has provided important institutional backing to the emphasis on sex-based biology. In 2000 the agency cosponsored a program, called Building Interdisciplinary Research Careers in Women's Health, that funds universities to recruit junior researchers to the study of medically relevant sex differences.[51] The following year, the ORWH advertised a new funding initiative, cosponsored by the NIH and the FDA for $11 million dollars per year for five years, the creation of "Specialized Centers of Research on Sex and Gender Factors Affecting Women's Health," designed to "develop a research agenda bridging basic and clinical research on sex/gender factors underlying a priority health issue."[52] Advocacy groups have kept up the pressure to institutionalize sex-based biology within the DHHS. For example, the SWHR has combed the database of NIH-funded grants to prepare a report on the funding of research into sex differences by the different NIH institutes, and it has used the findings to push for increased efforts by those institutes perceived as lagging.[53] In a noteworthy victory for the Society, the Senate Appropriations Committee, at the urging of the SWHR, placed "report language" in its version of the fiscal 2005 funding bill that urged the

NIH to "include sex-based biology as an integral part" of research conducted as part of a transinstitute initiative on brain research.[54]

As Peter Keating and Alberto Cambrosio have observed, "biomedicine does not have a stable division of labor corresponding to an unproblematic partition of the object of work, namely the human body." While many specialties are formed with reference to an organ or system, others are defined by bodily functions, life stages, occupation, or other criteria.[55] This variety of ways in which specialties may emerge and be defined leaves the door open for all sorts of medical innovations to become institutionalized over time. By midway through the first decade of the twenty-first century, there were many signs that sex-based biology was on its way to becoming, if not a full-fledged specialty, then at least an established and entrenched intellectual movement within the biomedical sciences and within the U.S. health research infrastructure. One indicator was the endorsement by the American Medical Association in 2000 not simply of increased research on women's health but also of the "sex-based analysis of data."[56]

Feminism, difference, and the new politics of women's health

One of the most striking aspects of the movement for sex-based biology is its unabashed embrace of a thoroughgoing conception of difference between women and men. A publicity video put out by the SWHR in 1998 opens with the voice of a teenage girl:

> When I was young, I didn't like boys very much. But now that I'm grown up, I know that men and women are just different. Boy, are they different! My mother says [Mother's voice], "Men are from Mars, and women are from Venus." My dad says [Father's voice], "Vive la différence!" But he doesn't even know how different we really are. Men and women may have been created equal, but we were not created alike. Our brains, our hearts, our immune systems, even our livers work differently. From conception to death, we live separate biological lives.[57]

This short segment does several bits of ideological work. It grounds the difference between the sexes in biology, even while establishing a domain of bodily difference far more extensive than the reproductive organs. It hastens to remind the viewer that "different" does not mean "unequal." It associates the new scientific findings with conventional wisdom from popular culture— "Men are from Mars, and women are from Venus," and "Vive la différence!" And it renders the fact of difference as something timeless, universal, and unchallengeable by its expression in the voices of parental authority and tradition.

Making the logic of sex-based biology comprehensible to a broader public by resting it on cultural stereotypes about gender difference is a common strategy in public representations of this scientific movement. According to the Web site of "Women's Health @ Stanford," "The differences between men and women are well-known: we think and act differently at almost every level. However, medical researchers are now realizing that those same sex differences extend to every cell in the human body."[58] One author, writing in the magazine *American Health for Women*, observed: "Everyone knows men and women have different shapes, hormones, and psyches. It seems obvious then that illnesses and medications would affect us differently too."[59] Here, phrases that gesture at an irrefutable common sense—"everyone knows" and "it seems obvious"—seek to root sex-based biology within an everyday discourse of gender essentialism, while at the same time laying the groundwork for a reformulation of that common sense in the language of modern biomedicine.

These strategic moves in the construction and public representation of sex-based biology raise important questions about the politics of women's health and about the broader feminist currents within which the women's health movement has swum. With the rise of second-wave feminism in the late 1960s, and throughout the 1970s, many women devoted considerable energy to preaching the philosophy of sameness, challenging gender stereotypes and demanding equal treatment in all walks of life. "Men and women are, of course different. But they are not as different as day and night, earth and sky, yin and yang, life and death," wrote the feminist theorist Gayle Rubin in a classic statement from the period that sought to rethink the conventional wisdom suggested by the ordinary, but very problematic, phrase "the opposite sex."[60] Many considered it important to argue that to the extent that women and men exhibited different behavioral characteristics or personalities in modern society, those differences were the product of nurture, not nature, and would largely disappear in an egalitarian society.[61] However, there also were strong expressions of "difference feminism" within the broader women's movement of the 1970s, including among those who valorized women's characteristics or even argued for women's innate superiority.[62] And by the 1980s, as the theorist Lise Vogel has analyzed, struggles in the domains of law and public policy around issues of particular concern to women, such as pregnancy and childbirth, had raised questions about whether a philosophy of sameness really made sense in the struggle for social justice: "Faced with the specificities of women's lives, equality suddenly appeared inadequate as a goal of social policy."[63]

Thus, at different moments and to varying degrees, feminists (like many other challenging groups) have pursued either "symmetric" or "asymmetric" approaches to the pursuit of social change: they either have insisted upon their fundamental sameness with the dominant group (and hence their right to be treated as equal), or they have emphasized their fundamental difference (and hence their special claim for attention or special grounding for social critique).[64] In recent years, the pendulum swing toward embracing difference has been pronounced. Some social commentators have tried to dislodge the dominant frame of Mars versus Venus. According to Katha Pollitt, for example, "It would be truer to say that men are from Illinois and women are from Indiana—different, sure, but not in ways that have much ethical consequence."[65] Yet it seems that whenever bodies and biology are brought into the discussion, the notion of the two sexes as "opposites" tends to win out.

Medically oriented proponents of the new wave of women's health research, like Bernadine Healy, the former director of the NIH, locate it broadly within the legacy of feminism—in Healy's historical reckoning, it constitutes the third stage of modern feminism, after the suffrage movement and women's liberation. In the two previous stages, explained Healy, women were obliged to present themselves as really just like men. But this time women "could acknowledge that they are different from men without giving up any of the rights gained."[66] As opposed to Healy's stage theory, perhaps a better way of classifying the current oscillation toward difference in women's health research advocacy would be to associate it with so-called postfeminism. That is, such views appear to reflect a perception that the fruits of previous feminist struggles are now being reaped, that those victories are safely entrenched, that women need no longer be concerned about establishing their claims to social equality, and, indeed, that "strident" discourse about "the patriarchy" and suchlike is counterproductive and passé. "It's safe to talk about sex differences again," was how Hara Estroff Marano expressed it in her essay on sex-based biology in *Psychology Today*. "Of course, it's the oldest story in the world. And the newest. But for a while it was also the most treacherous. Now it may be the most urgent. . . . Do we need to explain that difference doesn't imply superiority or inferiority?" Citing feminist icon Simone de Beauvoir's dictum, "One is not born a woman but rather becomes one," Marano effectively drew a separation from an earlier generation of feminism by asserting, "Science suggests otherwise, and it's driving a whole new view of who and what we are."[67]

Leaders of the sex-based biology movement have addressed the sameness/difference debate in somewhat more reflective terms than this, but also in ways that mark their distance from a previous feminist moment. Marianne Legato has written, "It is important to address the concerns of women who resist our concentrating on the differences between the genders, fearful that such an emphasis will once again define women as less fit and able than their male counterparts. In fact, it is important to tell women that our research does not prove them less competent than men. Quite simply, we are finding only that they are different."[68] Similarly, Sherry Marts, the scientific director of SWHR and a sociologist by training, noted the concern among feminists that claims about biological differences "seem to hearken back to that whole 'biology is destiny' thing." But, she added, "the thinking is that hopefully we've come far enough along now that it won't turn into another way to ghettoize women or to cast gender differences in concrete."[69]

In 2005 the question of the extent of innate differences between women and men burst into public consciousness again after Lawrence Summers, the president of Harvard University, was quoted speculating about the reasons why relatively few women were represented in the highest ranks of the sciences and mathematics. Perhaps it had something to do with innate differences, Summers suggested, to the consternation of many, not least among his own faculty.[70] While many commentators were outraged by the suggestion that this social outcome of gender inequality had biological causes, Legato embraced the controversy as an opportunity to advance the agenda of gender-specific medicine. Wrote Legato, "Despite the personal cost to Harvard's president, nothing could have been healthier for the new science of gender-specific medicine than the flurry of discussion his remarks provoked." Legato noted the divergence in public reaction between claims about biomedical differences and claims about differences in intellectual abilities, but her general message was that we should all put emotions aside and embrace the new science of sex:

> Saying that the ingredients and flow rates of our saliva differ as a function of sex is politically neutral; no one is going to be outraged by the fact that the salivary flow rates of males are higher and the sugar content lower than that of their female counterparts. But to point out the many sex-specific differences in brain anatomy and chemistry and in the systems involved in cognition is a different story. And to hypothesize that we are not equally gifted or that we at least excel at different things—and to say so—is the equivalent of loping across a minefield and expecting to reach the other side without incident. Despite the dangers of traveling this path, many institutions are investing huge sums of money and effort into expanding the whole realm of neurobiology—my own university, for one.[71]

Citing the furor that greeted past scientific heroes such as Darwin and Freud when they first proposed their new theories. Legato cast the new science of sex differences as a dragon-slayer that ultimately would succeed in displacing "old and entrenched systems."[72]

At a time when the broader women's health movement has become increasingly heterogeneous, the willingness—indeed, eagerness—to embrace findings or assertions of biological differences by sex is a characteristic way in which the new women's health research advocacy groups distinguish themselves from the politics of those organizations that emerged directly out of the feminist women's health movement of the 1970s and 1980s.[73] However, it is not the only such point of divergence. As Sheryl Burt Ruzek and Julie Becker have described, where groups like the Boston Women's Health Book Collective (the publishers of *Our Bodies, Ourselves*), the National Black Women's Health Project, and the National Women's Health Network have remained tied to other progressive movements for social change, the new advocacy groups have a narrower focus; where the earlier groups often sought to "demedicalize" women's experiences, the new advocacy, often led by women inside medicine and science, seeks to extend scientific scrutiny of their bodies; where the earlier activism sought to empower women as consumers and as patients, the newer advocacy embraces professionalism; and where the earlier activism steered clear of corporate ties (and mostly continues to do so), the new groups depend heavily on funding from the pharmaceutical industry.[74] (Confirming this last point, the SWHR's Corporate Advisory Council reads like a Who's Who of the drug industry, and the financial dues paid by these corporations to the SWHR provide that organization with a substantial part of its operating budget. In addition, Legato's research center at Columbia University was supported by a $2.5 million donation from Proctor & Gamble.[75])

Spokespersons such as Vivian Pinn, the director of the ORWH, are quick to credit the pivotal accomplishments of the feminist women's health movement of the 1970s and 1980s and to point out that "a focus on women's health didn't just start in 1990."[76] However, others have warned that this history is indeed in danger of being lost and its present-day descendants marginalized. According to feminist scholars of medicine Paula Treichler, Lisa Cartwright, and Constance Penley, "this new women's health agenda is founded upon a well-documented history of feminist politics and women's health activism; yet it achieved its present prominence only by obscuring or obliterating its problematic political roots in struggles over abortion, reproductive choice, patient autonomy, and egalitarian ideals of health access for women across class, race, and employment status."[77] A trenchant critique by Anne Eckman has linked the transmutation of women's health politics and the foreshortening of its history precisely to the new emphasis on the pervasiveness of sex differences and a corresponding de-emphasis on reproductive rights. According to Eckman, the shift in attention away from women's reproductive organs and toward bodily differences that are less obviously sex-linked—in the heart, the liver, and so on—"has ironically positioned women's reproduction . . . as peripheral to current efforts to secure equal health and health care for women."[78] At the same time, the presumption of pervasive biological difference between women and men has presupposed a forgetting of feminist critiques of much previous research into sex differences: "Biological sex, extended throughout the whole of a woman's body, has been repositioned as the foundational truth from which women's health research should start. . . . As a result, important questions about the construction of sexual difference as a category of analysis within research—questions at the heart of a well-elaborated feminist and radical critique of science . . . —have not been linked to the production of new biomedical knowledge."[79]

The nondebate over sex profiling

The ideological divides within the broader women's health movement and the concerns about the politics of sex-based biology suggest that there are political stakes in the questions that I posed at the outset of this chapter. Even if there is little public debate over the science of sex differences analogous to that over the science of racial differences, the topic of sex profiling in medicine does merit critical scrutiny. In what ways are the cases of racial profiling and sex profiling similar and in what ways are they different? In the last chapter, I developed six points of critique of racial profiling. In the remainder of this chapter, I consider the applicability of the same potential critiques to determine what we can learn about sex profiling.

The problems with profiling

Improper treatment

Much as with racial profiling, sex profiling poses the risk of improper medical treatment of a patient who doesn't conform to the stereotype that pertains to his or her group. It is noteworthy that so many claims in the sex-based biology literature are framed, at least rhetorically, as universal observations about all women and all men. Florence Haseltine has written that "the female body has more fat and less water"; Marianne Legato's book is called *The Female Heart*.[80] Representations of medically relevant sex differences in the popular press likewise use the language of blanket differences. According to *USA Today*'s magazine, "women are less active and consume less oxygen than men. Rib cages are smaller in women, resulting in lower lung capacity." Also, "Women say 'ouch!' to pain before men do, but tolerate the pain better."[81] At least at the level of rhetoric, such claims appear to divide the universe of human experience into two utterly separate camps, while thoroughly homogenizing all that which lies within each one. Because of the binary and either/or nature of the discourse on sex differences, such claims seem even more all-encompassing and less nuanced than those about racial and ethnic differences in medicine.

Certain sex differences, such as sex-linked traits linked to genes on the X chromosome, may indeed function to demarcate half of humanity from the other half—leaving aside, just for the moment, those individuals whose chromosomal sex is nonstandard. But most of the claims about sex differences are, once again, statements about differences between averages. Clearly it is not the case that all women have smaller rib cages than all men, or that all women say "ouch!" first. Just as the science of statistics has constructed diseases as racial, so statistical processes also result in the sexing of diseases. Stefan Hirschauer and Annemarie Mol have described how this process works using the example of anemia:

> There is nothing inherently sexed about this disease.... [A] normal hemoglobin level differs from one person to the next and has no sex.... Statistical practice turns anemia into a sexed disease. Statistical practice builds on the anatomical differentiation between the sexes and clusters hemoglobin levels of hundreds of people identified anatomically as either males or females. Two curves emerge. The median and cut-off point of the first are a little higher than those of the second. Thus "men" have a higher normal hemoglobin level than do "women."

As Hirschauer and Mol observed, "the sex generated in this way is not one of bodies but is one of populations."[82]

Particularly in the case of the pharmacokinetics and pharmacodynamics of medications, usually the best that can be claimed is a statement about probabilities. Raymond Woosley, the pharmacology expert who has researched the harmful effects of drugs that prolong the QT interval, noted that certain of those drugs affect men and women in strikingly different ways, while, with other drugs, "the most sensitive male [is] equal to the average female, so there is considerable overlap; ... it's a mean difference."[83] Thus, sex profiling in the clinic—drawing a decision about treatment based on knowledge of the patient's sex—may function quite reliably in certain circumstances, while in other circumstances it might raise, the familiar problem of taking statistical generalities about a group and applying them to individual cases. In other words, Hacking's claim, cited at the beginning of this chapter, that "many medical differences between males and females are uniform, but medical differences between races are almost always only statistical," fails to ask the crucial question of just how many medical differences between males and females are statistical as well.

As Judith Lorber has argued, the overriding mistake of so many "epistemologically spurious" studies of sex differences in both the biological and the social sciences is that they begin simply by assuming that "men" and "women" are the relevant groups to compare, look for differences between them, and then attribute whatever they find to the underlying sex difference. Lorber observed: "These designs rarely question the categorization of their subjects into two and only two groups, even though they often find more significant within-group differences than between-group differences."[84]

People and groups differ in an unlimited variety of ways. The problem here—as with race—is when we assume that the ways of differing that are most socially salient and "obvious" are necessarily the ones that carry the most explanatory weight.[85] In the context of clinical care, this becomes dangerous. The unavoidable risk is that some individuals might receive the wrong diagnosis or treatment if they are approached as a representative member of their social group. The hard-and-fast language of binary sex difference makes it particularly difficult to catch sight of this limitation, while the reliance on the group stereotype then serves to reinforce that "hardness" and "fastness."

The ideology of sexual binarism may have additional problematic consequences in the world of medical research. On one hand, it might function to obscure commonalities. In an example suggested by Barbara Hanson, it is not inconceivable that breast cancer and prostate cancer could have a causal factor in common, but the emphasis on studying women's and men's diseases separately makes it less likely that researchers would uncover it.[86] On the other hand, binary logic might work to obscure differences within each sex—by race, class, sexuality, age, or health status. As Sheryl Burt Ruzek, Adele Clarke, and Virginia Olesen have observed, "differences between groups of women may well be as salient as gender status itself in both the production and experience of health and healing."[87] While certain institutional actors within the inclusion-and-difference paradigm, such as the ORWH, are closely attuned to the diversity of women's experiences, many advocates of sex-based biology seem to privilege the universal category of female, while treating aspects of difference largely as an afterthought. For example, a book by the cardiologist Nieca Goldberg entitled *Women Are Not Small Men* makes many essentialist claims about women as a class—that their hearts are different, that they have different symptoms from men, and so on—but then devotes only two pages to "special considerations for women of color."[88]

Dubious associations between sex/gender and medical outcomes

Another way in which sex profiling could cause harm is by creating a tendency to routinely uncover questionable associations between sex/gender and medical outcomes. The arguments made in the previous chapter about race and ethnicity would seem to apply equally well here. As biostatisticians who are suspicious of an automatic turn toward subgroup analyses have argued, "the more questions asked of a set of data, the more likely it will yield some statistically significant difference even if the treatments are in fact equivalent."[89] With sex differences as with race differences, NIH and FDA policies calling for subgroup comparisons may inadvertently promote the generation of spurious findings that may bring about inappropriate or inferior medical care. In the process, the claim that women and men are utterly different becomes a self-fulfilling prophecy. Susan Leigh Star made this point in 1979, in relation to her study of sex differences in the brain: "The very fact of dividing subjects into male and female categories for research purposes may serve to reify and perpetuate a socially created dichotomy. The search for differences can help to create the differences; if you are looking for something you are likely to find it."[90]

Market incentives that may harm patients

Sex-based medicine also may create new opportunities for profit-making within the health sector, in ways that may work to the detriment of patients. In 2002 Zelnorm, a drug made by Novartis to treat irritable bowel syndrome, became the first of two drugs so far approved by the FDA for use only in women, for a condition that affects both sexes. The drug's advantages over a placebo in a mixed-sex population could not be demonstrated with statistical significance.[91] Is Zelnorm the "BiDil" of sex-based prescribing? Again, it is interesting that the advent of the first "ethnic drug" created a stir, while the marketing of the first "gender drug" went unnoticed—no doubt because so many other drugs, such as hormones and most contraceptives, have long been marketed only to women. For advocates of sex-based biology like Sherry Marts, the sex-based marketing of drugs like Zelnorm is a victory that validates their whole approach: if subgroup analyses had not been performed, a drug that brings demonstrable benefit to women would simply have been lost.[92] But of course, in the clinical trials that led to marketing, Zelnorm did not bring benefit to all women, while it did bring benefit to some men. One wonders, then, how often the ability to market to a subgroup will function primarily to provide a pharmaceutical company with a strategy for salvaging products that do not perform adequately in humans overall but, statistically, do so in subpopulations to some degree. If the drug truly brought benefit to women as a class, say, because of a difference related to sex chromosomes, then there would be no argument with sex-specific drug approvals. But if sex is merely a proxy—a crude way of distinguishing some of the drug responders from some of the nonresponders—then our enthusiasm to embrace such marketing might be diminished substantially.

Sex profiling as a permanent "temporary" solution

Just as with racial profiling, advocates of sex profiling describe it as a step on the way toward truly individualized medicine. "Researchers foresee a world in which they will be able to read a patient's DNA to gauge the likely course of the person's disease or response to drugs," wrote Viviana Simon, the Director of Scientific Programs at SWHR, in the special issue on women's health in *Science*: "Until that degree of individualization is possible, patients and doctors must continue to rely on the results of studies carefully designed and analyzed by patient type—including by sex—to obtain the clinical results that are useful and meaningful to the health of both women and men."[93] However, if indeed there are limitations with sex-based prescribing, then the future promise of pharmacogenomics is not guaranteed to mitigate the harm. Pharmaceutical companies are likely to be much more interested in marketing to a "niche" that constitutes half the population than to tiny, genetically distinct segments of the market. And to the extent that sex-specific drug development becomes institutionalized, it is highly questionable whether companies will want to abandon it in favor of more finely individualized treatment. In the meantime, while genetic screening remains unavailable and unaffordable to most people, the characterization of sex-based prescribing as the "next best thing" may endow the latter with a legitimacy that it does not deserve.

Inaccurate and problematic understandings of sex and gender

Yet another problem with sex profiling is that—like racial profiling—it disguises the problems of categorization. The result is to promote misleading views of the nature of sex. In the case of race, the problem of maintaining a stable scientific categorization system is obvious to many, and most will acknowledge it if pressed, even if in practice researchers and policymakers typically charge forward anyway, as if the meanings of categories were clear and settled. In the case of sex, the categorization problem is of a different order. Sex categories do have an obvious biological grounding in the body. But the precise ways in which sexed bodies correspond to our social categories—or fail to do so—are obscured by an overwhelmingly strong ideology of sexual dimorphism: the belief that males and females are utterly distinct, if not opposite, and that no middle ground exists. Thus, sex poses another sort of categorization problem, one that is less easily discernible than that resulting from our classifications by race and one that perhaps is even more deeply inscribed, both historically and cross-culturally.

In biomedicine as in our culture generally, sex is almost always treated as if it were a simple dichotomous variable. The presumptions are that one is either male or female and that the correct designation is not hard to determine—it can, in effect, be "read off" the body. But nature knows no absolute distinctions. There is no unambiguous dividing line between the two sexes, and every criterion of differentiation that might be invoked, from genitalia to hormones to chromosomes, fails to perform a strict demarcating function. According to Anne Fausto-Sterling:

> Are there *no* sex differences? I usually start by saying that there are reproductive differences, although even there the extreme borders get blurred. There are men who produce no sperm and women without ovaries. There are hermaphrodites who have some organs of each sex.... XY females and XX males may not abound, but they exist with a frequency high enough to worry the International Olympic Committee. They require chromosome tests of their female athletes, even though many believe these tests to be useless for telling male from female.[94]

Conventional notions of "male" and "female" fail to do justice to human variation—indeed, according to Fausto-Sterling, "no classification scheme could more than suggest the variety of sexual anatomy encountered in clinical practice."[95] Nor are intersexuals and hermaphrodites "really" just somewhere "in between" the natural poles of male and female.[96] Rather, as Alice Dreger has argued, modern scientific attempts to understand hermaphroditism were part of the process of defining biological sex in the first place.[97] Similarly, as Joanne Meyerowitz and Stefan Hirschauer both have shown, the medical creation and management of the transsexual has involved the practical transformation of the meaning of sex.[98]

Drawing on feminist analyses from the 1970s, social scientists sometimes think of "sex" as the biological bedrock and "gender" as a social and cultural edifice constructed on top of it—or, to use another metaphor, we imagine that sex provides the "raw materials" for the cultural work of defining and performing gender. However, as a range of feminist and science studies scholars have argued in the 1990s and since, cultural ideas about gender attributes have filtered into and shaped scientific conceptions of biological sex itself—in the process endowing sex with the strictly dichotomous character that we take for granted.[99] Nelly Oudshoorn's analysis of early research on sex hormones makes this point elegantly by showing how ideas about masculinity and femininity were attributed to sex hormones by scientists, and how those early-twentieth-century scientists were forced to grapple with the disconcerting realization that women also possessed "male" sex hormones and vice versa.[100] Thus, the classification of individuals into dichotomous sex categories inevitably involves cultural work made possible by a history of definitional acts.

Various authorities, from doctors who perform surgeries on intersexed newborns to the athletic committees referenced by Fausto-Sterling that debate whether athletes compete as male or female, perform the social control function of fitting individuals into categories. Yet the active labor that goes into making sex appear dichotomous is generally invisible to the broader society, or at least, rarely remarked upon. Despite the recent political agitation on the part of intersexuals insisting on their right not to be either male or female, and despite the emergence of surgical options to transform the sex of adults, this notion of clear and reliable sex differences endures.[101] Sex profiling, like racial profiling, both presumes and reinforces a problematic notion that each individual belongs to a category and can be diagnosed and treated accordingly.

*Dangerously inaccurate understandings
of the causes of health disparities*

By clouding the relationship between the biological and the social, sex profiling may interfere with our attempts to understand and eliminate health disparities. Nearly every point that I made about racial profiling applies equally well here—in particular, that the focus on biological differences encourages the inaccurate belief that health disparities by sex are mostly a function of biology and also disguises the role of cultural and social factors. Again, to avoid being misunderstood, it is important to clarify that the point is not that sex differences in health are really social and cultural rather than biological, or really environmental rather than genetic—any "either/or" formulation would be equally problematic and would misconstrue the tight interactive links and developmental loops connecting "nature" and "nurture."[102]

It also bears saying that, within the inclusion-and-difference paradigm generally, the increasing use of the "slash" concept of "sex/gender" (in place of the confused use of "gender" in the early years of the paradigm) functions to create space for research into both biological and social causes of men's and women's illnesses. For example, a 2003 call for funding proposals on "Women's Mental Health and Sex/Gender Differences Research" issued by the National Institute of Mental Health observed that the "pattern of disparities in the epidemiology of mental disorders in males and females provides indirect evidence of hormonal, biological, social, cultural and developmental factors in etiology and course."[103] Often, however, the research program of sex-based biology is as skewed toward the biological as the name would suggest. Yet there is good reason to insist on the serious limitations of biological explanations for health disparities between women and men—beginning with the fact that the most striking disparity of all, women's greater longevity in developed societies, is likely due significantly to social factors.[104] The fact that male "excess mortality" from cardiovascular disease appears to have emerged, in the United States and Britain, only in the 1920s should sound a further cautionary note about the growing tendency to attribute differences between "the male heart" and "the female heart" primarily to consequences of estrogen.[105]

To take another example from the cardiovascular arena, if women's heart attack symptoms are reported to be different from men's, why might this be so? Little discussion has focused on the possibility, supported by research conducted in Scotland, that "women were concerned that reporting their chest pain wasted the doctors' time."[106] Not only do accounts that privilege the biological often deflect our attention from the social organization of gender relations, but sometimes such accounts also serve to naturalize the conditions of gender inequality that in and of themselves may be bad for women's health and well-being.

Race, sex, and the politics of difference

Sex differences and race differences are *different differences*, and invocations of biological explanations in the two cases clearly do not pose precisely the same dilemmas. Nevertheless, my argument has suggested that many of the critiques of racial profiling apply to sex profiling as well, at least in some respects and to some degree. Indeed, although sex profiling is often more defensible then racial profiling, the extremity of many claims about sex differences—the glib imagery of Mars versus Venus, the presumption of fundamental difference at the level of every cell—is a particular point of concern. In my view, therefore, the tendency to engage in sharp boundary work between race and sex, and to accept sex profiling as "obviously" sensible in contrast to the problematic character of racial profiling, is both intellectually misguided and seriously mistaken in terms of health care interventions.

Why is it that, at the present moment in the United States, sex differences are thoroughly reified and naturalized in biomedical research, while the use of race as a proxy has been contested, within the research community and outside of it? Certainly some of the answer lies in the contrast between sex and race as kinds of difference, but perhaps some of the answer has to do with the broader political environments within which claims about sex and race circulate. My reflections on this latter point are necessarily speculative, so I will keep them brief. As I described, while an insistence on equality as sameness was a typical strategy of feminist movements in past decades, in more recent years notions of essential difference appear to provide a strategic wedge especially to certain sectors of the women's health movement. But which sectors? This particular wave of mobilization on women's health research reflects the professionalization of the women's health movement and the concomitant rise of some women (often white and middle-class) to positions of authority and influence within Congress, the Department of Health of Human Services, and biomedical research institutions. This was the constellation of forces that was positioned to press for measures such as the NIH Revitalization Act. For these women, whose relative social equality has been affirmed, conceptions of essential or biological difference appear to pose no substantial political risk. Instead, such essentialism serves as a foundation for their professional agendas.

By contrast, in an era of general retrenchment against affirmative action by race, advocates of biomedical research to benefit people of color stand in a less secure position. Especially given the historical suspicion of clinical research on the part of communities of color, it is not surprising that efforts to promote attention to minority health concerns through an emphasis on biological difference would war against profound concerns that difference will be construed in pejorative terms—indeed, as new justifications for racism. Finally, as social movements organize on behalf of multiracialism and as the discourses of multiracialism become more prevalent in popular culture,[107] racial categories gradually are coming to lose some of their obviousness and appear more arbitrary. Thus, it makes sense that the transposition of social categories of race into biological categories of difference would come under increasing scrutiny. By contrast, despite the efforts of intersexuals and transgender people to "queer" the meanings of "male" and "female," categories of sex and gender are rarely presented in the mass media and popular culture as anything but fixed and natural.

These reflections point to the importance of locating the policies, practices, and philosophies of the inclusion-and-difference paradigm within the broadest possible social and political context, in order to understand what is at stake in the changes that they represent. In the next chapter, I adopt a broad view in order to examine the likely future of the inclusion-and-difference paradigm.

Notes

1 Raymond Woosley, interviewed by author. Woosley maintains a list of pharmaceutical drugs linked to *torsades de pointes* at www.torsades.org. Many of them are associated with sex differences in risk. My account of the Seldane story also draws on Karen Young Kreeger, "The Inequality of Drug Metabolism," *Scientist* 16, no. 6 (March 18, 2002): 29. See also Woosley, Anthony, and Peck, "Biological Sex Analysis in Clinical Research," 933–34; Marietta Anthony, "Male/Female Differences in Pharmacology: Safety Issues with QT-Prolonging Drugs," *Journal of Women's Health* 14, no. 1 (2005): 47–52.
2 Jocelyn Kaiser, "Gender in the Pharmacy: Does It Matter?" *Science* 308, no. 5728 (June 10, 2005): 1572–74.
3 Viviana Simon, "Wanted: Women in Clinical Trials," *Science* 308, no. 5728 (10 June 2005): 1517.
4 Leslie Benet, interviewed by author. See also Benet's comments as quoted in Kaiser, "Gender in the Pharmacy," 1573.
5 Satel, *P.C., M.D.*, 125.
6 My searches for "sex profiling" and "gender profiling" in the National Library of Medicine's "PubMed" database retrieved null results. However, while this book was in production, I learned that Rebecca Young has used the phrase *sex profiling* from a critical perspective that is similar to my own. Rebecca Young, "Sexual Profiling: Contrasting Scientific Perspectives on Women's Health and the Embodiment of Marginality" (talk presented to the Barnard Center for Research on Women, New York City, April 2004).
7 However, Anne Fausto-Sterling is following up on a critical examination of the use of sex and gender categories in one domain of medical research (bone diseases) with a forthcoming article on the use of racial categories in the same domain. See Fausto-Sterling, "Bare Bones of Sex: Part 1."
8 Hacking, "Why Race Still Matters," 106.
9 Root, "Use of Race in Medicine," 1181.
10 For another example of the drawing of a clear distinction between sex and race in order to counter racial profiling in medicine, see Shields et al., "Use of Race Variables in Genetic Studies," 8. On boundary work in science, see the references in the introduction, n. 43.
11 Fausto-Sterling, "Five Sexes"; Anne Fausto-Sterling, "The Five Sexes, Revisited," *Sciences* (July/August 2000): 19–23. I expand on this point later in this chapter.
12 For a characteristic example, see Hara Estroff Marano, "The New Sex Scorecard," *Psychology Today*, July–August 2003, 38–46. On the debate over differences in brain function, see Angier and Chang, "Gray Matter and the Sexes." For critiques of biological reductionism in the understanding of male-female

differences, see Roger N. Lancaster, *The Trouble with Nature: Sex in Science and Popular Culture* (Berkeley: University of California Press, 2003); Harding and O'Barr, *Sex and Scientific Inquiry*; Anne Fausto-Sterling, *Myths of Gender: Biological Theories about Women and Men* (New York: Basic, 1992); Tavris, *Mismeasure of Woman*; Fausto-Sterling, "Five Sexes," 20–26; Wijngaard, *Reinventing the Sexes*; Fausto-Sterling, "Five Sexes, Revisited," 19–23; Anne Fausto-Sterling, *Sexing the Body: Gender Politics and the Construction of Sexuality* (New York: Basic, 2000); Fausto-Sterling, "Bare Bones of Sex."

13 Bob Beale, "The Sexes: New Insights into the X and Y Chromosomes," *Scientist* 23 (July 2001): 18.
14 Mary J. Berg, "Pharmacological Differences between Men and Women," in *Principles of Clinical Pharmacology*, ed. Arthur J. Atkinson et al. (San Diego: Academic Press, 2001), 265–75.
15 Monica Gandhi et al., "Sex Differences in Pharmacokinetics and Pharmacodynamics," *Annual Review of Pharmacology and Toxicology* 44, no. 1 (2004): 499–523.
16 Ibid., 511–12.
17 Ibid., 512–13.
18 "FDA Commissioner & SWHR Outline Critical Steps to Improve Women's Health," *Sex Matters*, fall 2003, 1.
19 See, for example, NIH, Office of Research on Women's Health, "Conference on Biologic and Molecular Mechanisms for Sex Differences in Pharmacokinetics, Pharmacodynamics, and Pharmacogenetics," May 5, 1999, www4.od.nih.gov/orwh/pharmacology.html.
20 Gail D. Anderson, "Sex and Racial Differences in Pharmacological Response: Where Is the Evidence? Pharmacogenetics, Pharmacokinetics, and Pharmacodynamics," *Journal of Women's Health* 14, no. 1 (2005): 25.
21 Rosaly Correa-de-Araujo, "Improving the Use and Safety of Medications in Women through Sex/Gender and Race/Ethnicity Analysis: Introduction," *Journal of Women's Health* 14, no. 1 (2005): 12.
22 "Medscape Women's Health eJournal: Instructions for Authors," www.medscape.com/viewpublication/128_guideline.
23 Doug Bowles, "A Radical Idea: Men and Women Are Different," *Cardiovascular Research* 61, no. 1 (January 2004): 5. See also Robert Preidt, "Nailing Down Differences in Heart Disease," HealthDayNews, December 16, 2003, www.healthscout.com/printer/1/516486/main.html.
24 Amanda Gardner, "The Gender Differences of Heart Disease," HealthScout News Service, February 21, 2004, www.healthday.com/printer.cfm?id=516951.
25 Denise Grady, "Many Women Face Hidden Risk of Heart Disease," *New York Times*, February 1, 2006.
26 Medscape, "Arrhythmias More Common in Men Than Women with Implanted Defibrillators," June 18, 2004, www.medscape.com/viewarticle/481325.
27 Michael E. Mendelsohn and Richard H. Karas, "Molecular and Cellular Basis of Cardiovascular Gender Differences," *Science* 308, no. 5728 (June 10, 2005): 1583–87.
28 Ridker et al., "Randomized Trial of Low-Dose Aspirin"; Mary Duenwald, "Aspirin Is Found to Protect Women from Strokes, Not Heart Attacks," *New York Times*, March 8, 2005, F5.
29 Richard I. Levin, "The Puzzle of Aspirin and Sex," *New England Journal of Medicine* 352, no. 13 (March 31, 2005): 1366. Levin did also observe that the Women's Health Study and the Physicians' Health Study were "not directly comparable," due to the time lag between them and the overall changes in mortality from cardiovascular causes in the interim (1367).

30 Marilynn Marchione, "Study: Aspirin Affects Sexes Differently," *San Diego Union-Tribune*, March 8, 2005, A1; Rob Stein, "Aspirin's Benefits Differ for Women," *Washington Post*, March 8, 2005, A1.
31 Theresa M. Wizemann and Mary-Lou Pardue, *Exploring the Biological Contributions to Human Health: Does Sex Matter?* (Washington, DC: National Academy Press, 2001), x.
32 Ibid., 178–79.
33 See the discussion in the preceding chapter.
34 "Sex Matters," *The NewsHour with Jim Lehrer*, PBS, April 25, 2001.
35 Robert Pear, "Sex Differences Called Key in Medical Studies," *New York Times*, April 25, 2001, A14.
36 Comments at "Science Meets Reality" workshop (author's field notes).
37 Five years later, the organization's president, Phyllis Greenberger, was named one of the one hundred "Most Powerful Women" in Washington, DC, by *Washingtonian* magazine. Society for Women's Health Research, "Society President Named One of 100 Most Powerful Women in Washington," June 6, 2006 www.womenshealthresearch.org/site/News2?page=NewsArticle&id=5808&JServSessionIdr002=6pgqjyjp23.app6b.
38 Florence B. Haseltine, conclusion to *Women's Health Research: A Medical and Policy Primer*, ed. Florence B. Haseltine and Beverly Greenberg Jacobson (Washington, DC: Health Press International, 1997), 331–36.
39 Florence Haseltine, interviewed by author.
40 Marianne J. Legato and Carol Colman, *The Female Heart: The Truth about Women and Coronary Artery Disease* (New York: Simon & Schuster, 1991); Marianne J. Legato, "Men, Women, and Brains: What's Hardwired, What's Learned, and What's Controversial," *Gender Medicine* 2, no. 2 (2005): 59–61.
41 Society for Women's Health Research, "What Is Sex-Based Biology?" www.womenshealthresearch.org/site/PageServer?pagename=hs_sbb.
42 Society for the Advancement of Women's Health Research, "Annual Update on Women's Health Research: Discoveries and Implications" (Eighth Annual Scientific Advisory Meeting of the Society for the Advancement of Women's Health Research, Washington, DC, November 2, 1998).
43 For a few years, the title was changed to the *Journal of Women's Health and Gender-Specific Medicine*.
44 Sherry Marts, interviewed by author.
45 Karen Young Kreeger, "X and Y Chromosomes Concern More Than Reproduction," *Scientist* 16, no. 3 (February 4, 2002).
46 Susan Brenna, "Women's Health: Sex Matters," *New York Magazine*, February 8, 1999.
47 See the Partnership's Web site at www.cumc.columbia.edu/dept/partnership/.
48 Marianne J. Legato, "Why Do We Need an *Association for Gender-Specific Medicine*?" *Journal of Gender-Specific Medicine* 6, no. 1 (2003).
49 See www.gendermedicine.com/default.asp.
50 See womenshealth.stanford.edu/research/.
51 Karen Birmingham, "NIH Funds Gender Biology Research," *Nature Medicine* 6, no. 9 (September 2000): 950.
52 NIH, "Specialized Centers of Research on Sex and Gender Factors Affecting Women's Health (RFA-OD-02-002)" (Washington, DC: U.S. Department of Health & Human Services, December 18, 2001).
53 Viviana Simon et al., "National Institutes of Health: Intramural and Extramural Support for Research on Sex Differences, 2000–2003" (Washington, DC: Society for Women's Health Research, May 2005), www.womenshealthresearch.org/site/DocServer/CRISPreport.pdf. The authors found that the percentage of

funding devoted to the study of sex differences varied significantly from one institute to another, with the highest percentage, nearly 8 percent, at the National Institute on Alcohol Abuse and Alcoholism.

54 Society for Women's Health Research, press release, "Senate Appropriations Committee Instructs the National Institutes of Health to Make 'Sex-Based Biology an Integral Part' of Research," September 20, 2004, www.womenshealthresearch.org/site/News2?page=NewsArticle&id=5477; Correa-de-Araujo, "Improving the Use and Safety of Medications," 13. Recommendations contained in "report language" from Congress are not legally binding, but government agencies tend to take them seriously as indications of strong congressional concern about a topic.

55 Keating and Cambrosio, *Biomedical Platforms*, 19. See also Rae Bucher, "On the Natural History of Health Care Occupations," *Work and Occupations* 15, no. 2 (May 1988): 131–47.

56 Council on Scientific Affairs, American Medical Association, "Featured CSA Report: Women's Health: Sex- and Gender-Based Differences in Health and Disease" (CSA Report 4, I-00, 2000, www.ama-assn.org/ama/pub/print/article/2036-4946.html. Another indicator was the announcement in 2006 of funding from the Fannie E. Rippel Foundation to support investigators performing "sex-difference biomedical research and gender-specific medicine." Fannie E. Rippel Foundation, "Rippel Scholars Program—2006 Competition," April 25, 2006, http://foundationcenter.org/grantmaker/rippel/scholars.pdf.

57 Society for the Advancement of Women's Health Research, *Vive La Différence!* [sic] *A Comprehensive Introduction to Gender-Based Biology*, videotape (Washington, DC: Society for the Advancement of Women's Health Research, 1998).

58 See http://womenshealth.stanford.edu/research/.

59 Elizabeth Shaw, "What Your Doctor Didn't Learn in Med School," *American Health for Women* 17, no. 6 (July/August 1998): 42.

60 Rubin, "Traffic in Women," 179.

61 Nancy Chodorow, *The Reproduction of Mothering: Psychoanalysis and the Sociology of Gender* (Berkeley: University of California Press, 1978).

62 See Echols, *Daring to Be Bad*.

63 Vogel, *Woman Questions*, 111. See also Vogel, *Mothers on the Job*.

64 On symmetric versus asymmetric approaches, see Vogel, *Woman Questions*, 113–18; V. Taylor, *Rock-a-by Baby*, 166–68. I return to the issue of the "equality versus difference" debate in the conclusion.

65 Katha Pollitt, *Reasonable Creatures: Essays on Women and Feminism* (New York: Knopf, 1994), 58.

66 Healy, "Challenging Sameness," 18.

67 Marano, "New Sex Scorecard."

68 Marianne J. Legato, "Gender-Specific Physiology: How Real Is It? How Important Is It?" *International Journal of Fertility and Women's Medicine* 42, no. 1 (1997): 26.

69 Marts, interview.

70 Angier and Chang, "Gray Matter and the Sexes."

71 Legato, "Men, Women, and Brains," 59. Legato did not entirely endorse Summers's remarks; she commented that "what Dr. Summers might have more accurately expressed is that when vast numbers of people are tested, there are well-documented differences in some abilities between the sexes" (60).

72 Ibid., 61. For a critique of claims of sex differences in brain anatomy, see Fausto-Sterling, *Sexing the Body*, 115–45.

73 On the U.S. women's health movement generally, see the references in chap. 3, n. 9.

74 Sheryl Burt Ruzek and Julie Becker, "The Women's Health Movement in the United States: From Grass-Roots Activism to Professional Agendas," *Journal of the American Medical Women's Association* 54, no. 1 (winter 1999): 7; Judy Norsigian, interviewed by author; Julia Scott, interviewed by author; Cynthia Pearson, interviewed by author. Another interesting difference is the increasingly gender-neutral framing of the political project mounted by the medically minded professionals: although clearly the new advocacy groups remain recognizably focused on health as a women's issue, the goal of sex-based biology is promoted in terms of its benefits to both sexes. Marianne J. Legato, "Research on the Biology of Women Will Improve Health Care for Men, Too," *Chronicle of Higher Education*, May 15, 1998, B5. It is worth noting the emergence of a men's sex-based biology movement, as reflected by the launch, in 2004, of the *Journal of Men's Health and Gender.*

75 On SWHR, see www.womenshealthresearch.org/about/corppart.htm; on Legato's Partnership, see Gigi Verna, "Partners to Study Gender Medicine," *American City Business Journal*, March 24, 1997.

76 Vivian Pinn, interviewed by author.

77 Treichler, Cartwright, and Penley, "Paradoxes of Visibility," 5.

78 Eckman, "Beyond 'the Yentl Syndrome,'" 145.

79 Ibid., 149.

80 Haseltine, conclusion to *Women's Health Research*, 333; Legato and Colman, *Female Heart*.

81 "Men and Women Are Different," *USA Today (Magazine)*, April 2003, 8.

82 Hirschauer and Mol, "Shifting Sexes, Moving Stories," 377.

83 Woosley, interview.

84 Judith Lorber, "Believing Is Seeing: Biology as Ideology," *Gender and Society* 7, no. 4 (December 1993): 571. See also Jeanne Mager Stellman and Joan E. Bertin, editorial, "Science's Anti-Female Bias," *New York Times*, June 4, 1990, A23; Joan E. Bertin and Laurie R. Beck, "Of Headlines and Hypotheses: The Role of Gender in Popular Press Coverage of Women's Health and Biology," in *Man-Made Medicine*, ed. Moss, 37–56. Such work draws on an earlier history of critique of scientific studies of sex differences; see, for example, Susan Leigh Star, "Sex Differences and the Dichotomization of the Brain: Methods, Limits and Problems in Research on Consciousness," in *Genes and Gender II*, ed. Hubbard and Lowe, 113–30; Harding and O'Barr, *Sex and Scientific Inquiry*.

85 On this point see Hanson, *Social Assumptions, Medical Categories*.

86 Barbara Hanson, "Gender Blind, Sex Bind: Sex Categories as Problematic to Cancer Research and Intervention" (Annual Meeting of the American Sociological Association, Chicago, August 1999).

87 Sheryl Burt Ruzek, Adele K. Clarke, and Virginia L. Olesen, "What Are the Dynamics of Differences?" in *Women's Health: Complexities and Differences*, ed. Ruzek, Olesen, and Clarke, 52.

88 Nieca Goldberg, *Women Are Not Small Men: Life-Saving Strategies for Preventing and Healing Heart Disease in Women* (New York: Ballantine, 2002). Missing from most of this literature is an understanding of the "intersectionality" of identities. See Crenshaw, "Mapping the Margins." Ironically, in her ethnographic work with sufferers of cardiovascular disease, Janet Shim discovered that understandings of intersectionality are alive and well among laypeople of color. Shim, "Race, Class, and Gender across the Science-Lay Divide." On the implications of intersectionality for health, see also Schulz and Mullings, *Gender, Race, Class, and Health*. On health activism on behalf of women of color, see Avery, "Breathing Life into Ourselves"; Grayson, "Necessity Was the Midwife of Our Politics."

89 Yusuf et al., "Analysis and Interpretation of Treatment Effects," 94.
90 Star, "Sex Differences and the Dichotomization of the Brain," 114–15.
91 Robert Temple, interviewed by author; Pollack, "Drug to Treat Bowel Illness Is Approved by the F.D.A.," A12.
92 Marts, interview.
93 Simon, "Wanted: Women in Clinical Trials," 1517.
94 Fausto-Sterling, *Myths of Gender*, 269.
95 Fausto-Sterling, "Five Sexes."
96 Fausto-Sterling, "Five Sexes, Revisited," 22.
97 Alice Domurat Dreger, *Hermaphrodites and the Medical Invention of Sex* (Cambridge, MA: Harvard University Press, 1998).
98 Hirschauer, "Performing Sexes and Genders in Medical Practices"; Meyerowitz, *How Sex Changed*.
99 J. Butler, *Gender Trouble*; Haraway, *Simians, Cyborgs, and Women*, 127–48; Oudshoorn, *Beyond the Natural Body*; Clarke, *Disciplining Reproduction*; Fausto-Sterling, "Bare Bones of Sex: Part 1," 1493–95.
100 Oudshoorn, *Beyond the Natural Body*; Nelly Oudshoorn, "The Birth of Sex Hormones," in *Feminism and the Body*, ed. Londa Schiebinger, 87–117 (Oxford: Oxford University Press, 2000).
101 Judith Lorber, "Beyond the Binaries: Depolarizing the Categories of Sex, Sexuality, and Gender," *Sociological Inquiry* 66, no. 2 (1996): 143–59; Hirschauer, "Performing Sexes and Genders in Medical Practices"; Kessler, *Lessons from the Intersexed*; Katrina Alicia Karkazis, "Beyond Treatment: Mapping the Connections among Gender, Genitals, and Sexuality in Recent Controversies over Intersexuality" (Ph.D. dissertation, Columbia University, 2002); Meyerowitz, *How Sex Changed*.
102 Krieger, "Embodying Inequality," 296; Fausto-Sterling, "Bare Bones of Sex: Part 1." For an integrated model for the study of biological and social aspects of men's and women's health, see Chloe E. Bird and Patricia P. Rieker, "Gender Matters: An Integrated Model for Understanding Men's and Women's Health," *Social Science & Medicine* 48, no. 6 (March 1999): 745–55.
103 NIH, "Women's Mental Health and Sex/Gender Differences Research (PA-03-143)." June 20, 2003, http://grantsl.nih.gov/grants/guide/pa-files/PA-03-143.html. This program announcement replaced a prior one that used the term *gender*, rather than *sex/gender*.
104 Karen Young Kreeger, "Sex-Based Longevity," *Scientist* 16, no. 10 (May 13, 2002): 34.
105 Sergey V. Nikiforov and Valery B. Mamaev, "The Development of Sex Differences in Cardiovascular Disease Mortality: A Historical Perspective," *American Journal of Public Health* 88, no. 9 (September 1998): 1348–53.
106 H. M. Richards, M. E. Ried, and G. C. Watt, "Why Do Men and Women Respond Differently to Chest Pain? A Qualitative Study," *Journal of the American Medical Women's Association* 57, no. 2 (spring 2002): 79–81.
107 Reynolds Farley, "Racial Identities in 2000: The Response to the Multiple-Race Response Option," in *The New Race Question*, ed. Perlmann and Waters, 33–61; Harris and Sim, "Who Is Multiracial?"

51
GENDER AND THE MEDICALIZATION OF HEALTHCARE

Susan E. Bell and Anne E. Figert

Source: E. Kuhlmann and E. Annandale (eds), *The Palgrave Handbook of Gender and Healthcare*, London: Palgrave, 2010, pp. 107–22.

Introduction

Medicalization is a key concept of modernity, ubiquitously used in the social and medical sciences since the 1970s. We begin by adopting what sociologist Peter Conrad calls its essential meaning: *'defining a problem in medical terms, usually as an illness or disorder, or using a medical intervention to treat it'* (Conrad, 2005: 3, emphasis in the original). In this large and growing field, scholars generally agree that medicalization was a critical – if not fundamental – transformation of the 20th century. As we will show in this chapter, scholars disagree about its definitions, its connection with the dynamics and conceptual apparatuses of modernity and a global economy, and its cultural situatedness.

There are dangers of writing critically about medicalization. One of the dangers, resulting from its conceptual origins, is to assume the binaries of men/women, femininity/masculinity and sex/gender. Another is to get stuck in a Eurocentric frame and to focus empirically on studies of its processes in North America, the UK and 'the west' more generally. This limits the development of medicalization theory. Just as medical anthropologists are increasingly examining US/western biomedicine as sites of ethnographic and cultural analysis, so should sociologists turn their gaze to more international and global concerns.

Although it is a gender-neutral term, the concept of medicalization historically has been linked to women. Most of the early work in sociology was about the medicalization of women's bodies; focused on the process by which conditions were defined and treated from a 'top down' perspective; and gave attention to Anglo-American settings. Recent feminist and gender scholarship has begun to re-imagine what medicalization is, to consider how medicalization affects men and women, and how gendered medicalization is more complicated than dichotomous views allow (Clarke et al., 2003). These reconsiderations reflect developments in sexuality scholarship and the turn in social science research to the study, of global processes.

This chapter incorporates specific examples in gender and sexuality studies to reflect upon the political and theoretical significance of medicalization in people's lives and the implications for global healthcare policy. We ask how men's bodies are medicalized and how this process is similar to or different from women's experience. When sexuality enters into the debate, how do we think about transgendered people and their bodies? How has categorical thinking about gender and sex limited understandings of gendered medicalization?

Much of the early research was guided by theories of professional dominance and/or social construction. Current scholarship has refocused our analytic gaze from the power and authority of the medical profession to consider the active participation of individual patients/consumers/users individually and collectively (Figert, 2010). Informed by this refocus we ask how medicalization occurs within the increasingly complex healthcare system, erosion of physician control and professional dominance, and the expansion of expert patients. What happens when medicalization is actively sought instead of challenged? How have patterns of direct-to-consumer advertising and risk trafficking in some economies (notably the USA and New Zealand), and the global circulation of pharmaceuticals and biomedicine, influenced policy and practice? Pharmaceuticalization, biomedicalization and geneticization are concepts developed to describe and explain these complexities.

Tracing medicalization

The process of medicalization has a long and varied history. Historians and anthropologists document its beginnings in 17th-century western modernization and the application of scientific knowledge (Lock, 2004). The location of medicalization within large-scale social processes, such as modernization, the rise of a positivistic framework for understanding social problems, public health programmes of the modern state, and the emergence of science and the professions, is echoed throughout the historical and anthropological literature. To simplify, medicalization is a process associated with modernity.

The term medicalization itself has its roots in mid- to later 20th-century scholarship in the social sciences and humanities. The early sociological work of the 1970s focused upon the technically competent power and authority of physicians in modern society to define and treat individual patients. At the macro-level, it was pointed out that physicians and their organizational representatives have the authority and professional power in modern society to define and control what is formally recognized as a disorder, sickness or deviance; sociological analyses traced the medicalization process from the top down (Conrad and Schneider, 1980; Zola, 1972). The concept of control was prominent, used to explain consumers' demand (to control and improve upon their physical bodies) as well as medical imperialism (to control deviance through surveillance and the rational application of science to everyday life) and the turn to treatment as opposed to incarceration or punishment for deviance and mental illness (Lock, 2004).

While successful in documenting the process of medicalization in modern medicine, the focus on deviance (from badness to sickness) and on authority and professional control resulted in gender being relatively absent from this early sociological work (Plechner, 2000). Supported by a burgeoning body of feminist scholarship on women's bodies and the concurrent rise of the Women's Health Movements in the USA and western societies, historians, anthropologists and sociologists focused upon the connections between women's bodies and the greater control/medicalization of them by a predominantly male medical profession and a gendered scientific knowledge base. This research initially focused upon gender-specific processes such as childbirth and women's reproductive cycles (Leavitt, 1984; McCrea, 1983).

Most of the sociological scholarship in the 1980s and 1990s continued to take more of a social constructionist approach to medicalization in its examination of the construction of diagnostic categories, professional process and social control of behaviours. Articles by Riessman (1983) and Bell (1987) are noticeable exceptions to the early medical sociology work on medicalization and were important in challenging the idea that medicalization is entirely a top-down process and that women were passive recipients (as opposed to active proponents) of medicalization by a primarily male medical profession. However, feminist work in medical sociology in this period continued to emphasize the unique ways in which women's bodies were more susceptible to medicalization than men's bodies through processes such as childbirth, premenstrual syndrome (PMS) and menopause (Figert, 1996; Plechner, 2000). The literature since the late 1990s has taken a more expansive view of sex/gender to include men's bodies and intersex/transbodies and of recent feminist thought – in particular intersectionality and attention to international, global and transnational processes. Thus Conrad writes:

> Men and masculinity have often been omitted from analyses of medicalization, in part because of the belief that men are not as vulnerable to medical surveillance and control (e.g., monitoring and intervention for medical conditions) as women. But . . . such a belief is no longer tenable.
>
> (2007: 43–4)

In Conrad's work, the absence of a specific mention about men's bodies does not mean that men were absent from the analysis. Men and male bodies were the focus of a few early medicalization studies in sociology, notably of Conrad's own research about hyperactivity and alcoholism, but these studies did not use gender as a lens for understanding (Conrad and Schneider, 2000).

Masculinities and medicalization

As the above statement by Conrad (2007) points out, medicalization studies are now turning their analysis to the male body in order to remedy the equation of gender with women in sociological work. Thus scholars no longer ask *whether* men's bodies are medicalized but how, why and under what circumstances (Riska, 2003). Just as earlier studies of women expanded their focus beyond the reproductive realm, studies of men and medicalization have moved away from the initial focus upon the definition and control over sexuality to address how boys and men are medicalized through attention deficit hyperactivity disorder (ADHD) pharmaceuticals, sexual dysfunction and post-traumatic stress disorder (PTSD) treatments, and the development of the diagnostic category of 'andropause' to apply to ageing male bodies (Rosenfeld and Faircloth, 2006). Scholarly attention to the medicalization of men's sexuality continues, but the focus is less on the definitions and professional control of homosexuality than on the medicalization of heterosexual male sexuality, specifically, pharmaceutical interventions for male erections (Loe, 2004). Annandale and Riska argue that:

> [a]lthough the empowerment of consumers and the increased importance of the pharmaceutical industry – the so-called medical industrial complex – have been identified as independent actors in the construction of disease categories in general and medicalization in particular ... the gendered implications of this development have been insufficiently realized to date.
>
> (2009: 127)

So where to go with this burgeoning field? All of these works on both men and women still assume sex and gender as categories of modernity. That is, studies distinguish sex from gender; they take for granted the biological category of recognized (and fixed) sex differences and the socially constructed categories of those we call men and women or homosexual and heterosexual. As Epstein points out:

> In biomedicine as in our culture generally, sex is almost always treated as if it were a simple dichotomous variable. The presumptions are that one is either male or female and that the correct designation is

not hard to determine – it can, in effect, be 'read off' the body. But nature knows no absolute distinctions. There is no unambiguous dividing line between the two sexes, and every criterion of differentiation that might be invoked, from genitalia to hormones to chromosomes, fails to perform a strict demarcating function.

(2007: 253)

Early studies in the field of sexuality unpacked the meanings of sex, sexuality and sexual identity and traced the social construction of the categories of homosexuality and heterosexuality. The contribution of these studies to understanding medicalization and masculinity is that they demonstrate the social construction of sexuality, sexual identity and homosexuality and begin to unpack the binaries of heterosexuality/homosexuality and man/woman.

Sexualities and medicalization

It is important to understand how and why men's bodies are also medicalized, but this area of scholarship does not necessarily problematize the sex of the human body. The work in the field of sexuality studies and the history of the medicalization of homosexuality which treats sex and the human body as problematic is foundational to our understanding of trans- and intersex today (Foucault, 1978).

Whereas homosexual behaviours are known to exist in the historical record and in all societies, and the category of homosexual was created and medicalized from the 19th century, transsexuals did not appear or were conflated with homosexuals before the 20th century. As Anne Fausto-Sterling (2000) argues, the 'modern' transsexual could not exist until the availability of hormones and surgery for changing bodies, and these technologies were developed and controlled by medicine. Before the availability of hormones and surgery for changing their bodies, women could pass as men (and vice versa) with clothing, appearance and performance. After the technologies were developed the possibility of 'transsexuals' emerged, but only by gaining access to these technologies. Access was secured when:

> ... transsexuals convinced their doctors that they had become the most stereo-typical members of their sex-to-be. Only then would physicians agree to create a medical category that transsexuals could apply in order to obtain surgical treatment.
>
> (Fausto-Sterling, 2000: 253)

Much like the early literature on women and medicalization, sexuality scholars are quick to point out that trans people were not 'medical dupes' (Rubin, 2006). Transsexuals were dependent on their medical care providers, but their use of the conceptual and material apparatus exemplifies how medicalization became a strategy for those wishing to become transsexuals (Rubin, 2006).

Harry Benjamin introduced the medical category of transsexual in the 1950s to advocate for and to treat people who wanted to permanently change their physical bodies into those of a different gender. Today 'gender identity disorder' is found in the latest version of the official diagnostic manual of the American Psychiatric Association (APA, 2000). A new generation of trans activists and mental health practitioners points out harmful effects of the medicalized (psychiatric) 'disorder'. Samons writes:

> In its current diagnostic form, only a small minority of transgender people benefit from the mental health diagnosis of gender identity disorder. Only a very few have [health] insurance that will pay for any kind of treatment [. . .] It is a dubious benefit that only a few receive but for which the entire population of transgender people pays the price: the social stigma that results from this labeling of transgender as a mental illness through the existence and use of this diagnosis.
> (Samons, 2009: xxvi)

To put it in terms of medicalization and gender, many transgender people are actively choosing not to pathologize or medicalize their bodies at the same time that they are actively challenging western and modern concepts of what it means to connect bodies with (sexual and gender) identities. 'Agnes' is one of the more famous cases of trans identity that was documented by the sociologist Harold Garfinkel in the 1960s. As told by Garfinkel (2006[1967]: 58), Agnes presented herself to the Gender Identity Clinic in Los Angeles as someone who was 'a girl' born in a male body that had 'spontaneously begun to feminize at puberty'. Agnes was diagnosed by the doctors at the clinic as having a rare intersexual condition, 'testicular feminization syndrome'. As a result of this diagnosis, Agnes was *allowed* to have a sex reassignment. It was later revealed that Agnes had deliberately lied to her doctors and had taken feminizing hormones before coming to the clinic in order to get past the diagnoses required for the operation (Garfinkel, 2006 [1967]).

While Agnes lied about her body, there are babies born every year with either ambiguous genitalia or where their genitalia are not consistent with their sex chromosomes. Estimates vary widely, but forms of intersexuality have always existed in the written human record (see Fausto-Sterling, 2000). Trans activists challenge the medical and scientific concept of sex and gender binarism, but as Preves points out, sexual surgery is not simply a practice resulting from medical imperialism: 'People who are sexually ambiguous and their families (may) also desire some semblance of normalcy in relation to social expectations of sex and gender' and seek sexual surgery to achieve 'gender binarism', and adopt medical language and categories to make sense of and talk about their experiences (Preves, 2003: 39). This acceptance of medicalized sexuality can make it difficult for intersex individuals 'to question medical opinion or authority, or to seek alternative care' (Preves, 2003: 45).

Expanding the medicalization frame: pharmaceuticalization, biomedicalization and geneticization

Today, scholars are questioning the usefulness of 'medicalization' as a sufficient framework 'in an age dominated by complex and often contradictory interactions between medicine, pharmaceutical companies, and culture at large' (Metzl and Herzig, 2007: 697). Physician power and authority (so important to early theories of medicalization) is changing in the west and indeed waning as a result of healthcare reforms and direct-to-consumer advertising of pharmaceuticals (in the USA and New Zealand) (Rose, 2007). Scholars are demonstrating the differential impact of biomedicalization and pharmaceuticalization across the globe such as found in demands for safe and cost-effective drug treatments for tuberculosis and HIV/AIDS (Petryna et al., 2006). To put it bluntly,

> some people are more medically made up than others – women more than men, the wealthy differently from the poor, children more than adults, and ... differently in different countries and regions of the world.
>
> (Rose, 2007: 700)

Whereas some populations in some areas of the world are (over)medicalized, other populations in other parts of the world are undermedicalized, and medicalization scholarship suffers from insufficient attention to these differences and their consequences for global health and healthcare. During their travels through the disciplines and among different sociological cultures, scholars have expanded the definition of medicalization and introduced new terms to capture its dynamics in more subtle and nuanced ways (Clarke et al., 2010). Notable among these terms are pharmaceuticalization (Biehl, 2004), biomedicalization (Clarke et al., 2003) and geneticization (Lippman, 1991), which overlap with and provide an analytical focus to particular strands in medicalization.

Pharmaceuticalization

Williams and colleagues have defined pharmaceuticalization thus:

> [it] refers to the transformation of human conditions, capacities or capabilities into pharmaceutical matters of treatment or enhancement. As such it overlaps with but extends far beyond the realms of the

medical or the medicalised, and serves further to blur the boundaries between treatment and enhancement.

(Williams et al., 2008: 850)

Pharmaceuticalization maps on to global patterns of wealth and poverty, power and inequality and extends the concept of medicalization beyond the influence of the medical profession on a person's health or body to include dynamics among states, NGOs and pharmaceutical companies (Busfield, 2006; Petryna et al., 2006). Attention to the global dynamics of pharmaceuticals is not new, although the dynamics have been transformed in the 50 years since feminist scholars and activists in Women's Health Movements looked critically at the development of the birth control pill and other reproductive technologies (Boston Women's Health Book Collective, 1973; Hartmann, 1987; Roberts, 1997). A recent study of the emergence and contested use of the human papillomavirus (HPV) vaccine for cervical cancer illustrates how the new pharmaceuticalization frame can be applied to understanding the permeation of sexual and reproductive technologies 'with meanings of sex/gender' and their role in the politics of gender and sexuality in social relations (Casper and Carpenter, 2008: 886). In richer countries, pharmaceuticalization combines

> the biological effect of a chemical on human tissue, the legitimacy of a condition as a disease, the willingness of consumers to adopt the technology as a 'solution' to a problem in their lives, and the corporate interests of drug companies. Together, these factors [transform] aspects of daily life into disease categories alongside the pharmaceutical agents that 'treat' them.
>
> (Fox and Ward, 2008: 865)

In these settings, pharmaceutical companies are either highlighting daily life choices, such as sleeping through the night, or publicizing new conditions and illnesses to gain more customers or consumers of their products (Fox and Ward, 2008). For example, the HPV vaccine is being widely marketed to girls and young women (but not boys or men) in the USA and UK, although most (80–85 per cent) of the annual deaths from cervical cancer are in developing countries (Casper and Carpenter, 2008). Direct-to-consumer advertising (DTCA) reflects global inequalities and contributes to medicalization in many ways. Conrad and Leiter state:

> Direct-to-consumer advertising for prescription medications has fuelled the medicalization that analysts noted as increasing in Western societies in the 1980s ... DTCA has become a major source of expanding medical markets and public engagement with medical solutions for life's conditions and problems.
>
> (2008: 829)

In addition, DTCA has 'changed the ways physicians and patients speak and listen to each other' (Metzl, 2007: 704). DTCA has also amplified, and in some cases changed, cultural expectations about illness and health, medication prescription and use and, in some ways, normalized the medicalization of the gendered body. Currently, television and radio broadcast advertising of prescription drugs or pharmaceuticals directly to consumers is permitted only in the USA and New Zealand. It is prohibited in the UK and most developed countries.

The globalization of pharmaceutical development has also produced new subjectivities through medicalization. The first is the creation of a need for pharmaceutically naïve subject populations to sustain clinical research and development and the expansions of markets (Petryna et al., 2006). This in turn opens the possibility for individuals and communities to gain access to resources and power and opportunities for citizenship. Other new subjectivities produced through pharmaceuticalization are 'pharmaceutical citizenship' or 'therapeutic citizenship', which can be tools for gaining access to resources and power (Biehl, 2004; Nguyen, 2005).

AIDS policy in Brazil illustrates how pharmaceutical citizenship through the medicalization of HIV/AIDS can be a new democratic tool for individuals, activist groups and states (Biehl, 2004). The Brazilian government joined with the World Bank in 1992 to create a National AIDS Program and by 1996 had begun to provide free antiretroviral drugs to all registered AIDS cases in the country. People with HIV/AIDS who were previously marginalized (noncitizens), claimed 'a new identity around their politicized biology, with the support of international and national, public and private funds' and through their social and biomedical inclusion became 'biomedical citizens' (Biehl, 2004: 122, 123). More importantly, AIDS activists successfully forced the Brazilian government to allow compulsory licensing of patented drugs during a declared public health crisis. In this respect, this therapeutic citizenship comes to represent a biomedicalized form of the state (Nguyen, 2005). Biological notions of citizenship – such as being HIV-positive – are used to ascribe an essentialized identity such as sex or race (Nguyen, 2005). An important effect of selective forms of biomedical citizenship such as the one in Brazil is that they systematically make some people visible and others invisible: 'bureaucratic procedures, informational difficulties, sheer medical neglect and moral contempt, and unresolved disputes over diagnostic criteria' all contribute to turning some people into 'absent things' (Biehl, 2004: 119).

Making visible these macro-processes and their gendered dimensions is key to disentangling how pharmaceuticalization and medicalization are connected, as well as to understanding how they can contribute to the creation of new democratic tools for individuals, activist groups and states and to new possibilities for entering into the grip of (medical) power. Because pharmaceuticalization has occurred so recently, we are just beginning to see how medicalization might work differently (or similarly) for global pharmaceuticalization processes and what the gender implications of this are.

Biomedicalization

Gender is inherently built into the framework of biomedicalization theory. The era of biomedicalization emerged in the mid-1980s along with changes in high-tech biomedical interventions designed not only for treatment but also for health maintenance, enhancement and optimization (Clarke et al., 2010). Biomedicalization regulates bodies not only by offering

> 'control over' one's body through medical intervention (such as contraception), but also by 'transformation of' ones' body, selves, health. Thereby new selves and identities (mother, father, walker, hearer, beautiful, sexually potent person) become possible.
> (Clarke et al., 2003: 182)

According to Clarke and colleagues, the addition of the prefix 'bio' to 'medicalization' produces a concept that encompasses

> the transformations of both the human and nonhuman made possible by such technoscientific innovations as molecular biology, biotechnologies, genomization, transplant medicine, and new medical technologies.
> (Clarke et al., 2003: 162)

A significant proportion of scholarship in this field takes a feminist approach to biomedicalization, in part because of the commitment to feminist health scholarship by those who developed the concept. As Mamo and Fosket put it, 'female corporeality and subjectivity are understood as constituted in and through (cultural) practices of (techno)science' (2009: 927). That is, bodies are simultaneously 'objects and effects of technoscientific and biomedical discourse' (Mamo and Fosket, 2009: 927). Biomedicalization has been employed to examine how gendered subjectivities and forms of embodiment are produced in lesbian practices of assisted reproduction, breast cancer prevention technologies, pharmaceutical interventions for male erections, and contraception/menstruation (see Fosket, 2004; Mamo, 2007).

Proponents of biomedicalization argue that, whereas gender is conceived of categorically in medicalization scholarship, gender is an effect of power, 'produced in relations'. This conception of gender is aligned with postmodern feminist scholarship in which gender is not a stable, given status but an outcome of performance. Gender is also not a privileged status, but one that is produced in intersections with race, 'class, sexuality, disability, and so on' as a result of 'selective and uneven biomedical efforts to transform, regulate, and optimize bodies and futures' (Clarke et al., 2010). Although the concept of biomedicalization does not necessarily privilege gender, it takes gendered bodies seriously. To date most scholarship in this field has given attention to the study of biomedicalization processes in the USA and is only beginning to look transnationally. Whereas pharmaceuticalization scholarship is de-emphasizing gender and emphasizing transnational processes, biomedicalization is inherently gendered but more western in its focus.

The challenge of biomedicalization for gender and medicalization studies is very persuasive. It came into being as process and concept along with postmodernity, and is capable of tracking multistranded workings of gendered power and knowledge. At the same time, because biomedicalization has begun to circulate so recently, maybe it is too soon to know how fully it captures what is going on in the postmodern world and to know whether it will take off and be taken up among scholars in the way medicalization has.

Geneticization

Geneticization is a concept proposed in the early 1990s by Abby Lippman to capture a new way of seeing and solving problems that reduces individual differences of race, gender and nationality to DNA codes:

> [It is] an ongoing process by which differences between individuals are reduced to their DNA codes, with most disorders, behaviors and physiological variations defined, at least, as genetic in origin. It refers as well to the process by which interventions employing genetic technologies are adopted to manage problems of health.
>
> (Lippman, 1991: 19)

Lippman observed that in popular discourse genetic variations were increasingly defined as problems for which there were medical solutions. At the time when she proposed the concept of geneticization, prenatal testing was the most widely used and familiar genetic activity; Lippman gave attention to women's stories about prenatal diagnosis to exemplify geneticization. This line of work has continued (Finkler, 2001) and its gender dimensions expanded to include men and men's stories about their responses to premarital carrier matching and other genetic tests (Raz and Atar, 2004).

Scholars disagree about the extent to which the processes of geneticization and medicalization overlap, but all of them agree that there are important differences between the two. Gusterson (2001: 252) argues that medicalization 'cannot convey the novelty and power' of the processes and a new way of seeing made possible by genetic research. Conrad distinguishes between medicalization, which does not 'require specific claims about cause, although the assumption is often biological' and geneticization, which 'is very specific about where at least part of the cause lies' (2000: 329). In a recent study of the relationship between medicalization and genetics in mental illness, homosexuality and susceptibility to chemical exposures, Shostak and colleagues (2008: S310) identify different patterns: 'genetic information does not always lead to geneticization, nor does geneticization inevitably lead to medicalization.' But where geneticization is a useful concept for us lies in its potential to link both gender and transnational processes of medicalization. For example, the development and circulation of Assisted Reproductive Technologies, so important in the development of geneticization as a concept within a US/western framework, has been recently studied in a range of different populations, from lesbians in the USA and UK, to Bedouin Muslim women in Israel, and throughout the world (Inhorn, 2006; Mamo, 2007; Raz and Atar, 2004).

Conclusion

We have argued in this chapter that medicalization is a capacious concept, but it does not fully capture the related but unique processes of biomedicalization, pharmaceuticalization and geneticization, especially when examining issues of sex, gender and sexuality in relation to health and healthcare. There is certainly a fair amount of overlap, but even such a powerful term as medicalization is not quite adequate to fully capture what is going on in the globalized world at the start of the 21st century precisely because its very definition is rooted in modernity and categorical thinking. At the same time, the concept of medicalization is worth holding on to. It is widely accepted and employed not only among scholars but also among the public. It wields cultural authority and can explain how control over medical phenomena is produced, accomplished, resisted and transformed. Its connection with modernity and modern processes of control, regulation, knowledge and power make its reach and impact partial. In a world where postmodern forms of knowledge and power circulate, medicalization as a process is too simple and as a concept too narrow for capturing the gendered circulation of pharmaceuticals, genetics and technoscience. We argue that we still need to use the concept of medicalization as our starting point or analytic wedge to explore the larger question of 'what has happened to gender?'

Early critiques of medicalization repeatedly demonstrated its gendered dimensions by pointing out how and why women's bodies, life cycles and experiences are more likely to be medicalized than men's. As we have argued, connections between women's health and medicalization continue to be a rich resource for scholarly work, but more recent critiques have expanded the category of gender to include boys, men and transgendered people.

In the social sciences and the history of women's health, there is a long and established tradition of explaining the medicalization of women's bodies. Women have been both active participants in this medicalization and the object of sexist, racist and class-based policies and practices, especially surrounding reproductive issues. These gendered concerns have continued and elaborated with the conceptual tools offered by pharmaceuticalization, geneticization and especially biomedicalization. In addition, gender scholars have pushed the binaries of sex/gender/sexuality, and their work has informed that of medicalization scholars. The real danger, however, arises if this expansion allows scholars to turn away from the study of women and the various ways that the new processes of biomedicalization, pharmaceuticalization and geneticization continue to impact women as well as men, and trans and intersex bodies. With the disintegration of categorical frameworks and the expansion of subjectivities, how can gender be privileged and women included?

Although scholarship about medicalization is generally sharply critical, medicalization is not always a bad thing. For example, for those women globally who want to become mothers, participation in medicine (technology, services, knowledge) can be a strategy to accomplish what they perceive to be in their best interests. Childbearing is a key practice; evidence repeatedly shows how, why and with what consequences women seek medical assistance to achieve (biological) motherhood. In this case, medicalization is strategic (Inhorn, 2006). Additionally, new subjectivities are produced through the processes of medicalization and the conceptual frameworks for understanding them. These include 'transsexual', 'naive subjects', and 'pharmaceutical or therapeutic citizenship'. As Lock relates,

> paradoxically, [the process of] medicalization has actually promoted ... reflection by presenting people with choice, although globalization rather than medicalization per se has no doubt been the major driving force for change. The result is that older hegemonies have crumbled, only to give way to new ones, most often in the form of knowledge that comes under the rubric of science.
>
> (2004: 119)

Medicalization is sometimes, but not always, the right tool for the job of understanding complicated, global, multi-sited processes of gendered biomedical transformations today. Gender shows us how and why we need to fine-tune our thinking when we try to understand, intervene in, and improve healthcare. By continually expanding the concept of medicalization we risk losing its power to capture the processes and consequences of defining problems in medical terms and using medical interventions to treat them. At the same time, without the nuance provided by concepts such as biomedicalization, pharmaceuticalization and geneticization, we also risk losing the ability to capture these very real processes. Medicalization is a capacious concept that is a beginning but not the end of understanding gender and the medicalization of health and healthcare.

Summary

- Medicalization theory has shifted away from the initial focus on professional dominance to include active participation of patients/consumers.
- Medicalization theory has expanded. It has moved away from its initial focus on women to include men and it has moved away from a dichotomous view, for example, of homosexuality/heterosexuality, to sexualities that include trans and intersex.
- Medicalization is now a global process.
- The processes of geneticization, pharmaceuticalization and biomedicalization overlap with and extend beyond the processes of medicalization.

Key reading

Busfield, J. (2006) 'Pills, Power, People: Sociological Understandings of the Pharmaceutical Industry', *Sociology*, 40 (2), 297–314.

Clarke, A., E. L. Mamo, J. R. Fishman, J. K. Shim and J. R. Fosket (2003) 'Biomedicalization: Technoscientific Transformations of Health, Illness, and U.S. Biomedicine', *American Sociological Review*, 68 (April), 161–94.

Conrad, P. (2007) *The Medicalization of Society: On the Transformation of Human Conditions into Treatable Disorders* (Baltimore: Johns Hopkins University Press).

Rosenfeld, D. and C. Faircloth (eds) (2006) *Medicalized Masculinities* (Philadelphia: Temple University Press).

Acknowledgements

We would like to acknowledge Allan Brandt, Ellen Annandale and Ellen Kuhlmann who gave us valuable comments on a draft of the chapter. Susan Bell is grateful for support from the Fletcher Research Fund, Bowdoin College.

References

APA – American Psychiatric Association (2000) *Diagnostic and Statistical Manual of Mental Disorders, Fourth Edition (DSM-IV)* (Washington, DC: American Psychiatric Association).

Annandale, E. and E. Riska (2009) 'New Connections: Towards a Gender-Inclusive Approach to Women's and Men's Health', *Current Sociology*, 57 (2), 123–33.

Bell, S. E. (1987) 'Changing Ideas: The Medicalization of Menopause', *Social Science & Medicine*, 24 (6), 535–42.

Biehl, J. (2004) 'The Activist State: Global Pharmaceuticals, AIDS, and Citizenship in Brazil', *Social Text*, 22 (3), 105–32.

Boston Women's Health Book Collective (1973) *Our Bodies, Ourselves* (New York: Simon and Schuster).

Busfield, J. (2006) 'Pills, Power, People: Sociological Understandings of the Pharmaceutical Industry', *Sociology*, 40 (2), 297–314.

Casper, M. J. and L. M. Carpenter, (2008) 'Sex, Drugs, and Politics: The HPV Vaccine for Cervical Cancer', *Sociology of Health and Illness*, 30 (6), 886–99.
Clarke, A., E. L. Mamo, J. R. Fishman, J. K. Shim and J. R. Fosket (2003) 'Biomedicalization: Technoscientific Transformations of Health, Illness, and U.S. Biomedicine', *American Sociological Review*, 68 (April), 161–94.
Clarke, A., J. Shim, L. Mamo, J. R. Fosket and J. R. Fishman (eds) (2010) *Biomedicalization: Technoscience and Transformations of Health, Illness and US Biomedicine* (Durham, NC: Duke University Press).
Conrad, P. (2000) 'Medicalization, Genetics, and Human Problems', in C. E. Bird, P. Conrad and A. M. Fremont (eds), *Handbook of Medical Sociology, Fifth Edition* (Upper Saddle River: Prentice Hall), 322–33.
Conrad, P. (2005) 'The Shifting Engines of Medicalization', *Journal of Health and Social Behavior*, 46 (1), 3–14.
Conrad, P. (2007) *The Medicalization of Society: On the Transformation of Human Conditions into Treatable Disorders* (Baltimore: Johns Hopkins University Press).
Conrad, P. and V. Leiter (2008) 'From Lydia Pinkham to Queen Levitra: Direct-to-Consumer Advertising and Medicalisation', *Sociology of Health and Illness*, 30 (6), 825–38.
Conrad, P. and J. Schneider (1980) *Deviance and Medicalization: From Badness to Sickness* (St Louis: Mosby).
Epstein, S. (2007) *Inclusion: The Politics of Difference in Medical Research* (Chicago: University of Chicago Press).
Fausto-Sterling, A. (2000) *Sexing the Body: Gender Politics and the Construction of Sexuality* (New York: Basic Books).
Figert, A. E. (1996) *Women and the Ownership of PMS* (Hawthorne: Aldine de Gruyter).
Figert, A. E. (2010) 'The Consumer Turn in Medicalization: Future Directions with Historical Foundations', in B. Pescosolido, J. Martin, J. McLeod and A. Rogers, (eds), *The Handbook of the Sociology of Health, Illness and Healing: Blueprint for the 21st Century* (New York: Springer).
Finkler, K. (2001) 'The Kin in the Gene: The Medicalization of Family and Kinship in American Society', *Current Anthropology*, 42 (2), 235–63.
Fosket, J. R. (2004) 'Constructing "High-Risk" Women: The Development and Standardization of a Breast Cancer Risk Assessment Tool', *Science, Technology and Human Values*, 29 (3), 291–313.
Foucault, M. (1978) *History of Sexuality, Vol. 1, An Introduction* (New York: Random House).
Fox, N. J. and K. J. Ward (2008) 'Pharma in the Bedroom . . . and the Kitchen . . . the Pharmaceuticalisation of Daily Life', *Sociology of Health and Illness*, 30 (6), 856–68.
Garfinkel, H. (2006 [1967]) 'Passing and the Managed Achievement of Sex Status in an "Intersexed" Person', in S. Stryker and S. Whittle (eds), *The Transgender Studies Reader* (New York: Routledge), 58–93.
Gusterson, H. (2001) 'Comment: The Kin in the Gene', *Current Anthropology*, 42 (2), 251–2.
Hartmann, B. (1987) *Reproductive Rights and Wrongs: The Global Politics of Population Control and Contraceptive Choice* (New York: Harper and Row).

Inhorn, M. C. (2006) 'Defining Women's Health: A Dozen Messages from More than 150 Ethnographies', *Medical Anthropology Quarterly*, 20 (3), 345–78.

Leavitt, J. W. (ed.) (1984) *Women and Health in America* (Madison: University of Wisconsin Press).

Lippman, A. (1991) 'Prenatal Genetic Testing and Screening: Constructing Needs and Reinforcing Inequities', *American Journal of Law & Medicine*, 17 (1&2), 15–50.

Lock, M. (2004) 'Medicalization and the Naturalization of Social Control', in C. W. Ember and M. Ember (eds), *Encyclopedia of Medical Anthropology: Health and Illness in the World's Cultures*, vol. 1 (New York: Lower Academic/Plenum Publishers), 116–24.

Loe, M. (2004) *The Rise of Viagra* (New York: New York University Press).

Mamo, L. (2007) *Queering Reproduction: Achieving Pregnancy in the Age of Technoscience* (Durham, NC: Duke University Press).

Mamo, L. and J. R. Fosket (2009) 'Scripting the Body: Pharmaceuticals and the (Re)Making of Menstruation', *Signs*, 34 (3), 926–49.

McCrea, F. (1983) 'The Politics of Menopause: The "Discovery" of a Deficiency Disease', *Social Problems*, 31 (1), 111–23.

Metzl, J. M. (2007) 'If Direct-to-Consumer Advertisements Come to Europe: Lessons from the USA', *The Lancet*, 369, 704–6.

Metzl, J. M. and R. M. Herzig (2007) 'Medicalisation in the 21st Century: Introduction', *The Lancet*, 369, 697–8.

Nguyen, V. (2005) 'Antiretroviral Globalism, Biopolitics and Therapeutic Citizenship', in A. Ong and S. J. Collier (eds), *Global Assemblages: Technology, Politics, and Ethics as Anthropological Problems* (Malden: Blackwell), 124–44.

Petryna, A., A. Lakoff and A. Kleinman (eds), (2006) *Global Pharmaceuticals: Ethics, Markets, Practices* (Durham, NC: Duke University Press).

Plechner, D. (2000) 'Women, Medicine, and Sociology – Thoughts on the Need for a Critical Feminist Perspective', *Research in the Sociology of Health Care*, 18, 69–94.

Preves, S. E. (2003) *Intersex and Identity: The Contested Self* (New Brunswick: Rutgers University Press).

Raz, A. E. and M. Atar (2004) 'Upright Generations of the Future: Tradition and Medicalization in Community Genetics', *Journal of Contemporary Ethnography*, 33 (3), 296–322.

Riessman, C. K. (1983) 'Women and Medicalization: A New Perspective', *Social Policy*, 14 (Summer), 3–18.

Riska, E. (2003) 'Gendering the Medicalization Thesis', *Advances in Gender Research*, 7, 61–89.

Roberts, D. (1997) *Killing the Black Body: Race, Reproduction, and the Meaning of Liberty* (New York: Vintage Books).

Rose, N. (2007) 'Beyond Medicalisation', *The Lancet*, 369, 700–2.

Rosenfeld, D. and C. Faircloth (eds) (2006) *Medicalized Masculinities* (Philadelphia: Temple University Press).

Rubin, H. (2006) 'The Logic of Treatment', in S. Stryker and S. Whittle (eds), *The Transgender Studies Reader* (New York: Routledge), 482–98.

Samons, S. (2009) *When the Opposite Sex Isn't: Sexual Orientation in Male-to-Female Transgender People* (New York: Routledge).

Shostak, S., P. Conrad and A. V. Horwitz (2008) 'Sequencing and its Consequences: Path Dependence and the Relationships Between Genetics and Medicalization', *American Journal of Sociology*, 114, S287–S316.

Williams, S. J., C. Seal, S. Boden, P. Lowe and D. L. Steinberg (2008) 'Waking Up to Sleepiness: Modafinil, the Media and the Pharmaceuticalisation of Everyday/ Night Life', *Sociology of Health and Illness*, 30 (6), 839–55.

Zola, I. (1972) 'Medicine as an Institution of Social Control', *Sociological Review*, 20 (4), 497–504.

52

GENDERING THE MIGRAINE MARKET

Do representations of illness matter?

Joanna Kempner

Source: *Social Science & Medicine*, 63 (2006), 1986–97.

Abstract

Migraine is a common, debilitating and costly disorder. Yet help-seeking for and rates of diagnosis of migraine are low. Drawing on ethnographic observations of pharmaceutical marketing practices at professional headache conferences and a content analysis of migraine advertising, principally in the USA, this paper demonstrates: (1) that the pharmaceutical industry directs its marketing of migraine medication to women; and (2) as part of this strategy, pharmaceutical advertisements portray women as the prototypical migraine sufferer, through representations that elicit hegemonic femininity. This strategy creates the impression that migraine is a "women's disorder", which, in turn, exacerbates gender bias in help seeking and diagnosis of migraine and reifies presumptions about the epidemiology of the disorder. I conclude that these pharmaceutical marketing practices have a paradoxical effect: even as they educate and raise awareness about migraine, they also create barriers to help seeking and diagnosis.

© 2006 Elsevier Ltd. All rights reserved.

Introduction

Migraine is a common, debilitating and costly disorder. Epidemiologists estimate that 23.6 million Americans over the age of 12 have a migraine each year, three quarters of whom are women (Lipton, Stewart, Diamond, Diamond, & Reed, 2001). Pain ranges from mild to severe, but even moderate migraines can leave people in bed for several hours. In severe cases, a migraine can incapacitate a sufferer for days or more (Ruiz de Velasco, Gonzalez, Etxeberria, & Garcia-Monco, 2003). This disability decreases quality of life (Terwindt, Launder, & Ferrari, 2000) and has significant economic effects. In the aggregate, migraine-related disability is estimated to cost about $13 billion a year due to missed workdays and impaired work function (Hu, Markson, Lipton, Stewart, & Berger, 1999). The World Health Organization (WHO) has ranked migraine as one of the top 20 disabling disorders in the world (Murthy et al., 2001).

Yet help-seeking for and rates of diagnosis of migraine are low (Lipton, Stewart, Celentano, & Reed, 1992; Lipton, Stewart, & Simon, 1998; Stang, Osterhaus, & Celentano, 1994). Fewer than half of those with migraine (according to the International Headache Society, 2003) seek treatment and, when they do, their physicians often do not diagnose it (Tepper et al., 2004). This is true for both sexes, but especially common among men. For example, a 1998 population survey of the USA found that 41% of women with migraine reported that they received a physician-diagnosis of migraine, compared to only 29% of men (Lipton et al., 2001). Although little is known about the causes of this discrepancy, it suggests a low agreement between diagnostic criteria and medical practice, as well as gender differences both in the application of migraine as a diagnosis and in help-seeking behavior. Given advances in treatment, there is great benefit to increasing help seeking within this population.

Drawing on ethnographic observations of pharmaceutical marketing practices at professional headache conferences and a content analysis of migraine advertising, largely in the USA, I demonstrate: (1) that the pharmaceutical industry directs its marketing of migraine medication predominantly to women; (2) as part of this strategy, pharmaceutical advertisements portray women as the prototypical migraine sufferer by eliciting familiar tropes of femininity and hegemonic feminine behavior. I argue that the pharmaceutical gendering of the migraine market is a powerful cultural force, which creates the false impression that migraine is exclusively a "women's disorder," thus ignoring the estimated 6 million men with migraine and exacerbating gender bias in help-seeking and diagnosis. In a culture that has not always valued the contributions of women or take women's illnesses as seriously as men's, the identification of migraine as a women's disease can influence how both physicians and patients understand the disorder. I conclude that these gendered pharmaceutical marketing practices have a paradoxical effect: even as they educate and raise awareness about migraine, they also create barriers to help seeking and diagnosis.

Background

The newly internationalized and consolidated pharmaceutical industry (Busfield, 2003) has a profound influence in the treatment and care of patients. According to a Kaiser Foundation (2004) report, the industry spent $25.3 billion for advertising in the US during 2003. Migraine medications are a lucrative market of interest for pharmaceutical companies. With a year-long prevalence rate of 12% for Americans adults, migraine provides a large market for treatment. In only the first half of 1997, GlaxoWellcome (now GlaxoSmithKline or GSK) spent $22.9 million on direct-to-consumer (DTC) advertising for its migraine medication Imitrex (Imigran in the UK) (Krajnak, 1998), one of GSK's highest selling drugs. (GlaxoSmithKline, 2004). A recent report from Reuter Business estimates that the migraine market is forecast to grow from $2.4 billion in 2001 to $3.5 billion in 2007.

The bulk of money used in marketing medications (approximately $22.1 billion) is directed toward physicians and invested in a diverse range of marketing tactics to brand pharmaceutical products. Advertising to physicians now extends far beyond the traditional office visits from sales representatives, direct mailings or advertisements in medical journals (Pines, 1999). Physicians are targeted at professional conferences, where companies sponsor meetings and, in return, receive the best booth positions and their logo imprinted on conference materials. Companies pay the travel expenses of researchers who speak about the efficacy and use of their drug. They arrange expert panels to speak at "Continuing Medical Education" (CME) sessions, where health care practitioners register for the credit necessary to maintain their board affiliations. Outside conferences, pharmaceutical companies fund the physicians who conduct clinical trials, and in the process choose which studies they want funded at all. While there is strong evidence that these strategies indirectly bias study outcomes (Bodenheimer, 2000; Cho & Bero, 1996; Lexchin, Bero, Djulbegovic, & Clark, 2003; Melander, Ahlqvist-Rastad, Meijer, & Beermann, 2003), pharmaceutical companies also intervene directly in clinical trials. It has been reported that companies review study articles before they are submitted to publication, draft findings, and even ghost write articles (Healy, 2004; Tierney & Gerrity, 2005).

In the USA, an additional $3.2 billion is spent on DTC advertisements, using a variety of media, including television, print and Internet advertising, as well as educational pamphlets and campaigns. The industry also uses subtle marketing tactics. For example, the industry hires celebrities and doctors to go on publicity tours and make mention of a particular drug on radio and television talk shows when they give interviews to reporters (Pines, 1999). The audience is often not told that these celebrities receive fees for their service (Goodman, 2002).

The pervasiveness of DTC advertising has caused grave ethical concerns. In theory, DTC advertising can provide important patient education and help reduce the gap between expert and patient (Basara, 1996). Critics argue that, in practice, DTC advertisements transform pharmaceutical treatments from medical therapies to commodities, marketed in the same ways as other goods. Subsequently, pharmaceutical marketing has successfully promoted not just its own drugs, but the acceptance of new disorders (see Clarke, Shim, Mamo, Fosket, & Fishman, 2003; Conrad, 2005). While DTC may encourage diagnosis and bring important knowledge and relief to patients, it may also promote overuse (Kravitz et al., 2005; Mintzes et al., 2003) and a lowered tolerance for the expression of otherwise normal human fragilities (Conrad & Leiter, 2004; Metzl & Angel, 2004).

Taken together, these diverse marketing practices disseminate widespread messages on health and illness. The information, tactics, metaphors, catch-phrases and images communicated via promotional schemes not only increase the visibility of those conditions for which drugs are advertised, they inject public discourse with a new set of meanings and symbols with which to understand diseases and disorders. When the American Senator Bob Dole and former football coach, Mike Ditka, speak on behalf of Viagra, they raise awareness about the drug, while reducing the stigma around "erectile dysfunction" (see Mamo & Fishman, 2001). When Pfizer runs advertisements for "Premenstrual Dysphoric Dysfunction," they are reconfiguring premenstrual syndrome (PMS) into a disorder that ought to be treated by Sarafem (previously known only as Prozac). And the appearances of a sportsman such as Magic Johnson in advertisements selling HIV treatments attempt to destigmatize HIV and AIDS. These advertisements draw on familiar tropes and shared cultural knowledge, such as the body as machine, the woman patient as emotive, and celebrity know-how (Lupton, 1993). En masse, these advertisements have the powerful ability to appear natural, no matter how staged or contrived Thus, it is increasingly important to analyze the messages disseminated by the pharmaceutical industry, as these marketing practices now serve as an important form of public health messaging that can influence help-seeking and diagnostic practices (Kravitz et al., 2005).

Gender in pharmaceutical advertisements

Images in medical advertising are an important site of analysis because they depict the normative patient, while contributing to the dominant discourses underpinning medical practice. Early research in this area was influenced by the burgeoning feminist movement and focused on representations of women in advertisements that appear in medical journals (Courtney & Whipple, 1983; King, 1980; Mant & Darroch, 1975; Smith & Griffin, 1977). Most of these early analyses found that women were over-represented in medical advertisements. In particular, women were more likely to be represented in advertisements, especially those for psychoactive medications. Men, however, were more often represented in drug advertisements for nonpsychoactive medications (Prather & Fidell, 1975). In addition, both men and women were portrayed as stereotypes, with men at work and women in social or domestic situations (Mant & Darroch, 1975). Similarly, the normative representation of men patients is that of a rational or mechanistic body, while the equivalent representation of women patients is depicted as emotive, self-obsessed, or (in the case of older women patients) even comical (Lupton, 1993).

The 1980s saw a rise in the number of men represented in advertising, however, advertisers continued to depict men and women in traditional gender positions (Hawkins & Aber, 1988). This trend continued in the 1990s, despite changes in social attitudes and the role of women in the workplace. Advertisements for hormone replacement therapies, for example, continue to use suggestive symbols to represent menopausal women as "out-of-control, grotesque, stressed, or confused and a threat to the idealized feminine" (Whittaker, 1998, p. 81).

Goffman's (1979) early analysis of gender and social rank in advertisements informs this research on the discursive structure of power and knowledge in advertisements. Goffman found, for example, that social status is often represented via the relative size of various characters; the character with valued social status is emphasized by virtue of enlargement or by being placed in an executive role (e.g., the male physician is positioned in the foreground, with the female nurse watching in the background). Women are portrayed as prostrate, sexually available, childlike, or in slanted postures, whereas men are shown as upright, rational protectors. Similarly, women more than men are pictured using their hands, holding and caressing objects, people, or themselves. Others (especially Bordo, 1993) have further developed Goffman's original guide to decoding advertisements. In this paper, I draw on these analyses to decode a diverse set of advertising data, asking: How do pharmaceutical advertisements depict the typical migraine patient? How do pharmaceutical companies use gender as a framework for their promotional strategies?

Methods

The data presented are drawn from a large, multi-method research study on the production of knowledge on headache. The materials were collected via ethnography at headache conferences and a sample of DTC advertisements collected from websites, in order to assess how advertisements depict the typical migraine patient and their care. This study emphasizes pharmaceutical advertising in the USA, although some data (described below) were collected in Italy and Japan.

Ethnography

From 2001 to 2005, I was a participant-observer in seven professional headache conferences sponsored by the American Headache Society (AHS, 2001, 2002, 2003, and 2005 annual meetings), the International Headache Society (IHC, 2001, 2003 and 2005 biennial meetings),[1] and the New York Headache Foundation (NYHF, 2005). These meetings took place in the USA, except for the IHC 2003, which was held in Rome, Italy and the IHC 2005, held in Tokyo, Japan. The manifest purpose of these meetings is the dissemination of new research. However, these meetings are also opportunities for pharmaceutical sponsors to market their products. From elaborate booths, drug representatives attract passersby with a bewildering array of merchandise, including pens, post-its, magnets, mugs, mouse pads, clocks, watches, laser pointers, toys, backpacks, pins, posters, radios, tape players, and books. Some companies offer separate lounge areas, where participants can check email, snack, and receive "educational" materials on medications. Large companies also sponsor satellite symposia (funded by unrestricted educational grants), at which physicians can receive professional credit. In the evenings, companies frequently hold expensive receptions at local tourist attractions. I collected hundreds of promotional materials and advertisements, including newsletters, pamphlets, patient package inserts to medications, television, radio and print advertisements, direct mailings to physicians, press releases, and educational materials produced for physicians.

Coding categories emerged from theoretical concerns about gender representation (see Bordo, 1993; Goffman, 1979; Metzl, 2003) and multiple close readings of the materials. This ethnographic approach to understanding pharmaceutical marketing allowed me to pursue the presentation of gender in promotional strategies without artificial boundaries, and to make connections between pharmaceutical funding of research studies, press releases and news stories on migraine.

Internet advertising

In order to produce descriptive statistics about gender ratios of people portrayed in migraine advertisements, I conducted a content analysis of images used in a discrete sample of pharmaceutical advertisements. The sample was collected in November 2003 from a cross-section of pharmaceutical websites that market headache medicine, and whose parent company rented booths at professional headache conferences (Table 1). For over-the-counter medications used to treat a variety of ailments, images were limited to those that specifically addressed migraine. Of these images, I retained those that would illuminate how marketing campaigns represent the migraine patient and health care workers. I kept all images of people, including both photographs of real people and illustrations or animated representations of people. I discarded all images of objects, such as medication or schematics demonstrating how a medication works. Multiple readings of each website aided analyses of images.

In total, 86 images were analyzed. Several depicted more than one person. The social characteristics of the people depicted were classified according to gender and number (male, alone; female, alone; multiple females; multiple males; mixed), race (white; black; Asian; other; unclear), setting (work—white collar; work—pink collar; work—blue collar; casual; family; clinic; romantic), pain status (pain; nonpain; metaphor for pain; mixed narrative; not-applicable),

Table 1 List of websites analyzed.

Pharmaceutical websites	Website Product name	Website
GlaxoSmithKline	Imitrex	www.migrainehelp.com
GlaxoSmithKline (educational)	Headachequiz.com	www.headachequiz.com
GlaxoSmithKline (educational)	HeadacheTest.com	www.headachetest.com
AstraZeneca	Zomig	www.zomig.com
Pfizer	Relpax	www.relpax.com
Pfizer (educational)	MigraineRelief	www.migrainerelief.com
Merck	Maxalt	www.maxalt.com
Ortho-McNeil	Axert	www.axert.com
Bristol-Meyers Squibb	Excedrin	www.excedrin.com
Health Assure	MigraHealth (herbal)	www.migrahealth.com
Ortho-McNeil	Motrin	www.motrin.com
Wyeth Consumer Healthcare	Advil Migraine	www.advil.com
MigreLief	MigreLief	www.migrelief.com
Weber and Weber	Petadolex	www.migraineaid.com

and status (patient; healthcare provider; expert; other). The location (homepage or not) and size (small, medium, or large) of images were also coded. All images were coded by the author and an independent coder trained in content analysis. Inter-coder agreement, calculated using a Kappa statistic, was 89.6% ($p = .019$). Disagreements were settled by the author.

Results

Who is the prototypical migraine patient?

Contemporary medical literature portrays migraine as a woman's disease (e.g., Phillips, 1998; Warshaw, Lipton, & Silberstein, 1998). This association comes from global epidemiological data that suggest that migraine is two or three times more common among women than men. In the USA, 18% of women have migraine, as compared to 6% of men (Lipton et al., 2001; Rasmussen, 1995; Stewart, Lipton, Celentano, & Reed, 1992). The gender difference in migraine prevalence is relatively consistent across cultures, even as prevalence estimates fluctuate. Further, the effects of migraine in women tend to be more severe and frequent than in men (Stewart, Schechter, & Lipton, 1994).

In addition to this basic statistical association, researchers cite the strong relationship between migraine incidence and hormonal milestones (Rasmussen & Stewart, 2000; Stewart et al., 1994). Girls and boys have similar rates of migraine until puberty, when rates in girls rise rapidly (Warshaw et al., 1998), and menopause brings relief to a substantial portion of women. However, the gender difference persists even at the age of 70, long after menopause, suggesting that hormonal cycles may not fully explain the variance in gender difference.

The basic epidemiological data on the gender difference in migraine in the USA are robust. These findings are drawn from large population-based studies using a standardized diagnostic algorithm for migraine, developed in 1988 by the IHS. The best of these epidemiological studies draw on self-reports of symptoms (i.e., presence of a one-sided headache; light and sound sensitivity; or nausea), rather than self-reported diagnoses. These diagnostic criteria draw a tight definitional boundary around migraine and may underestimate its prevalence. It is possible that the diagnostic criteria for migraine ought to be loosened, as migraine-specific drugs often work on a broad range of headache symptoms. However, these criteria have shown little of the "diagnostic creep" that has affected related diagnoses like depression (Metzl & Angel, 2004), perhaps because triptans are effective only in the treatment of headaches.

Even so, these statistical and hormonal associations do not constitute sufficient evidence for assigning migraine to the exclusive purview of women. An estimated 6% of American men have migraine and many experience great associated disability (Lipton et al., 2001). In fact, men experience migraine more than diabetes, diseases of the prostate, and ulcers (National Center for Health Statistics, 1996). Men tend to have other forms of headache at a similar rate to women; for example, in the USA 42% of men and 36% of women have episodic tension-type headache, (Schwartz, Stewart, Simon, & Lipton, 1998). If migraine diagnosis were broadened to include some tension-type headaches (a possibility, as migraine and tension-type headaches may be part of a spectrum disorder), then the relative rates of men with migraine would rise (Cady, Gutterman, Saiers, & Beach, 1997; Lipton et al., 2000; Marcus, 1992).

How is the typical migraine patient represented?

The 1993 release of Imitrex (sumatriptan) by GlaxoWellcome (now GSK) marked a revolution in the pharmacological care of migraine. For the first time, a therapy with few side effects aborted migraine symptoms in a majority of patients. To date, Imitrex maintains a dominant market share through name recognition, advertising, and its position as the first such medication on the market. However, several other medications in its class (referred to as *triptans*) have diversified the market. Although each triptan offers slightly different advantages and disadvantages, none have emerged as a clear leader in terms of efficacy (Ferrari, Roon, Lipton, & Goadsby, 2001). Their similarities increase companies, reliance on promotional strategies.

As part of its marketing campaign, GSK supports at least three US websites promoting Imitrex: www.migrainehelp.com, www.headachequiz.com, and www.headachetest.com (each accessed November 2003). The first website is dedicated to advertising Imitrex to people with migraine (migraineurs) and provides both general information about migraine and more specific information about the product. The latter two sites are primarily educational, so while labeled as GSK they do not mention Imitrex by name.[2] The overall message of these websites is designed to bring people with headache to the doctor. The main website (www.migrainehelp.com), for example, offers "tips on communicating with your doctor to get a treatment that's right for you". Readers are advised to *"Ask for IMITREX by name"* and the site suggests language to use when speaking to physicians: "I read that IMITREX targets your total migraine. If you think IMITREX is right for me, I'd like to try it". (Migrainehelp.com, accessed 2003).

The text is gender-neutral throughout the website. The patient is studiously referred to in the second person or a neutered third person. Most of the descriptions are short and—with the exception of those referring to the menstrual cycle—could apply to either a man or a woman with migraine. Yet on nearly every page, this text is accompanied by a visual depiction of a woman.

Few pages within each site provide more than a couple of lines of text. With so little information, the image creates a powerful signifier of the typical migraine sufferer. In the case of GSK's three websites dedicated to migraine, women are portrayed as patients 14 times more often than men. In contrast, GSK features two images of physicians, both of whom are white men. With an advertising campaign that limits male representation to physicians, the casual reader might infer that migraine is a condition of women.

GSK's website is typical. Migraine is represented as a women's condition across all of the websites included in the sample. Of the 86 images analyzed, 79 (85%) featured an image of a lay person with migraine. Of these 79 images, 55 (70%) had a female as the primary figure(s); 15 (19%) had a male as the primary figure; 4 (5%) featured both men and women; and, 5 (6%) featured a romantic couple. Because the representations of women with migraine dominate these images, pictures that portray both men and women read as though the woman in the image is the one who has the migraine. Of the 15 pictures of men, five depicted the same man in different postures on Bayer's aspirin website. In sum, only 10 different men are depicted as headache sufferers across all 14 websites.

Consistent with other feminist analyses of advertising, role portrayals of lay people conformed to gender stereotypes. For example, men were significantly (at $p < .01$) more often represented in work settings (40%) than women (12.7%). Women were as likely to be shown with children (12.7%), as they were to be shown at work. No men were portrayed as caretakers of children. There were, however, occasional gender role transgressions. The website for Axert (almotriptan) portrayed a black female physician caring for a white male patient, where the woman doctor is positioned only a little higher than the male patient. Another advertisement, posted on Relpax's (eletriptan) educational website, depicted two women speaking at work, where one appeared to be in a position of authority. These examples reflect a changing workplace where women and minorities play an increasingly important role, but these representations are rare. In GSK's website, for example, three images portray male physicians, two of which are speaking to female patients who appear smaller and shorter than their physicians. As Goffman (1979, p. 28) suggested, such differences in size and perspective connote the "social weight of power, authority, and rank".

Both patients and health care providers were usually portrayed as white and middle class. Sixty four (81%) of the patients were white. The race of an additional 6 (7.5%) was unclear, as each bore some subtle ethnic markers (e.g. an olive tone to the skin or features suggesting mixed race). Only 4 (5%) were clearly black. Class was more difficult to discern, though the vast majority of patients bore markers of affluence; most, for example, wore expensive clothes. With only three exceptions, workers held white-collar jobs, where they sat behind computers and wore business attire.

Representations on pharmaceutical websites exaggerate the epidemiological difference between men and women. As noted, women are represented in a ratio of about three and a half or four to one. The exaggeration may seem minor, but increases when one considers that Bayer's website accounts for a third of the male images. Generally, the prototypical migraineur was portrayed as a white, middle-class woman, attractive, with styled hair, expensive-looking clothing, jewelry and well-applied make-up. Most advertisements depicted a woman without pain, going about her day, whether at work, play, or in a relationship.

Images of men with migraine

The gendered portrayal of migraine is further exacerbated by the use and placement of male images, which obscure representations of male migraineurs. While images of women are prominently displayed on the homepages of websites, men are so embedded in the website that readers would need to click on several links to find them. This is true even in the rare case when the text refers to men with migraine. For example, Pfizer's website illustrates the following with an image of a man: although migraine was "once thought of as strictly a woman's disease, migraine affects a substantial number of men. In fact, 1 out of every 3 migraine sufferers on the job is a man" (Migrainerelief.com, accessed 2003b). Ironically, the website suggests elsewhere that representation of migraine as a women's disease might be responsible for the significant under-diagnosis and under-treatment of men with migraine: "Due to a misperception that people have about migraine being a woman's disease, many men may find it difficult to ask for help" (Migrainerelief.com, accessed 2003a). Here Pfizer includes one of its two representations of a man with migraine.

Female dominance exists even in those images that present men and women together as potential migraineurs. In these graphics, men are embedded within more dominant images of women, usually in a ratio that mimics the epidemiological distribution of migraine. Women typically outnumber men in these scenarios 2–3:1. I call this strategy an *epidemiological mosaic*. The advertiser incorporates men into the image, while reasserting the conventional wisdom that migraine is predominantly a woman's condition. For example, MigreLief's advertisements present the faces of six migraine patients. The top row depicts, in order, an older white woman, a young white brunette, and a young black man. The second row begins with a young Asian man, a young white woman, and an older black woman. The ratio in this design represents epidemiological data, depicting four women to two men. Women dominate the image in numbers, but also in design. The layout encourages the viewer's eye to begin in the top left corner of the montage, attracted in part by the top left-hand woman's bright yellow jacket. The eye then drifts to the center images, both of which are women. Men flank the image on the top right and bottom left of the photos, the two corners designed to be the least obvious.

Using a similar strategy, an image from Migra-Health portrays a tiled montage of people with migraine. The advertisement depicts a small photograph of a man with two additional photographs of women. But all of these images are overshadowed by a gray, transparent woman looming in the background. The imagery is again repeated in an advertisement for Frova (frovatriptan), which shows four people reading newspapers with large headlines about Frova. Here, too, there is a man flanked by three women, and he is positioned in the rear, framed as the smallest and least consequential of these potential patients. Given his position, he might be the concerned partner of a migraineur, rather than a migraineur himself. These advertisements best represent the phenomena of migraine as it is understood in the US today. While acknowledging that men do get migraines, they reaffirm the commonsense notion that women have them more often than men.

Gendered messages/gendered metaphors

Most advertisements for migraine medicine present a gender-neutral text, with pictures of women (and occasionally men) looking pain free. But this is not the only way in which drug companies find their target audience. Rather, they devise entire marketing campaigns designed to appeal to women. I describe two strategies that pharmaceutical companies use to capitalize on stereotypical interests of women to sell their medication: gendered metaphors and gendered narratives. While these strategies are analytically distinct, they are not mutually exclusive and, as described below, marketers often use them in conjunction with each other.

Gendered metaphors

The use of metaphor communicates latent meanings embedded in marketing strategies (Ettorre & Riska, 1995; Lupton, 1993). Metaphors work by connecting an abstract idea to something concrete and familiar (Lakoff & Johnson, 1980). Advertisements for antihistamines, for example, show fields of flowers in order to indicate that the drug will give the consumer a renewed ability to enjoy the natural world. Gender can strengthen the use of advertising metaphors, as when romance is used to sell diamonds and the promise of sex to sell alcohol. When metaphors work well, the product itself becomes a metaphor for these otherwise abstract notions.

Pharmaceutical companies use feminine metaphors to market their medications to women. For example, Pfizer's 2003 promotional campaign for their newly released migraine drug, Relpax, which used a metaphorical "spa experience" to convey the experience of migraine to consumers.

> According to coverage in Anonymous (2003a), "Pfizer turned a wing of New York's Grand Central Terminal into a 'soothing oasis dedicated to the five senses' in a consumer promotion last month for its migraine headache medication Relpax" . . .
>
> The one-day event, which began at 7am and continued until 8pm, attracted thousands of commuters. The spa area included a three-piece orchestra, yoga clinics, a free massage area, a Zen garden and a gourmet food sampling area . . .
>
> Consumers who filled out a short survey about migraines received a gift carton that included a Relpax pamphlet, tea sample, scented candle and a mini eyelid mask.
>
> (2003a)[3]

Pfizer also created a "virtual spa" on their website. The spa is a small pop-up window, which plays sounds of a rain forest, accompanied by images evocative of a spa vacation. The text uses the "spa experience" as a metaphor to describe relief from the pain of migraine. For example:

> **Imagine the fresh scent of a beautiful garden.** For some, even the most exhilarating fragrance can increase nausea when the pain of a full-blown migraine takes over.
>
> **Imagine the gentle touch of your dancing partner.** Even a soft touch that causes the slightest motion can become unbearable. Sometimes, that's how it feels when you're stopped in your tracks by headsplitting migraine pain.
>
> (www.relpax.com, accessed November 2003)

This advertising strategy limits its audience by carefully targeting a middle-class audience and a particular kind of urban, affluent woman. Marketers appeal to women rather than men, by distributing scented candles and mini eyelid masks in exchange for information about potential customers. Alternatively, masculine metaphors could have conveyed a similar message, for example, the troubling experience of developing a migraine during a sporting event.

Gendered messages

Another discursive tactic is to depict a narrative that draws on hegemonic and familiar tropes of femininity. In this section, I describe two such campaigns. Both feature women as migraine patients, each of whom are represented as caretakers, whose migraines interfere in their ability to nurture. Migraine medications are positioned as a solution to these narratives of pain, nurturing, and care.

The first campaign is run by GSK. Visitors to the Imitrex website who request a "free offer" of medication will receive, by mail, a "Migraine Action Guide" from GSK that provides information on Imitrex, how it differs from general analgesics, and how to ask a physician for the medication. This information is designed as a pamphlet with pages that turn like a book. Across from each page of information about the drug, the pamphlet portrays a series of pictures representing one person's recovery narrative. While the images correlate with the text (i.e. when the text refers to physicians, the image portrays a doctor–patient interaction), the text makes no specific comment on the story unfolding on the opposite pages:

The visual story features a young white woman. She is first presented to us on the cover of the guide, where she stands confidently next to a quotation: "Finally, a medicine that can target my total migraine!" On the inside cover, we see the woman dressed in a nurse's uniform, working in a hospital room full of newborn infants. But she is in pain. She grimaces, pressing her fingers into her temple and furrowing her brow. Her back is turned away from the babies, presumably because the intensity of the pain disables her and prevents her from performing her job. That the advertisers chose to represent their model migraineur as a neonatal nurse elicits feminine qualities of nurture and care.

On the top of the next page, she gives voice to her frustration: "I wish people realized how much a migraine disrupts my life." Imitrex is proposed as the appropriate solution: the text explains, that "general pain relievers are made for general kinds of pain ... IMITREX is different." Using a computer animated outline of a universal patient, the image depicts how Imitrex works. The universal patient model used here is a woman, rather than the typical "universal man" so often used to portray the medical norm (Riska, 2004). The spots on the first body demonstrate how diffuse general pain relief can be. The adjacent image demonstrates how Imitrex works differently, by "targeting" the pain. Shaped like a bullet, the pill shoots towards the source of the pain.

231

In the next image, the nurse, armed with new knowledge, approaches her physician for a prescription. As the story unfolds, we see an effective interaction with her physician. She gesticulates animatedly as she makes her points and the physician (a white male) appears to listen actively, his posture signifying relinquished authority and an attentive respect for the patient's medical insight. The two are positioned at nearly the same height, signaling shared power in the interaction.

The physician must have prescribed Imitrex, because in the next two images, she is free of pain and back to work. With Imitrex, the neonatal ward no longer carries the cold, institutionalized ambience of the earlier picture, and now looks more like a homey nursery. Warm, yellow walls with alphabet bordering indicates a change in atmosphere. The nurse's demeanor has changed as well. She now cradles and cares for a baby, tenderly smiling and cooing. She has a renewed capacity for nurture and work. The final image depicts her in plain clothes again, lounging on a sofa, while talking on a phone. Her face is bright and smiling. Not only has she returned to her work of caring for babies, she has returned to her social life, and is presumably telling her friends how Imitrex has cured her migraines. In short, the patient is a happy customer, brought back to life by GSK's medication.

This visual narrative appeals to the consumer by using images that draw on culturally resonant images of women at work. As many studies have shown, stories have more rhetorical force when they are relevant to beliefs already held by the audience (Gamson & Modigliani, 1989; Schudson, 1989). Advertisements that coincide with broadly held commonsense notions about the ways of the world appear to be natural and objective. By setting this narrative in a neonatal ward, the advertisement is designed to appeal to workers both at work and at home with their children. The manifest message is that the medication works and that those with migraine should request Imitrex at next doctor's visit. The latent message confirms that migraine is a women's disorder. In addition, GSK manages to usurp the patient's voice in their effort to create recognition with the public.

While pain-free women cradling children demonstrate good caring, pharmaceutical companies also use narratives that demonstrate just the reverse for women in pain. In a recent AstraZeneca advertising campaign of their migraine medication Zomig (zolmitriptan), women in migraine pain are depicted as bad mothers because they are prevented from giving their children the care they need. They appear to abandon their children, crippled by their migraine, literally turning their back on them, just as the GSK nurse turned her back on newborn babies in the neonatal ward.

Two Zomig advertisements are particularly effective at exploiting this narrative. One portrays a little boy standing in front of an open bedroom. His body language conveys utter dejection. Under one arm, he carries a baseball glove, and in the other a baseball. He is ready to play with his friends and is only missing the transportation. His mother, who we see languishing in the bedroom behind him, is too ill with migraine to take him to his game. The mother's posture suggests that the pain is intense—she is grimacing and her hand is pressed against her forehead. Her eyes are closed and her body contorts away from her son. The boy calls out to the reader as if asking for help: "Mama has another migraine." It is clearly not the first time that the mother has let her son down like this. The boy is dressed in crumpled clothing and his hat appears to be too big for him, as if his mother has not even been able to take him shopping recently, or that he had to dress himself that morning.

The second image presents a woman in pain on the bus. In this scenario, she is experiencing stress—both the stress of motherhood, but also the daily stress of running errands while caring for her son. Like the mother in the previous advertisement, her body is turned away from her child. Her right hand pressing against her temple may soothe the pain, but it also shields him from her sight. Her opposite hand reaches around the front of her body to hold on to his arm, perhaps signaling a residual desire to nurture. Yet the headline 'ESCAPE' evokes a more primal desire of liberation from an overwhelming day-to-day routine. One gets the sense that for this woman motherhood might be too much to bear. The advertisement suggests that Zomig can help with this predicament and mothers can return to their regular duties.

The power of these images is their ability to reflect and reconstruct familiar tropes. Together, these narratives put to work a normative notion of family and motherhood, in which the woman's primary duty is to care for children, which is represented as straightforward for healthy and pain-free women. Men are not represented as caretakers, nor are they represented as sufferers of migraine. This kind of marketing material provides a detailed and emotive social context in which women suffer from migraines, and in which their suffering has damaging effects on their loved ones. No similar context is imagined for men.

Conclusion

The pharmaceutical industry genders migraine advertisements using a variety of techniques: gendered images; gendered metaphors; and gendered messaging. In addition, the use of *epidemiological mosaics* allows marketers to include lesser demographics (in this case, men), without actually drawing attention to them. These representations of patients in DTC advertising serve to construct the typical patient for a general audience and disseminate important messages about gender and pain to the public.

Pharmaceutical companies market to women because they believe that women are their market. At least this is what they are being told by marketing trade journals, which consistently report that migraine affects many more women than men. For example, Anonymous (1999) report that "about 24 million Americans, most of whom are women, suffer from migraine".

Another journal reports that "about 28 million Americans—one in five women and one in 15 men—experience migraines" (Anonymous, 2003b). (Such inconsistencies in reporting epidemiology frequently appear in these journals.) Other trade articles suggest that pharmaceutical companies market to women because they believe women are an "underserved market." Mark Kreston, president of Bristol-Myers Squibb (BMS) Consumer Medicines, explains how BMS used migraine to create a new market among women: "By aligning the brand with female health experts and advocates, and focusing on aspects of the disease that impact women most, we have helped establish migraine as a serious women's health issue" (Anonymous, 2001).

That migraine is represented as more prevalent among women reflects a clinical reality: more women than men seek help for head pain. But as noted previously, more men experience migraine than diabetes, diseases of the prostate, and ulcers (National Center for Health Statistics 1996), all of which are described and constructed either as unisex or specifically male diseases. Marketers want to target women because women buy more of their medication. But by targeting migraine as a purely "women's health issue", drug companies may actually be constructing their audience rather than merely representing it, and in doing so, excluding many people who might suffer from the condition and who would benefit from their medication.

Just as importantly, the construction of migraine as a women's health issue evokes historical associations between pain, hysteria and neurotic women and may increase the stigma of both men and women in pain. Images of women in stereotypically gendered scenarios are effective marketing tools because they draw on familiar tropes regarding women, particularly with regards to motherhood and the ability to nurture. However, these images also reify these relationships and promote the false claim that these ideas are fundamentally connected.

Advocates of DTC advertising, in those countries where it is legally permitted, have argued that this advertising provides much needed education to health care consumers. This paper suggests that these pharmaceutical marketing practices actually have a paradoxical effect: even as they educate and raise awareness about migraine, they also create barriers to help-seeking and diagnosis. It is beyond this study to assess whether these advertisements directly affect the exchange between physicians and patients and more research is needed to understand the links between representation, help-seeking and diagnosis.

Acknowledgements

The author thanks Charles Bosk, Joseph Drury and Jason Schnittker for their revisions; Michelle Kempner and Ezra Golberstein for their assistance; and the Robert Wood Johnson Foundation and the Otto and Gertrude K. Pollak Research Fellowship for their support.

Notes

1. AHS and IHS co-sponsored a meeting in New York in 2001.
2. The pharmaceutical industry uses so-called "educational" advertisements that do not mention the name of the marketed drug to avoid federal restrictions on advertising in the US. This form of advertising is extremely effecting. For example, in 1993, an unbranded advertising campaign recommending that people talk to their doctors about a "surprisingly effective" new treatment for migraine generated approximately $22 million in new and refill prescriptions (Basara, 1996).
3. Ironically, scents, especially perfumes, are a major trigger of migraine headaches.

References

Anonymous (1999). Maxalt-MLT. *R&D Directions, 5*(3), 51.
Anonymous (2001). Manufacturers have an eye for the ladies. *Drug Store News, 23*(16), 24.
Anonymous (2003a). Pfizer gives its new Relpax drug the spa treatment. *Medical Marketing & Media, 38*(7).
Anonymous (2003b). Migraine. *Medical Advertising News, 22*(2), 81.
Basara, L. R. (1996). The impact of a direct-to-consumer prescription medication advertising campaign on new prescription volume. *Drug Information Journal, 30*(3), 715–729.
Bodenheimer, T. (2000). Uneasy alliance—clinical investigators and the pharmaceutical industry [Health Policy Report]. *The New England Journal of Medicine, 342*(20), 1539–1544.
Bordo, S. (1993). *Unbearable weight: Feminism, western culture, and the body* (pp. 1–42). Berkeley: University of California Press.
Busfield, J. (2003). Globalization and the pharmaceutical industry revisited. *International Journal of Health Services, 33*(3), 581–605.
Cady, R., Gutterman, D., Saiers, J., & Beach, M. (1997). Responsiveness of non-IHS migraine and tension-type headache to sumatriptan. *Cephalalgia, 17*, 588–590.
Cho, M. K., & Bero, L. (1996). The quality of drug studies published in symposium proceedings. *Annals of Internal Medicine, 124*(5), 485–489.
Clarke, A. E., Shim, J. K., Mamo, L., Fosket, J. R., & Fishman, J. R. (2003). Biomedicalization: Technoscientific transformations of health, illness, and U.S. biomedicine. *American Sociological Review, 68*(2), 161–194.
Conrad, P. (2005). The shifting engines of medicalization. *Journal of Health and Social Behavior, 46*(1), 3–14.
Conrad, P., & Leiter, V. (2004). Medicalization, markets and consumers. *Journal of Health and Social Behavior, 45*, 158–176.
Courtney, A. E., & Whipple, T. W. (1983). *Sex stereotyping in advertising*. Lexington, MA: Lexington Books.
Ettorre, E., & Riska, E. (1995). *Gendered moods: Psychotropics and society*. London and New York: Routledge.
Ferrari, M. D., Roon, K. I., Lipton, R. B., & Goadsby, P. J. (2001). Oral triptans (serotonin 5-HT1B/1D agonists) in acute migraine treatment: A meta-analysis of 53 trials. *The Lancet, 358*(9294), 1668–1675.
Gamson, W., & Modigliani, A. (1989). Media discourse and public opinion on nuclear power. *American Journal of Sociology, 95*(1–37).

GlaxoSmithKline. (2004). *Annual Report*, 2003. London.
Goffman, E. (1979). *Gender advertisements*. Cambridge, MA: Harvard University Press.
Goodman, L. (2002). Celebrity pill pushers. *Salon.com*. San Francisco.
Hawkins, J. W., & Aber, C. (1988). The content of advertisements in medical journals: Distorting the image of women. *Women & Health, 14*, 43–59.
Healy, D. (2004). *Let them eat Prozac: The unhealthy relationship between the pharmaceutical industry and depression*. New York: New York University Press.
Hu, X. H., Markson, L., Lipton, R., Stewart, W., & Berger, M. L. (1999). Burden of migraine in the United States: Disability and economic costs. *Archives of Internal Medicine, 159*(8), 813–818.
IHS, Classification Committee of the International Headache Society. (2003). International classification of headache disorders, 2nd ed. *Cephalalgia, 24*(Suppl. 1), pp. 1–150.
Kaiser. (2004). *Prescription drug trends* (pp. 10–22). Menlo Park, CA: Kaiser Family Foundation.
King, E. (1980). Sex bias in psychoactive drug advertisements. *Psychiatry, 43*, 129–137.
Krajnak, M. (1998). Glaxo Wellcome: Marketing strategy without bounds. *Pharma Business*, May.
Kravitz, R. L., Epstein, R. M., Feldman, M. D., Franz, C. E., Azari, R., Wilkes, M. S., et al. (2005). Influence of patients' requests for direct-to-consumer advertised antidepressants: A randomized controlled trial. *JAMA, 293*(16), 1995–2002.
Lakoff, G., & Johnson, M. (1980). *Metaphors we live by*. Chicago: University of Chicago Press.
Lexchin, J., Bero, L. A., Djulbegovic, B., & Clark, O. (2003). Pharmaceutical industry sponsorship and research outcome and quality: Systematic review. *British Medical Journal, 326*(7400), 1167–1170.
Lipton, R. B., Stewart, W. F., Cady, R., Hall, C., O'Quinn, S., Kuhn, T., et al. (2000). Sumatriptan for the range of headaches in migraine sufferers: Results of the spectrum study. *Headache, 40*(Suppl.), 783–791.
Lipton, R. B., Stewart, W. F., Celentano, D., & Reed, M. (1992). Undiagnosed migraine headaches: A comparison of symptom-based and reported physician diagnosis. *Archives of Internal Medicine, 152*(6), 1273–1278.
Lipton, R. B., Stewart, W. F., Diamond, S., Diamond, M. L., & Reed, M. (2001). Prevalence and burden of migraine in the United States: Data from the American Migraine Study II. *Headache, 41*, 646–657.
Lipton, R. B., Stewart, W. F., & Simon, D. (1998). Medical consultation for migraine: Results from the American Migraine Study. *Headache, 38*, 87–96.
Lupton, D. (1993). The construction of patienthood in medical advertising. *International Journal of Health Services, 23*(4), 805–819.
Mamo, L., & Fishman, J. R. (2001). Potency in all the right places: Viagra as a technology of the gendered body. *Body & Society, 7*(4), 13–35.
Mant, A., & Darroch, D. B. (1975). Media images and medical images. *Social Science & Medicine, 9*, 613–618.
Marcus, D. A. (1992). Migraine and tension-type headaches: The questionable validity of current classification systems. *Clinical Journal of Pain, 8*(1), 28–36 (discussion 37–28).

Melander, H., Ahlqvist-Rastad, J., Meijer, G., & Beermann, B. (2003). Evidence b(i)ased medicine—selective reporting from studies sponsored by pharmaceutical industry: Review of studies in new drug applications. *British Medical Journal, 326*(7400), 1171–1173.
Metzl, J. M. (2003). *Prozac on the couch: Prescribing gender in the era of wonder drugs.* Durham and London: Duke University Press.
Metzl, J. M., & Angel, J. (2004). Assessing the impact of SSRI antidepressants on popular notions of women's depressive illness. *Social Science & Medicine, 58,* 577–584.
Migrainehelp.com. (accessed 2003). *Let Your Doctor Know The Facts.* GlaxoSmithKline.
Migrainerelief.com. (accessed 2003a). *Toughing it out: wondering what other think.* Pfizer.
Migrainerelief.com. (accessed 2003b). *Who suffers: An office snapshot.* Pfizer.
Mintzes, B., Barer, M. L., Kravitz, R. L., Bassett, K., Lexchin, J., Kazanjian, A., et al. (2003). How does direct-to-consumer advertising (DTCA) affect prescribing? A survey in primary care environments with and without legal DTCA. *Canadian Medical Association Journal, 169*(5), 405–412.
Murthy, R. S., Bertolote, J. M., Epping-Jordan, J., Funk, M., Prentice, T., Saraceno, B., et al. (2001). *The World Health Report: Mental health: New understanding, new hope.* Geneva, Switzerland: World Health Organization.
Phillips, P. (1998). Migraine as a woman's issue—Will research and new treatments help? *JAMA: Medical News & Perspectives, 280*(23).
Pines, W. L. (1999). A history and perspective on direct-to-consumer promotion. *Food and Drug Law Journal, 54,* 489–518.
Prather, J., & Fidell, L. S. (1975). Sex differences in the content and style of medical advertisements. *Social Science & Medicine, 9*(1), 23–26.
Rasmussen, B. K. (1995). Epidemiology of headache. *Cephalalgia, 15*(1), 45–68.
Rasmussen, B. K., & Stewart, W. F. (2000). Epidemiology of migraine. In J. Olesen, P. Tfelt-Hansen, & K. M. A. Welch (Eds.), *The headaches* (2nd ed., pp. 227–233). Philadelphia: Lippincott Williams & Wilkins.
Riska, E. (2004). *Masculinity and men's health: Coronary heart disease in medical and public discourse.* Lanham, MD: Rowman & Littlefield.
Ruiz de Velasco, I., Gonzalez, N., Etxeberria, Y., & Garcia-Monco, J. C. (2003). Quality of life in migraine patients: A qualitative study. *Cephalalgia, 23*(9), 892–900.
Schudson, M. (1989). How culture works: Perspectives from media studies on the efficacy of symbols. *Theory and Society, 18,* 153–180.
Schwartz, B. S. M., Stewart, W. F., Simon, D. M. S., & Lipton, R. B. (1998). Epidemiology of tension-type headache. *Journal of the American Medical Association, 279*(5), 381–383.
Smith, M. C., & Griffin, L. (1977). Rationality of appeals used in the promotion of psychotropic drugs. A comparison of male and female models. *Social Science & Medicine, 11,* 409–414.
Stang, P., Osterhaus, J., & Celentano, D. (1994). Migraine: Patterns of healthcare use. *Neurology, 44*(6(Suppl. 4)), S47–S55.
Statistics, N. C. f. H. (1996). *Current estimates from the National Health Interview Survey, 1996.* Hyattsville, MD: National Institutes of Health.

Stewart, W., Lipton, R., Celentano, D., & Reed, M. (1992). Prevalence of migraine headache in the United States: Relation to age, income, race and other sociodemographic characteristics. *Journal of the American Medical Association, 267*, 64–69.

Stewart, W. F., Schechter, A., & Lipton, R. B. (1994). Migraine heterogeneity: Disability, pain intensity, and attack frequency and duration. *Neurology, 4*, S24–S39.

Tepper, S. J., Dahlof, C. G., Dowson, A., Newman, L., Mansbach, H, Jones, M., et al. (2004). Prevalence and diagnosis of migraine in patients consulting their physician with a complaint of headache: Data from the Landmark Study. *Headache, 44*(9), 856–864.

Terwindt, G., Launder, L., & Ferrari, M. (2000). The impact of migraine on quality of life in the general population. *Neurology, 2000*(55), 624–629.

Tierney, W. M., & Gerrity, M. S. (Eds.). (2005). Editorial: Scientific discourse, corporate ghostwriting, journal policy and public trust. *Journal of General Internal Medicine, 20*(6), 550–551.

Warshaw, L. J., Lipton, R. B., & Silberstein, S. D. (1998). Migraine: A "woman's disease?". *Women & Health, 28*(2), 79–99.

Whittaker, R. (1998). Re-framing the representation of women in advertisements for hormone replacement therapy. *Nursing Inquiry, 5*(2), 77–86.

53

THE INFLUENCE OF PATIENT AND DOCTOR GENDER ON DIAGNOSING CORONARY HEART DISEASE

*Ann Adams, Christopher D. Buckingham,
Antje Lindenmeyer, John B. McKinlay, Carol Link,
Lisa Marceau and Sara Arber*

Source: *Sociology of Health and Illness*, 30 (2008), 1–18.

Abstract

Using novel methods, this paper explores sources of uncertainty and gender bias in primary care doctors' diagnostic decision-making about coronary heart disease (CHD). Claims about gendered consultation styles and quality of care are re-examined, along with the adequacy of CHD models for women. Randomly selected doctors in the UK and the US (n = 112, 56 per country, stratified by gender) were shown standardised videotaped vignettes of actors portraying patients with CHD. Patients' age, gender, ethnicity and social class were varied systematically. During interviews, doctors gave free-recall accounts of their decision-making, which were analysed to determine patient and doctor gender effects. We found differences in male and female doctors' responses to different types of patient information. Female doctors recall more patient cues overall, particularly about history presentation, and particularly amongst women. Male doctors appear less affected by patient gender but both male and especially female doctors take more account of male patients' age, and consider more age-related disease possibilities for men than women. Findings highlight the need for better integration of knowledge about female presentations within accepted CHD risk models, and do not support the contention that women receive better-quality care from female doctors.

Introduction

Improving the early detection and management of coronary heart disease (CHD) remains a key health improvement target across the developed world (*e.g.* UK Department of Health (DH) 2005, US National Center for Chronic Disease Prevention and Health Promotion (NCCD) 2005). While evidence suggests that health promotion and screening strategies are having a positive effect (DH 2005, NCCD 2005), the decline in CHD has been greater for men than women (Peltonen *et al.* 2000). Twice as many women as men aged 45–64 have undetected or 'silent' myocardial infarctions, suggesting later diagnosis (McKinlay *et al.* 1996, Mikhail 2005); and women also have a poorer post-infarction prognosis than men, even after adjusting for clinical covariates (NCCD 2005, Mikhail 2005). To understand why these gender differences persist, it is important to focus attention on primary care where CHD is first diagnosed. The need for research investigating the dynamics of the initial CHD diagnostic process amongst women is recognised as particularly urgent (Raine 2001, Richards *et al.* 2000, Mikhail 2005).

One explanation for persistent gender differences in the diagnosis, treatment and management of CHD is that knowledge about female presentations is not yet sufficiently integrated into received medical wisdom about what is 'normal' in CHD (Lorber 2000). Further, in the US Lorber contends that women receive better quality care for CHD at the hands of female compared with male doctors. This is based upon evidence about different consultation styles used by male and female doctors, which have also been identified by others (*e.g.* Roter, Lipkin and Korsgaard 1991, Hall *et al.* 1994). This paper re-examines these claims using a novel analytic approach which combines sociological and psychological perspectives. Much previous research has focused on how patient and doctor characteristics affect *outcomes* of clinical decision-making. Arber *et al.* (2006) identified significant gender differences in doctors' treatment and management decisions for patients presenting with symptoms of CHD, finding that doctors had greater diagnostic certainty in relation to male compared with female patients. In this paper we elucidate these findings by an analysis of complementary, qualitative data to determine how patient and doctor gender affects doctors' *cognitive processes* during consultations, to shed light on gendered sources of diagnostic uncertainty and bias.

We have argued elsewhere that different theories of decision-making and approaches to decision analysis can usefully be encapsulated within a psychological model of classification (Buckingham and Adams 2000a, 2000b). This psychological model (described below) is used to analyse primary care doctors' accounts of decision-making about older and middle-aged patients presenting with symptoms of CHD. It enables us to focus on the micro-processes of doctors' clinical decision-making, and to explore the effects of patient and doctor gender on them.

First, we review relevant literature on gender and heart disease. The concept of clinical decision-making as classification is then introduced, followed by a description of our analytic model and study methods. A number of hypotheses are derived and presented for empirical testing. Findings are discussed in the context of identifying sources of clinical uncertainty and potential gender bias, and in the light of Lorber's (2000) claims about the better treatment of women by female doctors than by male doctors.

Patient gender and heart disease

Coronary heart disease is the most common cause of death for women both in the UK and the US (DH 2005, NCCD 2005), killing 10 times more women than breast cancer (NHS Confederation Press Summaries 6 September 2005). It was only in the mid-nineties, however, that it was recognised by the medical profession as an 'equal opportunity killer' (Wenger 1994), or indeed, as is now suggested, more deadly for women than for men in Europe (NHS Confederation Press Summaries 6 September 2005). Consequently, numerous studies have set out to determine gender effects on the diagnosis, treatment and outcomes associated with CHD, and researchers have found a systematic gender bias in secondary care. In the US and UK women were less likely to be admitted to cardiac units, even though they were generally in a worse condition on admission than men (Clarke et al. 1994), and less likely to be re-vascularised (DeWilde et al. 2003). Similar patterns were found in Australia (Sayer and Britt 1996), Ireland (Bennett, Williams and Feely 2002), Sweden (Agvall and Dahlstrom 2001), and Austria (Hochleitner 2000).

Less is known about the influence of gender in primary care however, where CHD is first diagnosed. Lorber's (2000) contention about knowledge of female presentations being not yet sufficiently integrated into received medical wisdom about what is 'normal' in CHD may be particularly influential here. Generalist primary care doctors are less likely to be aware of subtle gender differences in presentation than cardiac specialists. This is borne out by evidence that women are less likely than men to receive a diagnosis of CHD in primary care (Wenger 1994, Richards et al. 2000) because doctors are less certain about the accuracy of this diagnosis in women, particularly mid-life women (Arber et al. 2006). As a consequence, women may not be so thoroughly investigated. They are less likely to have CHD risk factors recorded, or to receive secondary prophylaxis; and if they do receive lipid lowering drugs, they are treated less 'aggressively' than men (Hippisley-Cox et al. 2001, Corbelli et al. 2003, Mikhail 2005). This, in turn, leads to difficulty in referral for appropriate tests (see for example Richards et al. 2000, Bennett, Williams and Feely 2002, Arber et al. 2006). In particular, women are less likely to be referred for echocardiography (Agvall and Dahlstrom 2001), or for evaluation of left ventricular function (Burstein et al. 2003). When they are referred, women may be further disadvantaged because the exercise

ECG, the most reliable diagnostic tool for CHD, functions better in relation to detecting CHD in men than in women (McKinlay 1996, Wong *et al.* 2001).

Prevalent stereotypical conceptualisations of CHD as a male disease also remain important, particularly amongst women themselves (Guilleman 2004, Ruston and Clayton 2002). People generally recall heart disease as being a sudden, dramatic collapse in male relatives, but a slow decline associated with normal ageing in female relatives, with stereotypical male presentations being more readily remembered (Emslie, Hunt and Watt 2001). The observations made by Martin, Gordon and Lounsbury (1998) and Lockyer and Bury (2002), that women are more in danger than men of having their symptoms of CHD interpreted as being of psychosomatic origin, is another indicator of a lack of integration of knowledge about women within prevalent conceptualisations of what is normal in CHD.

Explanations for differences in doctors' decision-making behaviour vary. Lorber's (2000) argument is in part predicated on the fact that there is an andro-centric gender bias that runs throughout much of medical knowledge and practice (Healy 1991, Hayes and Prior 2003), which pays insufficient attention to the distinctiveness of disease presentation amongst women. For example, women are under-represented in CHD-related medical trials (Rosser 1994, Mikhail 2005); at best they receive a 'gender-neutral' assessment of their symptoms, but care based on the needs of male patients, which could significantly disadvantage them (Borzak and Weaver 2000, Bandyopadhyay, Bayer and O'Mahony 2001, White and Lockyer 2001).

Indeed, there is growing evidence that women often have different clinical presentations of CHD compared with men (see *e.g.* Philpott *et al.* 2001, Mikhail 2005), which has led others to dispute that an inappropriate gender bias exists (Roeters van Lennep 2000, Wong *et al.* 2001). For example, women being treated less aggressively than men could rightly reflect real clinical differences in women's CHD profile, where their target lipid levels are different from men's (Wild 2001). Others contend that there is a gender bias in the opposite direction, arguing that men are generally over-treated (Kitler 1994). Unravelling the extent to which inappropriate, stereotypically-gendered thinking affects the diagnosis, treatment and management of CHD is highly important, yet complex to execute. Our study methods (described below) explain how we have sought to understand how this affects diagnosis, by controlling for clinical presentation, social interaction and behavioural differences within consultations.

Gender differences in the treatment of CHD are also confounded by the influence of other variables, such as age, socio-economic status (SES) (Lawlor, Ebrahim and Davey Smith 2002a, 2002b) and ethnicity (Schulman *et al.* 1999). Our own work (Arber *et al.* 2004, 2006), has highlighted the importance of age and gender interaction, suggesting significant under-investigation of CHD in middle-aged women in particular. In this paper we examine gender differences amongst mid-life and older patients, while simultaneously controlling for the effects of ethnicity and social class, and compare how doctors locate male and female patients' symptoms according to age-related disease expectations.

The influence of doctors' gender

An apparent lack of awareness of CHD in women amongst many healthcare professionals has recently been noted as a worrying phenomenon (Mikhail 2005), and is important to examine in terms of doctors' gender. While there is considerable evidence about the impact of *patients*' gender on the treatment and management of CHD (demonstrated above), much less is known about the impact of *doctors*' gender, and particularly about how it affects diagnostic decision-making in primary care.

Available literature about the effects of doctor gender tends to focus on differences in consultation styles and interaction patterns between male and female doctors with their patients. Women doctors encourage patients to talk more and develop fuller history narratives, to be involved in decision-making, demonstrate more supportive non-verbal communication, conduct longer consultations and are more likely to perform female prevention procedures (Lorber and Moore 2002, Lorber 2000, Roter, Lipkin and Korsgaard 1991, Hall *et al.* 1994). Based on her examination of existing research evidence, Lorber (2000) contends that 'women patients . . . do not get the best treatment for heart disease nor do they get good preventive care . . . unless they have a woman doctor' (2000: 45). Women use primary care services more than men (Hayes and Prior 2003), and with more women choosing to see female doctors (Franks and Bertakis 2003), and a steady growth in the numbers of women entering primary care medicine, it is timely to re-examine this claim.

In summary, we aim to investigate the influence of both doctors' and patients' gender on doctors' cognitive processes during clinical decision-making, and to identify sources of uncertainty in the diagnosis of CHD. We are particularly concerned with unravelling the extent to which inappropriate, stereotypically-gendered thinking gives rise to inequity in the early stages of women's care, and how this is influenced by patients' age. The next section describes our approach to investigating these cognitive processes for clinical decision-making.

Clinical decision-making as classification

Building on earlier work (Buckingham and Adams 2000a, 2000b), we have developed a detailed psychological model of clinical decision-making within consultations, which interprets it as three linked, iterative classification tasks (diagnosing, assessing potential outcomes and making intervention decisions – see Figure 1). In this paper we focus on the first task of diagnostic decision-making only, since the literature review suggests that this is the stage requiring most urgent investigation (Raine 2001, Richards *et al.* 2000, Mikhail 2005).

When making a diagnosis, the 'raw materials' doctors work with is a set of patient attributes and those pertaining to the healthcare context (*e.g.* health setting, cost of interventions, availability of tests). Referring to Figure 1, doctors select from this material what they believe to be relevant patient cues (*e.g.* gender but not eye colour from the whole set of patient attributes), and contextual information for making a diagnosis. The relevant cues then enter the psychological classification process, having been given a psychological interpretation if appropriate (*e.g.* a specific age might be interpreted as 'elderly'). The different cues are then integrated to determine their combined influence on differential diagnostic classes. Each class is paired with the certainty that the doctor believes the patient belongs to it. The classification process is iterative, with cues bringing to mind particular diagnostic classes, which then suggest further cues to be sought, and so on.

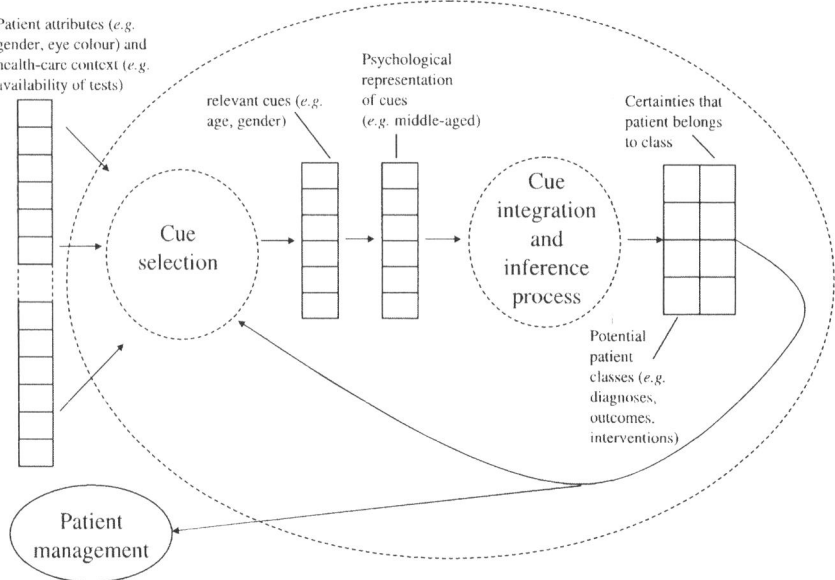

Figure 1 Psychological model of clinical decision-making (CDM) based on classification. The same process applies to all three CDM tasks: classification of diagnoses, potential outcomes, and interventions. The arrow from the classes and certainties leading back to the cue selection process illustrates the cyclical nature of CDM: the outputs of each stage can be input to the next stage, with iteration of stages as required.

By deconstructing the diagnostic processes into constituent parts, a mechanism is provided for revealing the different psychological components of clinical decision-making, the potential influences on them, and how they affect resulting diagnostic decisions. It suggests a number of areas where decision-making may be prone to gender bias: the number and nature of cues influencing classification; the knowledge structures used by doctors (explained later); and how doctors process cues and knowledge structures to estimate the certainty that the patient has a particular diagnosis. We refer to each of these areas where variation may occur as a decision-making component. The classification model is used to derive questions about the different components that can be tested for gender-related bias, which will be explained below after we describe the study methods that generated the required data.

Study methods

The qualitative data about primary-care doctors' decision-making analysed in this paper were collected within the context of a large cross-national study with a factorial experimental design (Cochran and Cox 1957), permitting control for the effects of doctor, patient and health service characteristics. The study was conducted simultaneously in the United States (Massachusetts) and the United Kingdom (Surrey/South West London and the West Midlands) in 2001–2002, to estimate the un-confounded effects of patient characteristics on different types of decisions made by primary care doctors. These included diagnostic, test ordering, treatment and referral decisions, when presented with patients manifesting symptoms strongly suggestive of CHD or depression. In this paper, we focus only on decision-making related to CHD. A full factorial of $2^4 = 16$ combinations of patient age (55 versus 75), gender, race (white versus black: African American in the US or Afro-Caribbean in the UK) and SES (lower versus higher social class – a cleaner/janitor versus a teacher) was used for the video scenarios. One of the 16 combinations was shown to each physician for each medical problem (two videos per physician structured such that half saw the CHD vignette last). Eight strata of physician (gender, years of clinical experience [<12 or >22 years]) and country (US/UK) characteristics were defined, to generate a total of $16 \times 2 \times 8 = 256$ physicians required to complete the experimental design.

Professional actors were used to create realistic videotaped portrayals of primary care consultations, which incorporated key symptoms for CHD. Such methods have been used successfully by the team in previous research examining primary care decision-making (McKinlay *et al.* 1997, 2002, McKinlay, Potter and Feldman 1996), and by others (*e.g.* McKinstry 2000). Scenarios were taped repeatedly, systematically varying the 'patient's' age, race, gender, SES and accent (UK v. US, Table 1).

Measures were taken to ensure the ecological and external validity of the scenarios for both countries, and to ensure identical clinical information

Table 1 Combination of patient characteristics in the experiment.

Patient characteristics	Values	
Age	55 years	75 years
Gender	Male	Female
Race	White	Black (Afro-Caribbean)
Social class/occupation	Janitor/cleaner	School teacher

$2^4 = 16$ Videos (combinations of patient characteristics).

portrayal by each 'patient'. For example, doctors were shown scenarios in their surgeries during normal working hours, were instructed to view video patients as one of their own, and to ground subsequent care decisions within existing local constraints (doctors were also asked at interview how typical scenarios were, and 92 per cent said either 'reasonably' or 'very' typical). The videos were shown to 256 primary care doctors, stratified by country (US v. UK), gender, and years of clinical experience (see Table 2). US doctors were randomly sampled from the Massachusetts Medical Society list and UK doctors from Surrey/South West London and West Midlands Health Authority lists. The sample of 256 doctors represents response rates of 65 per cent and 60 per cent of eligible doctors initially approached in the US and UK respectively.

After viewing each video scenario, doctors were asked about diagnosis and treatment decisions. Then, after viewing both scenarios, they were invited to give a free recall, unprompted account of their decision-making processes about the video scenario they had seen last (half or 128 physicians saw the CHD scenario last). The doctors' instructions were: 'I would like you to think back to the beginning of the second consultation and to describe your thoughts as they occurred during it. I am particularly interested in when a possible diagnosis

Table 2 Number of Primary Care Doctors in the Experiment by Gender, Year Completed Medical Training and Country.

	Location			
Doctor characteristics	Massachusetts, USA	Surrey & South East London	Midlands	Total
Male				
older (1965–1979)*	32	16	16	64
younger (1989–1996)*	32	16	16	64
Female				
older (1965–1979)*	32	16	16	64
younger (1989–1996)*	32	16	16	64
Total	128	64	64	256

* Year completed medical training.

first entered your mind and how the diagnoses developed on the way to your final conclusions. Starting at the beginning then, can you replay the tape in your mind and tell me what your thoughts were about the patient?'

This approach allows doctors to articulate thoughts based on their chronological genesis, thereby providing information not usually available about what, in their minds, was most significant about the video presentations, and about how their thoughts developed on the way to reaching their conclusions about diagnoses. Analysis of these data, referred to as the 'cognitive' data, is the focus of this paper. This free recall opportunity was followed by semi-structured questions designed to elicit information about uncertainty representation and doctors' knowledge structures. Due to missing and incomplete data, 112 (out of 128) accounts were analysed. These were provided by 56 doctors in each country, elicited in response to equal numbers (n = 56) of male and female patient presentations, thus constituting a balanced dataset according to the variables of interest.

Cognitive data were tape-recorded and transcribed verbatim by project support staff in both countries. Analysis was undertaken by one researcher (AA) in the UK, comprising thematic analysis using QSR NVivo 1.4 software, reflecting the components of the classification model of clinical decision-making. This involved an iterative process of developing a coding framework that embraced not only all of the important theoretical decision-making components, but also ensuring sufficient flexibility to identify additional concepts arising from the data. (See Appendix for a list of codes and examples.) Inter-rater reliability of coding (undertaken by AA and CDB) reached 90 per cent agreement when applied to the free recall data.

The next section describes how we investigated gender-related bias and the results. It provides more specific detail about the codes used and how they were applied to the data, with analysis of variance used to test all relationships in the data. The study design consisted of seven factors: four patient factors (gender, age, race, SES), two physician factors (gender, level of experience), and country. The analysis of variance model focused on the main effects and interactions of gender. In the absence of missing data, all effects would be orthogonal but due to missing 16 out of 128 responses, Type III sums of squares were used. All analyses were conducted using SAS version 9.1. Least square means (adjusting for the other variables in the model) and associated 95 per cent confidence intervals are given in Tables 3 and 4. Two-tailed tests were used because the mechanisms by which micro-cognitive processes are affected by gender are unknown, and because differences in either direction are of interest.

Testing for gender bias

The three components of our classification model of clinical decision-making that relate to diagnosis will be investigated with respect to gender effects.

Table 3 Results of testing differences between patients' and doctors' gender.

Decision-making component	Patient Gender (mean scores)			Doctor Gender (mean scores)		
	Male	Female	Sig. level	Male	Female	Sig. level
Component 1: number of cues considered						
(a) Unique general patient cues of all types	11.02	12.02	ns	10.61 (9.28–11.94)[b]	12.61 (11.28–13.94)[b]	p = 0.037
(b) Psychological cues	1.09 (0.67–1.52)[b]	1.72 (1.32–2.11)[b]	p = 0.036	1.22	1.60	ns
(c) Presentation cues	0.98	1.20	ns	0.90 (0.60–1.90)[b]	1.33 (1.03–1.62)[b]	p = 0.040
(d) Medical history cues	0.42	0.63	ns	0.50	0.55	ns
(e) Age cue mentioned for patients	0.81 (0.70–0.92)[b]	0.63 (0.52–0.73)[b]	p = 0.018	0.73	0.70	ns
Component 2: diagnostic inferences						
(f) All inferences	4.73	4.70	ns	4.81	4.63	ns
(g) Age-related inferences	1.00 (0.79–1.21)[b]	0.50 (0.30–0.70)[b]	p = 0.001	0.69	0.81	ns
Component 3: knowledge structures used by doctors						
(h) Use of prototypes	1.38	1.86	ns	1.44	1.80	ns
(i) Use of exemplars	0.44	0.56	ns	0.55	0.45	ns
(j) Use of probabilistic information	0.30	0.55	ns	0.58	0.27	ns

[b] 95% confidence intervals.
ns = p > 0.05.

Table 4 Significant interaction effects between patients' and doctors' gender.

Doctor Gender	Male (mean scores)		Female (mean scores)		Significance Level
Patient Gender	Male	Female	Male	Female	
Component 1: number of cues considered					
(a) Presentation cues	1.03 (0.60–1.46)[b]	0.75 (0.34–1.16)[b]	0.94 (0.50–1.38)[b]	1.72 (1.32–2.11)[b]	p = 0.014
(b) Age cue mentioned for patients	0.72 (0.56–0.88)[b]	0.75 (0.60–0.90)[b]	0.91 (0.75–1.07)[b]	0.50 (0.35–0.65)[b]	p = 0.007
Component 2: diagnostic inferences					
(c) Age-related inferences	0.78 (0.48–1.08)[b]	0.59 (0.30–0.88)[b]	1.22 (0.91–1.52)[b]	0.41 (0.13–0.68)[b]	p = 0.036

[b] 95% confidence intervals.
ns = p > 0.05.

Each comprises one or more micro-processes that will be analysed in turn to identify any influences of doctor and patient gender. Interaction effects will also be considered, but only the significant ones will be reported due to the number of potential interactions. Each micro-process is described, and outcomes associated with potential gender bias considered. Results of the analysis are presented in Tables 3 and 4. Table 3 shows independent influences of patient and doctor gender, and Table 4 shows significant interaction effects.

Component 1: The number of unique cues considered by doctors

Every mention of a patient cue was coded and the distinct cues were counted because the number of clinical, biographical, social or psychological pieces of data has implications for the number and range of diagnostic hypotheses entertained by doctors. Consideration of fewer patient cues may lead to fewer and less well-developed diagnostic hypotheses, with the potential to miss important ones (*e.g.* CHD). If there are systematic differences in the number considered for either male or female patients, this indicates less attention to their case and the potential for doctors to miss significant influences affecting diagnoses and subsequent care. However, the mean number of cues recalled for male and female patients was 11.02 and 12.02 respectively, which was not significantly different.

We went on to examine differences between the numbers of unique cues recalled by female doctors compared with male doctors, and found the mean number of cues recalled to be 12.6 and 10.6 respectively. This is a statistically significant difference ($p = 0.037$), occurring in the absence of any systematic differences in the lengths of male and female doctors' free recall accounts. It indicates that female doctors may be more open to a wider set of potentially influential factors than male doctors.

These differences could be associated with the direction of reasoning, where forward or data-driven reasoning gathers cues and uses them to suggest a range of diagnoses, whereas goal-driven or backward reasoning tries to find data associated with a particular diagnosis. Consultations always iterate between the two directions, but to varying degrees. If backward reasoning predominates, there may not be enough cues gathered to generate a full set of differential diagnoses, and focusing on the most likely ones will tend to generate a smaller set of confirming cues rather than ones suggesting alternative diagnoses. It may even lead to confirmation bias (Klayman 1995), when people try to prove the truth of ideas instead of disproving them. If it was taking place in this study, male doctors should have greater certainty of CHD than female doctors, but quantitative data collected from 256 doctors as part of the wider study did not show a significant difference. It is possible, though, that the type of cue is more influential than the numbers, which we explore next.

Systematic differences in the type of cues considered for either male or female patients may indicate over-sensitivity to some types of information and blindness to others. To test for it, cues recalled by doctors were coded into psychological, social, presentation, and medical history categories, described below.

Psychological cues relate to doctors' comments about a patient's state of mind (see Appendix). The overall mean number recalled was 1.4, with 1.7 considered for women and 1.1 for men, which is a statistically significant difference (p = 0.036, Table 3, row b). These findings support previous research (*e.g.* Emslie, Hunt and Watt 2001, Martin, Gordon and Lounsbury 1998, Lockyer and Bury 2002) by indicating that doctors are more likely to tune into psychological cues and to search for psychological explanations for women's symptoms than they are for men. There was no significant difference between doctor gender for these cues, though, which means both male and female doctors are equally prone to the behaviour.

Presentation cues concern the manner in which patients present their history and symptoms (see Appendix). Female doctors were found to recall significantly more presentation cues compared to their male counterparts (mean scores of 1.33 compared with 0.90 respectively, p = 0.040, Table 3, row c). A significant interaction between patient gender and doctor gender (p = 0.014) shows that the main cause of the difference between male and female doctors is due to how female doctors interact with female patients (Table 4, row a). Women doctors recall more presentation cues for female than male patients (mean cues of 1.72 compared with 0.94), whereas the difference for male doctors is less marked, albeit in the opposite direction, favouring men (mean cues of 0.75 and 1.03 for female and male patients respectively). These findings suggest that doctors are more attuned to the way in which patients of their own sex present their history, and that this is enhanced in the case of women doctors consulting with female patients, as Lorber and Moore (2002) suggest.

Patient medical history cues relate to pieces of information about past or present diseases, illnesses, and medical events affecting either the patient or their family, which may influence patients' current or future health (see Appendix). No significant effects of patient or doctor gender were found on the number of medical history cues recalled.

Our previous work showed interesting effects of patient age on diagnostic behaviour (Adams *et al.* 2006), but without specifically identifying how it influences decision-making about male and female patients. To find out whether age is noted more for women or for men, its influence on decision-making was recorded as a binary value, 'yes' if age was mentioned at all and 'no' otherwise. This exposed a significant difference between patient genders (p = 0.018), with 81 per cent of doctors mentioning age in relation to males but only 63 per cent in relation to females (Table 3, row e). These findings corroborate the influence of age, suggesting it is a more important 'anchor' for doctors in terms of considering potential diagnoses for men than it is for women, and possibly underpinning Healy's (1991) contention that most medical knowledge reflects a male gender bias.

Examination of interactions between doctor and patient gender (Table 4, row b) reveals that female doctors mention age more for male patients than for female patients (91% of the time versus 50%), whereas male doctors treat them roughly the same (72% versus 75%, male to female). This indicates that the gender effect is really down to the different behaviour of female doctors, suggesting that while female patients' presentation of history and symptoms resonates more with female doctors, female doctors are simultaneously less likely to be attuned to the clinical significance of their age when it comes to making diagnostic decisions.

Component 2: Doctor's diagnostic inferences

Figure 1 shows that the inference process for linking cues to diagnostic classes is an integral part of clinical decision-making. Component 2 examines these inferences, which are any inferred attributes of the patient, such as diseases (*e.g.* CHD) or non-medical attributes such as social isolation (see Appendix). Increased inferences indicate a more open mind to different diagnostic possibilities, and an increased likelihood that the correct diagnosis will be present within a doctor's set of differentials. This is especially important during the early stages because Barrows *et al.* (1982) showed that only 14 per cent of physicians will eventually identify the correct diagnosis if it is absent from the initial differential set.

The mean number of diagnostic inferences was 4.70, showing no significant gender differences, either between doctors or patients (Table 3, row f). It was seen above, however, that gender differences were found with respect to mentioning the age cue (Table 3, row e), so it is pertinent to explore whether age is also having an impact on gender with respect to diagnoses, by examining age-related inferences. An example is a doctor saying a patient is just the right age and type of person to have CHD. In this analysis, age has to be explicitly associated with an inference, testifying to its specific influence on decision-making rather than simply being noted as a patient attribute (see Appendix).

Given that age is more often mentioned with respect to male patients (see above), it is not surprising to see this is repeated for the association of age with diagnostic inferences. Male patients received an average of one inference associated with age (Table 3, row g), twice as many as the number for females (0.50, $p = 0.001$). Furthermore, the difference is again mostly linked to female doctors ($p = 0.036$, Table 4, row c), whose number of age-related inferences is 1.22 for males and 0.41 for females, compared to the smaller difference of male doctors (0.78 versus 0.59, for male and female patients respectively). These findings underline the importance of age as an influence on gender differences in diagnostic behaviour: it is mentioned more often by female doctors and is more influential on their diagnoses, but only with respect to male patients.

The increased number of age-related inferences for male patients seems to be having a real effect on diagnostic accuracies because there was a significant difference according to patient gender ($p = 0.031$) when the 256 doctors were asked for their certainties of CHD in the quantitative part of this study (reported by Arber *et al.* 2006). The doctors estimated their certainties of CHD to be 57 per cent certain for men, compared with 47 per cent for women, which correlates with better accuracy because the scenarios were supposed to indicate CHD as the correct diagnosis.

Component 3: Knowledge structures used by doctors

The analysis of gender effects has concentrated so far on cue selection and their relationship to inferences for diagnostic classes. We now turn to how cues relate to each other within the knowledge structures doctors possess.

In terms of psychological classification, there are two fundamental models for representing knowledge about classes (see Hampton 1993): the prototype model, which represents a class by a single, most typical member; and the exemplar model, which represents classes by all their known members. Prototypes do not directly hold information about disease frequencies, whereas the exemplar model does, because it stores all the members, and thus incorporates class sizes. The difference is important because failing to take account of class sizes means that the existing evidence base for prior probabilities of diseases and outcomes is potentially ignored, which, in terms of gender issues, would mean doctors failing to take account of the frequencies of CHD within male and female populations, and over-reliance on matching patients to disease stereotypes when making diagnoses.

The second difference between prototypes and exemplars is that the exemplar representation holds more information on variability amongst class members by retaining all the different manifestations and their particular combinations in each member. This may enable more unusual symptom patterns to be correctly matched to a doctor's disease representation, such as women's different descriptions of angina compared with men's (Philpott *et al.* 2001, Mikhail 2005), and thus facilitate more accurate diagnoses. If women do not present with typical CHD symptoms, then they may be disadvantaged by doctors' over-reliance on prototypes.

Our coding scheme (see Appendix) enabled us to test three important relationships between gender and the use of knowledge structures, namely, between gender and the use of prototypes; the use of exemplars; and the use of explicit probabilistic information (given by the disease frequency or probability code). Analyses failed to detect any significant gender effects, which means gender differences in diagnostic accuracy are not caused by the way knowledge is structured or how probabilistic information is integrated.

Summary and conclusions

Through the use of novel analytic methods combining sociological and psychological perspectives, this paper aimed to provide new insights into sources of uncertainty and gender bias in primary care doctors' diagnosis of CHD. In particular, it re-examined three important contentions in medical sociological literature: that there are differences in male and female doctors' consulting styles; that knowledge about female presentations is not yet sufficiently integrated into received medical wisdom about what is 'normal' in CHD; and that women receive better-quality CHD care from women doctors.

Our findings confirm the importance highlighted by others (Raine 2001, Richards *et al.* 2000, Mikhail 2005) of investigating gender differences in the initial diagnostic process for CHD. However, we failed to find evidence of differences due to variations in the knowledge structures used by male and female doctors, indicating that doctors' diagnoses were not inappropriately influenced by gender-stereotypical thinking, or failure to integrate probabilistic information. Instead, we found differences in the way male and female doctors respond to patient information, particularly in their perceptions of cue relevance and salience for potential diagnoses. Compared with their male colleagues, female doctors recall more patient cues and pay more attention to the way in which patients present their verbal histories, particularly in the case of female patients. These findings confirm differences in male and female doctors' consulting styles, with female doctors being particularly interested in patient narratives, as described by others (*e.g.* Roter, Lipkin and Korsgaard 1991, Hall *et al.* 1994, Lorber 2000, Lorber and Moore 2002).

Paying attention to the significance of women's age is not however reflected in female doctors' interest in women's histories. By contrast, both male and female doctors, but especially females, took particular account of male patients' age when diagnosing, and generated a greater number of age-related diagnostic hypotheses for them than for women. More focus on men's age may, in part, reflect the historical male bias in medical knowledge, arising out of women's under-representation in CHD-related medical research. Our findings therefore support Lorber's (2000) conclusions, that knowledge about female presentations is not yet sufficiently integrated into received medical wisdom about what is 'normal' in CHD. On the other hand, the greater focus on men's age may reflect more documented concern about the higher rates of mortality from CHD associated with increasing age amongst men compared with women (Lawlor, Ebrahim and Davey Smith 2002b).

There may however be something else going on in addition to clinical uncertainty. It has already been noted that prevalent stereotypical conceptualisations of CHD as a male disease remain important amongst women (Guilleman 2004, Ruston and Clayton 2002), suggesting a reluctance amongst women to accept that they are equally prone to CHD as they get older. This reluctance may translate into female doctors having a higher age threshold over which they will recognise potential CHD amongst women compared with men. Something akin to this is described by Bernard (1998), who examines female nurses' responses to caring for older women compared with older men. She identifies that nurses' discomfort with caring for their own sex, and comparative greater ease in caring for men, is associated in part with wishing to remain 'blind' to their own ageing, and the likely ill-health and role change consequences associated with it. On the other hand, due to the long-standing male bias in medical knowledge and clinical research, male doctors may be more accepting of the potential for CHD amongst their own sex.

Whatever is the explanation for less attention being paid to the significance of women's age as a risk factor for CHD, a key question remains: Do the identified gender differences have clinical significance, causing biases with potentially detrimental clinical consequences for patients? To determine this, it is necessary to re-consider population trends for CHD. Although new evidence about a change in trend is coming to light (NHS Confederation Press Summaries, 6 September 2005), to date, the known prevalence of, and mortality from, CHD has been higher amongst men than women (DH 2005, NCCD 2005). Despite standardisation of patient presentations, this received knowledge of population base rates may legitimately affect doctors' diagnostic certainty, as discussed above. Nevertheless, the patient presentations in our video-taped vignettes contained a high number of cardinal symptoms, universally recognised as being strongly suggestive of CHD. This means that doctors' certainty about a CHD diagnosis should have been high, irrespective of patient gender, raising some concern about the significant difference found between male and female patients in the quantitative part of this study (57% versus 47%, Arber *et al.* 2006). This was the case for doctors of both genders, casting doubt on Lorber's (2000) contention, that women receive better CHD care from female doctors. Indeed, our study makes this seem more unlikely given that female doctors pay significantly less attention to patients' age for women than men, when male doctors showed no difference. This has significant implications because: women are greater consumers of primary healthcare than men; numbers of female doctors are increasing in the primary care workforce; and female patients are more likely to choose to be seen by them (Franks and Bertakis 2003). It highlights the need for better developed risk and diagnostic models of CHD for women, particularly with respect to the influence of age, which was the main source of gender differences between patients.

Compared to female doctors, males work with fewer patient cues and appear to be less influenced by patients' gender when making diagnostic decisions. Results for them demonstrate more similarity in their dealing with information about male and female patients, except where both male and female doctors demonstrate gender bias, in relation to recalling more psychological cues about female patients. However, it may be that the observed gender neutrality of male doctors in diagnostic decision-making disadvantages men, if there are good clinical reasons for treating them differently from women, as suggested by others (*e.g.* Roeters van Lennop 2000, Wong *et al.* 2001).

The validity of our results resides in the rigour of our research methods. These involved a meticulously designed factorial experiment, generation of stratified random samples of primary care doctors in each research locality, and the use of ecologically valid video vignettes of simulated patients as stimuli for data collection. Doctors' unstructured ruminations on their thoughts about patients were then analysed according to the component parts of our classification model of diagnostic decision-making, through the rigorous application of the associated coding scheme we have developed. We are thus confident that our findings can be generalised.

A limitation of the study is the timing of the collection of the 'cognitive data', which followed structured questions about the scenarios. In order to capture doctors' dynamic reasoning processes, data should ideally be collected both during, and immediately after, watching video-taped scenarios, thus providing no opportunity for post-hoc justification (Ericsson and Simon 1993). This was not possible in the current study, but we will do this in future work, and compare the results. Another limitation relates to the use of standardised video-taped scenarios for controlling for variation in patient presentation. These inevitably remove naturally occurring variation in the ways in which men and women present during consultations, which may have influenced doctors' decision-making. Furthermore, the use of videos prevents interaction of the doctors with the patients, thereby removing any impact of their particular consultation styles. However, without standardising presentations and controlling for confounding variables, we should not have been able to present our results with confidence: no solution is perfect.

In summary, there may be doubt about whether differences between male and female patients' CHD diagnoses are based on reliable clinical evidence, but there should not be variations in the *process* of clinical decision-making simply because of the doctor's gender. Patients are entitled to expect the same quality of care whichever gender attends to them, but our research has demonstrated that this may not necessarily be the case. More research is needed into the causes of these doctor gender differences and how they can be counteracted to ensure equality of care, in addition to investigating disparities in CHD diagnoses between men and women.

Acknowledgements

The research was funded by the National Institutes of Health, National Institute of Aging, Grant no. AG-16747. The authors are grateful to Amy

O'Donnell and Sue Venn for facilitating all aspects of the project in the US and UK, to our interviewers – Sam Colt and Cathie McColl, and to Nathan Hughes for data entry. We are also grateful to Alan Goroll, MD, Ted Stern, MD, John Stoeckle, MD (Massachusetts General Hospital), David Armstrong, PhD, FFPHM, FRCGP and Mark Ashworth, MRCP, MRCGP (United Medical and Dental Schools of Guys, Kings and St Thomas's, London) and Diane Ackerley, MBBS (Guildford and Waverley Primary Care Trust). We thank all the 256 doctors who gave up an hour of their valuable time to participate in this research.

Ann Adams is funded by a Department of Health NCCRCD Primary Care Career Scientist Award.

Appendix: Coding scheme and examples of codes

I Patient Cues are any descriptive attributes of the patient, (including their age or gender); any symptoms offered by the patient; or any direct observations of a patient's behaviour by the doctor *e.g.*:

she was <u>rather thin</u>
he reported <u>frequent headaches</u>
she seemed <u>very debilitated</u>.

Psychological Cues are a subset of patient cues, where the above attributes, symptoms and observations are of psychological origin *e.g.*:

He seemed <u>very low</u>
She said she felt <u>very depressed</u>.

Presentation cues are also a subset of patient cues, representing doctors' observations about the manner in which patients present their history, *e.g.*:

<u>he doesn't give a very cogent history</u>
<u>She's a passive victim, something about the tone that suggested that</u>

Medical history cues are also a subset of patient cues, and relate to pieces of information about past or present diseases, illness and medical events affecting either the patient or their family, which may influence patients' current or future health *e.g.*:

He has been a <u>diabetic for 2 years</u>
She suffered from <u>depression in the past</u>
His <u>father died of a heart attack at age 50</u>.

II Doctors' Inferences are any inferred attributes of the patient, which may be potential diseases or patient attributes that are being inferred from lower-level data *e.g.*

I think he is suffering from coronary heart disease
he has no family or friends and no regular social activities which makes me think he is socially isolated.

Age-related inferences are a subset of doctors' inferences, where a doctor says a patient is just the right age and type of person to have a certain condition. Age has to be explicitly associated with an inference, testifying to its specific influence on decision-making rather than simply being noted as a patient attribute, *e.g.*:

At 45 she is in the right age group for a gall bladder problem
at his age, cancer has to be considered

III Disease frequency or probability statements relate to doctors' statements about the likelihood and how often a disease may be present within certain groups of people *e.g.*:

there is a higher than average incidence of coronary heart disease in elderly black males type 2 diabetes is more likely in people over 50.

IV Disease knowledge (prototypical information) is applied to statements that go beyond just the normal association of patient cues with inferences. The code is applied to any statement providing additional information about causal, probabilistic, or other more complex relationships existing between cues and inferences, which are clearly related to those inferences in general, not just how they apply to the particular patient in the consultation. This is akin to a classic textbook description of a disease *e.g.*:

She had all the features of typical angina
insomnia, loss of appetite, early morning waking and general lack of interest in life are all common manifestations of depression.

V Knowledge from **previous patients** (exemplar information) is applied to statements where doctors specifically refer to previous patients they have seen or where the information they are using comes from their experience of treating previous patients *e.g*:

I have been caught out in the past by missing stomach cancer
A patient I saw last week had exactly these same symptoms of headache and rash.

References

Adams, A., Buckingham, C., Arber, S., McKinlay, J. B., Marceau, L. and Link, C. (2006) The influence of patients' age on clinical decision-making about coronary heart disease in the US and the UK, *Ageing and Society*, 26, 2, 303–21.

Agvall, B. and Dahlstrom, U. (2001) Patients in primary health care diagnosed and treated as heart failure, with special reference to gender differences, *Scandinavian Journal of Primary Care*, 19, 9–14.

Arber, S., McKinlay, J. B., Adams, A., Marceau, L., Link, C. and O'Donnell, A. (2004) Influence of patient characteristics on doctors' questioning and lifestyle advice for CHD: a UK/US video experiment, *British Journal of General Practice*, 54, 673–8.

Arber, S., McKinlay, J. B., Adams, A., Marceau, L., Link, C. and Black, A. (2006) Patient characteristics and inequalities in doctors' diagnostic and treatment strategies related to CHD: a US/UK comparison, *Social Science & Medicine*, 62, 103–15.

Bandyopadhyay, S., Bayer, A. J. and O'Mahony, M. S. (2001) 'Age and gender bias in statin trials', *QJM: Monthly Journal of the Association of Doctors*, 94, 127–32.

Barrows, H. S., Norman, G. R., Neufeld, V. R. and Feightner, J. W. (1982) The clinical reasoning of randomly selected physicians in general medical practice. *Clinical and Investigative Medicine*, 5, 49–55.

Bennett, K. E., Williams, D. and Feely, J. (2002) Inequalities in the prescribing of secondary preventative heart therapies for ischaemic heart disease in Ireland. [Abstract only]. *Irish Medical Journal*, 95, 169–72.

Bernard, M. (1998) Backs to the future? Reflections on women, ageing and nursing, *Journal of Advanced Nursing*, 27, 633–640.

Borzak, S. and Weaver, D. (2000) Sex and outcome after myocardial infarction: a case of sexual politics? *Circulation*, 102, 2458–9.

Buckingham, C. D. and Adams, A. (2000a) Classifying clinical decision making: a unifying approach, *Journal of Advanced Nursing*, 32, 4, 981–9.

Buckingham, C. D. and Adams, A. (2000b) Classifying clinical decision making: interpreting nursing intuition, heuristics and medical diagnosis, *Journal of Advanced Nursing*, 32, 4, 990–8.

Burstein, J., Yan, R., Weller, I. and Abramson, B. L. (2003) Management of congestive heart failure: a gender gap may still exist, *BMC Cardiovascular Disorders*, 3, e-publication.

Clarke, K. W., Gray, D., Keating, N. A. and Hampton, J. R. (1994) Do women with acute myocardial infarction receive the same treatment as men? *British Medical Journal*, 309, 563–6.

Cochran, W. G. and Cox, G. D. (1957) *Experimental Designs*, 2nd Edition. New York: John Wiley and Sons.

Corbelli, J. A., Corbelli, J. C., Bullano, M. F., Willey, V. J., Cziraky, M. J. and Banks, L. D. (2003) Gender bias in lipid assessment and treatment following percutaneous coronary intervention, *Journal of Gender-Specific Medicine*, 6, 21–6.

Department of Health (2005) *Coronary Heart Disease National Service Framework: Leading the Way – Progress Report*. London: HMSO.

DeWilde, S., Carey, I. M., Bremner, S. A., Richards, N., Hilton, S. R. and Cook, D. G. (2003) Evolution of statin prescribing 1994–2001: a case of ageism but not sexism? *Heart*, 89, 417–21.

Emslie, C., Hunt, K. and Watt, G. (2001) Invisible women? The importance of gender in lay beliefs about heart problems, *Sociology of Health and Illness*, 23, 2, 203–33.

Ericsson, K. A. and Simon, H. A. (1993) *Protocol Analysis: Verbal Reports as Data*. Revised Edition, Cambridge, MA: MIT Press.

Franks, P. and Bertakis, K. (2003) Doctor gender, patient gender, and primary care, *Journal of Women's Health*, 12, 73–80.

Guilleman, M. (2004) Heart disease and mid-age women: focusing on gender and age, *Health Sociology Review*, 13, 1, 7–14.

Hall, J. A., Irish, J. T., Roter, D. L., *et al.* (1994) Gender in medical encounters: an analysis of physician and patient communication in a primary care setting, *Health Psychology*, 13, 382–92.

Hampton, J. (1993) Prototype models of concept representation. In Mechelen, I. V., Hampton, J., Michalski, R. S. and Theuns, P. (eds) *Categories and Concepts – Theoretical Views and Inductive Data Analysis*. San Diego: Academic Press.

Hayes, B. C. and Prior, P. M. (2003) *Gender and Health Care in the United Kingdom: Exploring the Stereotypes*. Basingstoke: Palgrave Macmillan.

Healy, B. (1991) The Yentl syndrome, *New England Journal of Medicine*, 325, 274–5.

Hippisley-Cox, J., Pringle, M., Crown, N., Meal, A. and Wynn, A. (2001) Sex inequalities in ischaemic heart disease in general practice: cross sectional survey, *British Medical Journal*, 322, 1–5.

Hochleitner, M. (2000) Coronary heart disease: sexual bias in referral for coronary angiogram. How does it work in a state-run health system? *Journal of Women's Health and Gender-Based Medicine*, 9, 29–34.

Kitler, M. E. (1994) Coronary disease: are there gender differences? [systematic literature review, abstract only], *European Heart Journal*, 15, 409–17.

Klayman, J. (1995) Varieties of confirmation bias. In Busemeyer, J., Hastie, R. and Medin, D. L. (eds) *Decision making from a Cognitive Perspective: Volume 32. The Psychology of Learning and Motivation*. New York: Academic Press.

Lawlor, D. A., Ebrahim, S. and Davey Smith, G. (2002a) A life course approach to coronary heart disease and stroke. In Kuh, D. and Hardy, R. (eds) *A Life Course Approach to Women's Health*. Oxford: Oxford University Press.

Lawlor, D. A., Ebrahim, S. and Davey Smith, G. (2002b) Role of endogenous oestrogen in aetiology of coronary heart disease: analysis of age related trends in coronary heart disease and breast cancer in England and Wales and Japan, *British Medical Journal*, 325, 311–12.

Lockyer, L. and Bury, M. (2002) The construction of a modern epidemic: the implications for women of the gendering of coronary heart disease, *Journal of Advanced Nursing*, 39, 432–40.

Lorber, J. (2000) *Gender and the Social Construction of Illness*, New York: AltaMira Press.

Lorber, J. and Moore, L. J. (2002) *Gender and the Social Construction of Illness* 2nd Edition. New York: AltaMira Press.

Martin, R., Gordon, E. I. and Lounsbury, P. (1998) Gender disparities in the attribution of cardiac-related symptoms: contribution of common sense models of illness, *Health Psychology*, 17, 346–57.

McKinlay, J. B. (1996) Some contributions from the social system to gender inequalities in heart disease, *Journal of Health and Social Behaviour*, 37, 1–26.

McKinlay, J. B., Potter, D. A. and Feldman, H. A. (1996) Non-medical influences on medical decision-making, *Social Science & Medicine*, 42, 5, 769–76.

McKinlay, J. B., Burns, R. B., Durante, R., Feldman, H. A., Freund, K. M., Harrow, B. S., Irish, J. T., Kasten, L. E. and Moskowitz, M. A. (1997) Patient, physician and presentational influences on clinical decision-making for breast cancer: results from a factorial experiment, *Journal of Evaluation in Clinical Practice*, 3, 1–69.

McKinlay, J. B., Lin, T., Freund, K. and Moskowitz, M. (2002) The unexpected influence of physician attributes on clinical decisions: results of an experiment, *Journal of Health and Social Behaviour*, 43, 92–106.

McKinstry, B. (2000) Do patients wish to be involved in decision making in the consultation? A cross-sectional survey with video vignettes, *British Medical Journal*, 321, 7265, 867–71.

Mikhail, G. W. (2005) Coronary heart disease in women, *British Medical Journal*, 331, 467–8.

National Center for Chronic Disease Prevention and Health Promotion (2005) *Heart Disease and Stroke, Healthy People 2010, Focus Area 12*, http://www.cdc.gov/cvh.

Peltonen, M., Lundberg, V., Huhtasaari, F. and Asplund, K. (2000) Marked improvement in survival after acute myocardial infarction in middle-aged men but not in women. The Northern Sweden MONICA study 1985–94, *Journal of Internal Medicine*, 247, 5, 579–87.

Philpott, S., Boynton, P. M., Feder, F. and Hemingway, H. (2001) Gender differences in descriptions of angina symptoms and health problems immediately prior to angiography: the ACRE study, *Social Science & Medicine*, 52, 10, 1565–75.

Raine, R. (2001) Clinical decision making is not necessarily guided by prejudice, [Letter], *British Medical Journal*, 323, 400.

Richards, H., McConnachie, A., Morrison, C., Murray, K. and Watt, G. (2000) Social and gender variation in the prevalence, presentation and general practitioner provisional diagnosis of chest pain, *Journal of Epidemiology and Community Health*, 54, 714–8.

Roeters van Lennep, J. E. (2000) Gender differences in diagnosis and treatment of coronary artery disease from 1981 to 1997: no evidence for the Yentl syndrome, *European Heart Journal*, 21, 874–75.

Rosser, S. V. (1994) Gender bias in clinical research: the difference it makes. In Dan, A. J. (ed.) *Reframing Women's Health*. London: Sage.

Roter, D., Lipkin, M. and Korsgaard, A. (1991) Sex differences in patients' and physicians' communication during primary care medical visits, *Medical Care*, 29, 1083–93.

Ruston, A. and Clayton, J. (2002) Coronary heart disease: women's assessment of risk – a qualitative study, *Health, Risk and Society*, 4, 2, 125–37.

Sayer, G. P. and Britt, H. (1996) Sex differences in morbidity: a case of discrimination in general practice, *Social Science & Medicine*, 42, 257–64.

Schulman, K. A., Berlin, J. A., Harless, W., Kerner, J. F., Sistrunk, S. and Gersh, B. J. (1999) The effect of race and sex on doctors' recommendations for cardiac catheterisation, *New England Journal of Medicine*, 1999, 618–26.

Wenger, N. K. (1994) Coronary heart disease in women: gender differences in diagnostic evaluation, *Journal of the American Medical Women's Association*, 49, 181–6.

White, A. and Lockyer, L. (2001) Tackling coronary heart disease: a gender sensitive approach is needed, *British Medical Journal*, 323, 1016–7.

Wild, S. (2001) Designating sex specific total cholesterol targets may be useful, [Letter], *British Medical Journal*, 323, 400.

Wong, Y., Rodwell, A., Dawkins, S., Livesey, S. A. and Simpson, I. A. (2001) Sex differences in investigation results and treatment in subjects referred for investigation of chest pain, *Heart*, 85, 149–52.

54

CONTINUITY AND CHANGE IN THE GENDER SEGREGATION OF THE MEDICAL PROFESSION IN BRITAIN AND FRANCE

Rosemary Crompton and Nicky Le Feuvre

Source: *International Journal of Sociology and Social Policy*, 23:4 (2003), 36–58.

Abstract

It is a well established fact that the entry of women into higher-level professional occupations has not resulted in their equal distribution within these occupations. Indeed, the emergence and persistence of horizontal and vertical gender segregation within the professions has been at the heart of the development of a range of alternative theoretical perspectives on both the 'feminisation process' and the future of the 'professions' more generally. Through an in-depth comparative analysis of the recent changes in the organisation and administration of the medical profession in Britain and France, this paper draws upon statistical data and biographical interviews with male and female general practitioners (GPs) in both countries in order to discuss and review a variety of approaches that have been adopted to explain and analyse the 'feminisation' process of higher-level professions. Our conclusions review the theoretical debates in the light of the evidence we have presented. It is argued that, despite important elements of continuity in respect of gendered occupational structuring in both countries, national variations in both professional and domestic gendered architectures lead to different outcomes as far as the extent and patterns of internal occupational segregation are concerned. Both female and male doctors are currently seeking—with some effect—to resist the pressures of medicine on family life.

Introduction

The entry of women into previously male-dominated occupations such as medicine raises a series of issues of interest to social scientists and policy makers. Past discussions of women's entry into medicine have tended to be dominated by a model of gender exclusion, reflecting the *actual* exclusion of women from prestigious occupations since their initial emergence as identifiable groupings in the nineteenth century (Witz 1992). These formal barriers have been largely removed, but nevertheless, intra-professional occupational segregation is still widespread. In part this reflects the persistence of masculine exclusionary practices—even though these are likely to be informal rather than formal in nature. However, patterns of occupational distribution within professions also reflect the (re)production of the gender division of labour within the professions as well as in the wider society.[1] Women still retain the major responsibility for domestic and caring work, and as we shall see, the intra-professional distribution of medical specialties in both Britain and France reflects this.

The increase in women's levels of employment is associated with a number of social trends and societal changes. Contemporary theoretical discussions emphasise the growing significance of lifestyle choices and identities in 'reflexively modern' societies. Some commentators have interpreted these trends as evidence of a growing individualism reflecting the marketisation of ever more areas of social life (Giddens 1992; Giddens, Beck and Lash 1994; Beck and Beck-Gernsheim 1995). An emphasis on the significance of individual choice is also found in Hakim's (2001) contentious argument that women are clustered in family-compatible feminised niches within occupations and organisations because the majority of women—even the well-educated—'choose' to put their family lives before their employment careers.

However, we shall argue that, rather than simply focus on the individual, it is important to examine the national, contextual and institutional implications and outcomes of changes in the gender division of labour of which the growth of women in the professions is but one aspect. The entry of women into occupations from which they were previously excluded—such as medicine—not only has implications for the profession and its practitioners. In a wider context it also impacts on state policies relating to the organisation and delivery of health care, as well as the national 'gender context' within which these changes are taking place. In this paper, therefore, we will explore the implications of the changing division of labour between men and women, both within the medical profession and also within 'work' in its wider sense, with reference to general practitioners (GPs) in Britain and France.

'Work' involves not only paid work but also domestic labour, which can often intermingle with paid work (Glucksmann 2000).[2] Patterns of market 'work' cannot be comprehensively grasped and understood without reference to patterns of unpaid domestic and caring work. By convention, women have assumed the major responsibility for this unpaid work but increasingly, women are participating in market work and (although to a lesser extent) more men are participating in unpaid domestic work (Sullivan 2000). These generalisations, of course, obscure the very wide variations in the distribution of market work and domestic labour between households, and between individual men and women in different countries. In comparison to Britain, the French state (and French employers) has historically offered more support to families, particularly in respect of childcare, and this has been associated with a higher level of full-time work amongst French women (Hantrais 1990). The contrasting organisation and delivery of healthcare in France and Britain also has consequences for the way in which doctors in Britain and France organise their 'care time' and 'working time', with rather different outcomes for the internal differentiation of the medical profession in the two countries.

In this paper, our object will be to shift the terrain on which discussions of 'women in the professions' have been situated. Previous discussions have tended to focus on women and men as *categories*, with a corresponding emphasis on the individual or collective effects of 'masculine' or 'feminine' behaviour within the profession. Whilst maintaining a focus on the individual, in this paper we will also emphasise the *context* within which individuals are located. We will see that universalistic theories relating to topics such as 'women' and 'the professions' need to be tempered by an appreciation of the sensitivity of these concepts to their national and local contexts.

Doctors

Medicine was once the epitome of a male-dominated, high status, profession (Witz 1992; Davies 1996). Medical training is long, and so, by tradition, are the hours worked by doctors, especially whilst in training positions in a hospital setting. Nevertheless, in nearly all industrialised countries, women are now the majority of those training in medicine. However, comparative research on women's entry into medicine in Britain, France and Norway has shown that, despite the increase in women's representation in the profession, they are still largely absent from some male-dominated specialties such as surgery. Perhaps even more importantly, women tend to cluster in those specialties in which it is possible to achieve some control over working hours (Crompton, Le Feuvre and Birkelund 1999). Thus the medical profession remains male dominated, and women are not represented in the most prestigious specialties in their due proportion.

In our recent comparison of the employment and domestic trajectories of doctors and bank managers in Britain, France and Norway (see Crompton 1999), we found that women doctors, despite being gender pioneers in their chosen profession, were nevertheless rather more likely to be relatively conventional as far as their domestic arrangements were concerned. They also tended to have more children than women bankers. We explained this tendency with reference to the capacity of women doctors to select, if they wished, professional options that gave them some control over their working time. This might mean either working less than full-time (whether salaried or self-employed), or choosing a specialty with regular and predictable hours of work.[3] Most women doctors had made these choices whilst still in training, in the expectation that they would assume the major responsibility for any future home and family—which they did. These choices reproduce somewhat conventional gender roles in the home and reinforce the sexual division of labour within the profession.

Our subsequent interviews with male doctors suggested that most male doctors with children had partners who took the major responsibility for childcare and domestic arrangements. However, we interviewed three male doctors (one in each country studied) who had *chosen* to share childcare with their wives. In each country, their approach to their careers and decision-making was very similar to that of the women doctors who had chosen their specialties in order to mesh an employment and family 'career'—although the career options chosen by family-oriented male medics were different in each country. In Britain, general practice had been chosen, whereas in France, the doctor was in a salaried position. As this paper will show, this difference is a significant one. The biographical information given in the table below makes a very simple point. If male doctors give priority to family compatibility when making their occupational decisions, then they will 'choose' options similar to those 'chosen' by like-minded women. Thus, the career consequences of caring responsibilities, whether conventionally imposed or freely chosen, will be the same for both sexes.

In this paper, we will be focusing on general practitioners in Britain and France. In both countries, GPs are self-employed independent contractors. However, there are important differences in the delivery of primary health care in the two countries (Crompton and Le Feuvre 1997). In Britain, GPs are remunerated by the National Health Service (NHS) according to a complex formula that incorporates an amount for each patient registered with their practice. Joint practices are prevalent (70% of all GP practices have two or more doctors) and doctors do not receive a fee for individual patient consultations. In France, on the other hand, patients are not required to register with a particular GP or GP practice and doctors receive a fee for each consultation. Joint practices are less common than in Britain. Given the high density of medical practitioners in France,[4] particularly in urban areas, competition between GPs for patients is widespread (Hassenteufel 1997; DREES 2001c).[5]

The British case

In Britain, the great majority of qualified doctors work either in hospitals (either in training positions or as specialists in particular branches of medicine), or in the community as GPs.[6] Doctors working in hospitals are salaried, although specialists often carry out private practice on a fee basis, in addition to their work for the National Health Service.

Family-oriented male doctors

Britain	Norway	France
Born: 1966, married,	Born: 1964, married.	Born: 1959, married
3 children (1994, 1995, 1997)	2 children (1994, 1996)	2 children (1989, 1992)
GP: part-time partner	GP: municipal health centre	Salaried *médecin du travail*
Childcare: during training used nursery, now shared equally with wife who also works part-time. "In my view, family's more important than work—and in my view, if there is a balance there—if you have to go home to your family then... you have to go home to your family and someone else will carry the can."	Childcare: alternating emphasis with wife, he took extended childcare leave (6 months, 18 months) to be full-time carer. "I chose general medicine, largely on account of my family. I have better work times now, and fewer night calls... I work only with women here—they understand my family needs... my ambitions are less important now."	Childcare: shared with wife. "In my family life my wife and I are interchangeable, when the children were young we each did every other night, we each did every other weekend, there is no doubt that we have reached equality between the sexes... I'm a bit of a nonconformist and traditional family life really gets on my nerves." Moved job (to salaried) because of children.

Although GP principals are self-employed, as a group they have resisted competition (between individuals or between different practices) and have drawn heavily on the ideology of 'professionalism' in their contractual negotiations with governments. In the case of medicine, as Shuval and Bernstein have argued, 'professionalism' involves an: "... all-encompassing devotion to work characterised by total personal involvement that focuses on the intrinsic rewards of work, transcends the monetary rewards and spills over to invade the professionals leisure time leaving little space for extra-occupational concerns" (cited in BMA 1998).

In the 1950s, the translation of this ideal into general practice in Britain was expressed as follows: "... the essence of general practice is to live amongst your patients as a definite cog in the whole machine, knowing them so well in both health and sickness, and from birth until death, that [...] the patient is so familiar to his family doctor that he of all people can be in the best position to give an accurate diagnosis, prognosis and treatment most suitable to the patient's way of life" (cited in Lewis 1997).

The stereotype of the dedicated professional, working very long hours, was, therefore, once commonplace in general practice, as well as in hospital medicine. The language of professionalism was prominent in the negotiations surrounding GP contracts up until the early 1990s. GPs strongly resisted the idea of a salaried service, as they claimed that this would compromise their autonomy as professionals. Indeed, as Lewis (1997:14) has argued, they sought to use the status of independent contractor to protect professional values, rather than as a means of securing a more business-like contract. In 1965, GPs in Britain drew up a Charter that emphasised professional standards and professional autonomy, and mass resignations from the NHS were threatened unless their demands were met.[7] These demands were accepted by the government of the day.

The claims to professionalism amongst GPs were also a reflection of the unease, in this section of the medical profession, concerning their status in relation to hospital consultants (specialists), considered by many to represent the apex of the medical profession. Indeed, within the profession the GP's representatives followed a classic 'pr-ofessionalisation' strategy, promoting the relative importance and significance of primary health care, and advocating and developing vocational education within general practice (Lewis 1997:19).[8] In the 1980s and 90s, however, the conservative government of the day sought to bypass these professional claims and to increasingly approach GPs as independent contractors—which, of course, they had always been in any case.

A series of government papers in the 1980s advocated good practice allowances, the contractual specification of services to be provided by GPs, increasing patient choice, and the promotion of competition by giving patients the right to 'shop around'. These proposals were furiously debated and some modifications achieved, but in 1989/90 the then Secretary of State (Kenneth Clarke) imposed a new contract on GPs that made doctors more accountable, gave patients more choice, encouraged competition and made pay more performance related. These changes to the GP contract were taking place at a time when the NHS itself was being reorganised along quasi-market lines. As Lewis has summarised this recent history: "Historically, GPs have seen negotiations over their contract as a means of defending professionalism, but in the 1990s the contract has become seen by government as part of a move towards the introduction of market principles and thus as an instrument for securing greater efficiency, quality, choice and accountability" (Lewis 1997:30).

During this period, the numbers of women training for and entering the medical profession was steadily increasing. A disproportionate number of women have always chosen to specialise in general practice and in 1998, women were 58% of GP registrars (i.e., GPs in training, e.g. Sibbald and Young 2001). One reason for the choice of general practice amongst women is that, as independent practitioners, GPs have been more able (than hospital doctors) to control their working hours. There is a direct parallel here with the situation in France, where women are over-represented amongst salaried and independently practising specialists for the same reason (Crompton, Le Feuvre and Birkelund 1999). Recent developments in general practice have further improved the capacity for control over working time by GPs. There has been a substantial increase in group practices and the use of deputising services (paid out-of-hours cover by locums). Since 1995, GPs have been encouraged to enter into out-of-hours co-operatives, which dramatically reduce the amount of time 'on call' during weekends and evenings. In 1998, personal medical services (PMS) pilots were introduced, which include GP salaried posts involving less administration and increased clinical content. 'NHS Direct'—a government-funded help-line for minor illnesses—was also introduced in the same year.

A number of parallel processes, therefore, were under way in general practice during the 80s and 90s. There has been a shift in emphasis away from the ideology of vocationalism, and more emphasis placed on the GP's status as individual contractors. Patients have become more critical of their doctors—a trend that Sibbald and Young attribute to "... the rise of consumerism within society which has made patients more demanding ... and less respectful of medical professionals" (Sibbald and Young 2001:3). Perhaps in response to the increased emphasis upon their contractual status, GPs have themselves sought to put a limit on their working hours and the extent of their contractual obligations.

As noted earlier, women are over represented amongst GPs in Britain and it would be widely accepted that an important reason for this is the control of working time that can be achieved in general practice. For example,

"I decided after I married and was doing house jobs that I didn't want to stay in the rat-race that was hospital medicine ... so I decided that, as I wanted to have a family, I would become a GP so that I could work part-time."

   Britain, female GP, born 1949, married (consultant), 3 children

"In the end we both [husband and respondent] decided to do general practice because we thought that we would stand a better chance of staying together ... I didn't want a family and no medicine. I was determined I was going to do both, so I kept on thinking: how can I do both, how can I do both?"

   Britain, female GP, born 1958, married (GP), 3 children

Family considerations, therefore, loom large in the 'lifestyle choices' of doctors entering general practice in Britain. Our interviews indicate that male GPs also stress the importance of giving space to family life that general practice offers. For men and women, other life-style choices may also be involved in making an occupational choice:

"There are lots of other things I wanted to do with my life than just work and it became obvious that general practice would be the way that I would be able to work part-time and fit in all the other things I wanted to do."

   Britain, female GP, no children

"I did six months in general practice ... I didn't like the idea of doing on-call for the rest of my working career, so I looked at hospital medicine ... Then I had the career crisis, so I thought I'd better have another look at general practice, which I did do. I realised there had been changes in general practice. Most places at that point had out-of-hours covered."

   Britain, male GP, 1st child expected

Of course, many GPs, particularly those in sole practice, do work very long hours, and complaints about workloads associated with governmental bureaucracy are legion. Nevertheless, doctors in general commented on changing attitudes to time commitments in medicine:

[Speaking of interviewing new partners] "They want to work less than full time, quite a few of them, if they could. They don't want to be on call. They don't want to work bank holidays, etc. etc. They would rather take less money and do less work."

   Britain, male GP, born 1953, married (GP), 2 children

Contractual changes, together with changes in the attitudes of patients and within society more generally, have all, without doubt, had an impact on attitudes to medicine as a 'vocation', with its emphasis upon a long hours and its work-centred culture. It is also very possible that an (unspecified) part of this shift in time preferences is a consequence of the increase in the employment of women doctors, who still bear the major responsibility for their families. They might therefore be anticipated to have more of a stake in the increase in flexible, shorter hours, working.

Detailed figures on the number of hours worked are not available for doctors in Britain. What evidence there is, however, suggests that GPs, on average, work shorter hours in Britain than in France, and that the trend is downwards. The Doctor and Dentists Remuneration Review (1991) reported that in 1989–90 GPs spent an average of 41 hours a week on general medical services (GMS) and six hours on non-GMS activity. An additional 26 hours were spent on-call. In 1998, the Review Body on Doctors' and Dentists' Remuneration reported that GPs averaged 39 hours per week. It should be remembered that these data do not include hours spent on-call, but, as we have seen, our information suggests that this is the area in which the most effective time reductions have been achieved in the recent past. These figures will also include part-time GPs, so the *actual* hours worked by full-time GPs in Britain will be greater than those given here.[9]

In line with these figures, our interview data suggests that amongst GPs, time is often valued more than money by both women *and* men. This is confirmed by a UK survey that reported that 91% of GP registrars saw having leisure time as the most important factor in their career choices, and another survey of GP leavers that found that the most important reason (after retirement) for leaving a GP principal post was that more personal and leisure time was wanted. The significance of this reason did not differ between men and women (Young et al. 2001). There has been an increase in the proportion of male doctors seeking part-time employment. In 1999, amongst applicants for part-time GP Principal posts, men represented 60% of all applications for job-shares, 46% for half time and 63% for three quarter time posts—although they were not recruited in due proportion to their applications and are still more likely to enter full-time posts (Sibbald and Young 2001).[10]

Non-principals (i.e., locums, assistants, retainers) form an increasing proportion of the GP workforce, and a survey of all GPs qualifying in 1986, 1991 and 1996 showed that the proportion of non-principals rose from 22% in 1986 to 45% in 1996 (ibid:21). A recent study of GP leavers showed that, although women were more likely than men to reduce their job commitments to meet family responsibilities, the "... most striking result of their study [was] not the difference but the similarity among men and women GPs" (Lees et al. 2001).

The French case

As in Britain, GPs represent about a half of the total medical profession (49%) in France. However, as we shall see, in France it is widely recognised that being a GP (*omnipracticien*) offers limited opportunities for part-time work without substantial financial penalties. Because of the long hours worked by *omnipracticiens*, French women doctors have been historically under-represented in general practice (Herzlich et al. 1993) and have tended to specialise more than their male counterparts and to work either in a hospital setting or as independent practitioners in *cabinets de ville*. This has often been explained by the fact that, in some particularly highly feminised specialties (medical gynaecology, dermatology, etc.), being on-call at weekends can generally be avoided.

Figures for 2000 show that 72% of all French GPs are in private practice (DREES 2001a:3). The remaining GPs are employed in public or private hospitals (15%) or in Community and Public Health Medicine (13%). Women make up 36% of all GPs, but only 27% of those in private practice. Although only 28% of French GPs (as against 50% of all doctors) are in salaried positions, women make up almost 60% of this category. They represent half the GPs working in hospitals and two-thirds of those in Community and Public Health Medicine (DREES 2001a:3). Of the self-employed GPs, only 39% work in joint practices and female GPs are even less likely to belong to a joint practice (35%) than their male counterparts (40%) (DREES 2001a:3). In addition, joint practices tend to be smaller in France than in Britain.

French GPs declare the longest working hours within the French medical profession (an hour a week more than specialists in private practice, three hours more than hospital based specialists and almost four hours more than non-hospital based salaried specialists). (DREES 2001b) Thus, many French GPs work very long hours, often to the detriment of family life:

> "The whole of family life is organised around my profession and my wife complains about this often enough. The practice is in the house, and work necessarily comes first. Last Sunday was my daughter's 16th birthday and we had arranged a celebration, I was just in the kitchen opening the oysters, someone knocked on the door and I was gone for half an hour and my daughters were very angry."
> France, male *omnipracticien*, born 1956,
> married (part-time nurse), 2 children

Furthermore, avoiding general practice is often cited as a strategy for gaining some kind of control over working time by male and female doctors in France. This can be illustrated by the case of a male GP who, under pressure from his second wife, decided to take a full-time salaried position in occupational health (*médecine du travail*):

> "As far as my personal life was concerned, I left the prison of general practice for the castle of occupational health: one could play sports, go out, I was free to have all the leisure time I wanted and

that I hadn't had during the time I was a GP. That's what occupational health is about, it doesn't take more than 8 hours a day of your time."

France, male salaried occupational health doctor,
born 1942, twice divorced, 4 children

"As a woman, I couldn't imagine becoming a GP, because I thought that it was alright for a man to be on call day and night, but, although at the time I didn't have a family, I thought that that would come eventually and that it would be much better to be a specialist, to be able to consult by appointment only."

France, female radiologist, born 1957, divorced, 1 child

It is important to remember that although the long hours and other time constraints on GPs in France are widely recognised, this does not mean that doctors are not generally in a position to choose medical specialties that enable them to control their working hours.

"There are numerous possibilities in medicine for anyone who wants to reserve some of their time for family life. I don't think its incompatible, it just requires more organisation, working in a group practice and it's totally feasible."

France, male *anigiologue*,
born 1965, married (doctor), 1 child

Nevertheless, the latest figures from a recent study of doctors self-declared working time in France suggest that the average length of their working week has actually increased over the past 8 years—from 48 hours per week in 1992 to 51 in 2000. During this time, there has been no reduction in the difference in doctors' working time by sex. Women doctors consistently work 6 hours a week less than their male counterparts. The length of their average working week has thus increased in the same proportion as that of male doctors. However, 25% of women doctors work part-time (as against 2% of the men). Part-timers work 29 hours a week on average. Thus, full-time doctors work 16 hours a week more than part-timers (DREES 2001b).

French doctors have increased their weekly working time by an average of 21 minutes per year since 1992. This increase has affected almost all categories of doctors, even the most feminised. Women full-time salaried hospital doctors now work an average of 4 hours a week more than they did in 1992 and even 5 hours a week more when they are in non-hospital salaried posts. Even full-time women GPs have increased their working time to an average of 50 hours a week, although the increase for full-time male GPs has been more spectacular—from 55 hours per week in 1992 to 58 in 2000 (DREES 2001b).

Explaining Franco-British differences

Here, we are faced with an apparent paradox. In both countries, doctors are aware of the possibilities of controlling their working hours but, whereas British doctors would seem to be taking advantage of these possibilities, in France working hours in the medical profession are increasing. Additionally, whereas in Britain general practice is regarded as the sector of the medical profession where it is easiest to control one's hours, in France this is not the case. We would suggest that a major factor that explains these differences is the contrast between the delivery of health care in the two countries.

As noted above, whereas in Britain rates of consultation have no direct effect on the level of GP remuneration, in France these are crucial.[11] The revenue of French GPs depends entirely on their ability to attract and retain patients. Thus, only by increasing the number of consultations, particularly those that command the highest fees, can income levels be raised. This leads to widespread competition between GPs.

> "Oh yes, there is a feeling of competition, a very strong feeling, there always has been, but I was particularly aware of that during the first five or six years of the practice, much less so now, because I have a pool of patients who keep coming back and others who I never see again, so that doesn't really matter any more."
> France, male *omnipracticien*, born 1952, married (full-time nurse), 1 child

In the days before the NHS, British doctors were in a similar position of competition for fees. For example, a British GP who had taken over his father's medical practice vividly recalled the time when his father ridiculed him for not charging a patient a fee for a prescription for the contraceptive pill:

> "Oh my God, you're giving things away, you've lost a fee there, my boy. You youngsters have got no idea at all."
> Britain, male GP, born 1946, divorced (remarried) 3 children

Of course, some GPs in France may decide to reduce their consultation hours and/or to refuse to do home visits or out-of-hours consultations, but they are then likely to earn much less than their colleagues:

> "For the out-of-hours consultations, I'm involved in an informal pool, there are four of us and we get on very well together, there were three men originally and they asked me to join them. When one of us has a problem, the others are there to help out. It's very useful in the evenings. It's true that we see things a bit differently, because they are all men, they have families to support, whereas I'm

a doctor because that's what I enjoy. If I ever decide that I've had enough, I know that I can just shut the practice, because I have my husband and with his job we would be able to manage anyway."

France, female *omnipracticien*, born 1958,
married (computer engineer), 3 children

"... there are some female GPs who work in joint practices and adopt a particular mode of working. I know one who doesn't do any home visits for example. She is married to a doctor so she doesn't have any financial problems and she organises herself accordingly. She does the odd consultation, a bit of psychology, and plays at being a high-class childminder [i.e. to *her own children*]."

France, male dermatologist, born 1956,
married (teacher), 2 children

In both countries, therefore, doctors can choose work and career options that allow them some control over the family-employment interface. General practice clearly offers reasonable opportunities for time sovereignty in Britain and women are proportionately over-represented in this area of health care. In France, on the other hand, women (and men) who wish to control their working hours will tend to gravitate towards independently practising specialties where patient demands can be controlled (such as dermatology), or towards salaried positions.

Discussion and conclusions

To return to the issues raised in the introduction, we would suggest that when looking at the possible consequences of the feminisation of the medical profession, it is not sufficient to refer to the behaviour of 'women' as such as the primary explanatory factor for gender segregation within the medical profession—either as potentially transforming the professional ethos from within (Davies 1996) or as reproducing the gendered medical hierarchy through their 'choices' (Hakim 2001).[12] There is considerable internal diversity within the medical profession in each country, and indeed, doctors have been identified amongst those occupations most able to take advantage of reflexive 'postmodern lifestyles' (Taylor and Field 1997, cited in BMA 1998).

As individuals in possession of considerable human capital resources, doctors have more power than most other occupational groups to make choices about which job slots they will occupy. However, as we have illustrated above, men and women doctors make these choices within the context of specific constraints and opportunities.

In particular, we have argued that when both male and female doctors make their career decisions, they most frequently do so with simultaneous reference to their actual or anticipated employment and family arrangements.

Thus, it would be misleading to describe these kinds of career decisions as straightforward expressions of their *individual* life-style preferences (Giddens 1992).

In both of the countries studied here, women's career aspirations are increasing. Thus, the improvement in women's educational levels, their rising economic activity rates and their access to the economic and social resources offered by a medical career are undermining their willingness to devote significant proportions of their working life solely to the domestic sphere. These changes, along with the general decline of the underpinnings of the 'male breadwinner' model in both these countries, are making it increasingly problematic for male GPs—and indeed, for professionals generally—to maintain the traditional one dimensional, 'vocational' relationship to their medical careers.

However, the actual outcomes of these changes are not identical in the two national contexts. We suggest that this is in part because the overall contours of the gendered division of labour in France and Britain are somewhat different. Although French women have a more extensive history of full-time, continuous employment than their British counterparts, French men's participation in the domestic sphere is, if anything, below that of British men. This has been explained by the fact that French men have been able to avoid increasing their domestic participation because of the historic and relatively high level of state support for working mothers in France (Gregory and Windebank 2000; Crompton and Le Feuvre 2000). Indeed, Windebank (2001:287) has suggested that: "... the greater flexibility in labour markets and traditional lack of state support in Britain is leading to a more equal gender division of domestic labour in [Britain] than in [France] because both partners need to be involved in caring for children in order to liberate the labour power of the woman".

In Britain, the opportunities for time sovereignty offered by the development of group practices, deputising services and salaried practice, have made it possible for GPs to achieve some control over their work levels according to the other potential demands on their time. In the absence of external time management resources, the adoption of shorter working hours has become a common strategy for male and female GPs. They have not necessarily had to accept a significant drop in income to do this, given that the larger part of their income depends on the number of patients registered, rather than the number of consultations achieved. At the same time, the British male doctors who can rely (or who choose to rely) on the availability of their spouses for childcare and home management are more likely to gravitate towards the most 'time hungry' sectors of the medical profession, in this case, hospital medicine and the most prestigious specialties such as surgery.

Indeed, it could be argued that a national context (such as France) characterised by a long history of state support for child-care combined with the more recent development of subsidised domestic services to high income households (Le Feuvre and Parichon 1999) actually places less pressure on individual medical practitioners to reduce their working time. In combination with the competitive nature of general practice and the more direct relationship between working time and income, these societal characteristics are conducive to a distinctive time management polarisation of the medical profession along gender lines. Because of the competitive environment in which they work, French GPs find it harder to strike a balance between maximising their income through long working hours and enhancing their 'time sovereignty'. Our evidence suggests that, contrary to the British case, the men and women who enter private practice as full-time GPs in France are those in a position to transfer most of their domestic responsibilities to a third party. This is usually a spouse, who, with potential support from the state-funded child-care and domestic services, may not necessarily have to abandon the labour market completely in order to fulfil this task. Thus, although the societal context means that women doctors in France can adopt relatively continuous employment profiles without having to mobilise too much of their partners' time, this strategy requires them to cluster in those sections of the medical profession where 'time sovereignty' is most easily achieved. This is evidently the case in salaried positions (as hospital GPs or specialists) and in certain private practice specialties, but much less so in full-time GP practice.

It therefore follows that, although aggregate levels of occupational feminisation might appear as very similar in different countries, national variations in professional and domestic architectures may lead to different outcomes as far as the extent and patterns of internal occupational segregation are concerned. In France, the 'fee for service' system for GPs goes a long way towards explaining the long hours worked by *omnipracticiens*. However, following the argument developed by Gregory and Windebank (2000), the extensive childcare support historically provided by the French state may serve to alleviate the pressures put on male doctors (principally by their working wives) to reduce their working time in accordance with family and domestic demands. This second consequence is obviously more likely to reinforce the pattern of the 'gender arrangements' (Pfau-Effinger 1993; 1999) of French GPs along 'modified male breadwinner' lines. In the British case, it is hospital medicine, particularly at consultant level, that offers the most restricted contextual opportunities for the adoption of 'time sovereignty' strategies and that is, therefore, the most conducive to the exclusion of women and to the replication of a 'modified male breadwinner' model of gender relations amongst the hospital doctors.

Finally, we would argue that individuals with substantial occupational power, such as the doctors discussed in this paper, are able to devise their own ways of combining employment with caring and family life, and, as we have seen, this is the case for both men and women. Particularly in the case of the British GPs, such individuals would indeed seem to be in the process of constructing their 'reflexive biographies' in ways that can impact on and re-shape the institutions within which they are making their choices. However, their ability to do this will nevertheless depend on the opportunities available within a particular professional context in a given country. Furthermore, it must be stressed that individuals with this level of power—women and men—represent only a small minority of all national populations.

Notes

1 Some authors have suggested that as more women enter the professions, then 'professionalism' itself (which is claimed to be essentially 'masculine') will be transformed as a direct consequence of feminisation (Davies 1996). For a critique of this approach, see Crompton, Le Feuvre and Birkelund 1999.
2 Glucksmann describes this as the 'total social organisation of labour' (TSOL). This concept "... refers to the manner by which all the labour in a particular society is divided up between and allocated to different structures, institutions, activities and people" (Glucksmann 2000:19).
3 In fact, because of the different manner in which medical services are organised in the three countries, the particular specialties chosen varied.
4 In 1999, France had a medical density of 331 doctors per 100 000 inhabitants, as against 175 in Britain in 1997 (DREES 1999:2 and DREES 2001c:6).
5 Patients are free to consult any number of GPs or specialists in the same week (or even day) and to have the consultation fees reimbursed through the Social Security system. Recent government attempts at curbing health spending in France, which involved 'capping' the number of consultations and making individual doctors pay back any fees received in excess of their targets have been strongly resisted by the medical profession.
6 In Britain, 45% of doctors are in hospital medicine, 50% are GPs, and the remainder work in Community and Public Health Medicine. These figures do not include junior doctors in training.
7 The majority of GPs submitted undated resignations which were held by the BMA.
8 In fact, recent developments within medicine in respect of diagnosis and treatment (for example, of diabetes), have strengthened the clinical position of GPs.
9 Hospital doctors work much longer hours. A survey of 515 Senior House Officers found that 60% worked more than 56 hours a week and 15% typically worked 80 hours or more. Following the EC Directive on Working Time, the NHS is currently engaged in measures to reduce the hours worked by hospital doctors.
10 The BMA 1995 cohort study of medical graduates showed that 58% (of which 47% were men and 53% were women) believed that doctors deserved a decent family life and leisure time, and 29% (of which 46% were men and 54% were women) thought that the practice of medicine must be organised in a way that allowed doctors to balance their family and other interests. Only 1% (3 men) believed that medicine was a vocation (BMA 1998).
11 As is, of course, the consultation fee that each type of doctor can charge patients. This is defined annually by the Ministry of Health, in consultation with the professional representatives on the board of the Social Security system. A higher consultation fee is negotiated for home visits and out-of-hours consultations. Doctors retain the right to charge patients more than the legal fee ('dépassement d'honoraires'), but these extra fees only represented 6% of GPs income in 1998, as against 12% of the annual revenue of French specialists (see DREES 2000:7).
12 For a critique of these perspectives, see Le Feuvre 1999.

Bibliography

Beck, U. and Beck-Gernsheim, E. (1995) *The normal chaos of love*, Cambridge: Polity Press.
BMA (British Medical Association) (1998) *The workforce dynamics of recent medical graduates*, BMA: Health Policy and Economic Research Unit.
Crompton, R. and Le Feuvre, N. (1997) Choisir une carrière, faire carrière: les femmes médecins en France et en Grande-Bretagne, *Les Cahiers du Gedisst* 19: 49–75.
Crompton, R. (ed) (1999) *Restructuring gender relations and employment: the decline of the male breadwinner*, Oxford: Oxford University Press.
Crompton, R., Le Feuvre, N. and Birkelund, G. (1999) The restructuring of gender relations in the medical profession, in R. Crompton (ed) *Restructuring gender relations and employment: the decline of the male breadwinner*, Oxford: Oxford University Press: 179–200.
Crompton, R. and Le Feuvre, N. (2000) The realities and representations of equal opportunities in Britain and France, *European Journal of Social Policy* 10 (4): 334–348.
Davies, C. (1996) The sociology of the professions and the profession of gender, *Sociology* 30 (4): 661–678.
DREES (Direction de la recherche, des études, de l'évaluation et des statistiques) (1999) Les effectifs et la durée du travail des médecins au 1er Janvier 1999, *Etudes et résultats* 44, Paris: Ministère de l'emploi et de la solidarité.
DREES (2000) L'évolution du revenu libéral des médecins en 1998, *Etudes et résultats* 89, Paris: Ministère de l'emploi et de la solidarité.
DREES (2001a) Les médecins omnipraticiens au 1er Janvier 2000, *Etudes et Résultats* 99, Paris: Ministère de l'Emploi et de la Solidarité.
DREES (2001b) Le temps de travail des médecins: l'impact des évolutions sociodémographiques, *Etudes et Résultats* 114, Paris: Ministère de l'Emploi et de la Solidarité.
DREES (2001c) La régulation démographique de la profession médicale en Allemagne, en Belgique, aux Etats-Unis, au Québec et au Royaume-Unie (étude monographique), *Etudes et résultats*, 120, Paris: Ministère de l'emploi et de la solidarité.
Giddens, A. (1992) *The transformation of intimacy*, Cambridge: Polity Press.
Giddens, A., Beck, U. and Lash, S. (1994) *Reflexive modernization*, Cambridge: Polity Press.
Glucksmann, M. (2000) *Cottons and casuals: the gendered organisation of labour in time and space*, Durham: Sociologypress.
Gregory, A. and Windebank, J. (2000) *Women's work in Britain and France*, Basingstoke: Macmillan.
Hakim, C. (2000) *Work-lifestyle choices in the 21st century*, Oxford: Oxford University Press.
Hantrais, L. (1990) *Managing professional and family life: a comparative study of British and French women*, Aldershot: Dartmouth.
Hassenteufel, P. (1997) *Les médecins face à l'Etat: une comparaison internationale*, Paris: Presses de la Fondation de Sciences Politiques.
Herzlich, C., Bungener, M., Paichler, G., Roussin, Ph. and Zuber, M.-Ch. (1993) *Cinquante ans d'exercice de la médecine en France: Carrières et pratiques des médecins français 1930–1980*, Paris: Editions INSERM/Doin.

Lees, R. et al. (2001) National Primary Care Research and Development Centre, Manchester: University of Manchester.

Le Feuvre, N. (1999) Gender, occupational feminisation and reflexivity: a cross-national perspective, in R. Crompton (ed) *Restructuring gender relations and employment: the decline of the male breadwinner*, Oxford: Oxford University Press: 150–178.

Le Feuvre, N. and Parichon, C. (1999) *Employment, family and community activities: a new balance for women and men in France*, Report to the European Foundation for Improving Working and Living Conditions, Dublin: Project 0202.

Lewis, J. (1997) *Independent contractors*, National Primary Care Research and Development Centre, Manchester: University of Manchester.

Pfau-Effinger, B. (1993) Modernisation, culture and part-time employment: the example of Finland and West Germany, *Work, Employment and Society* 7 (3): 383–410.

Pfau-Effinger, B. (1999) The modernisation of family and motherhood in Western Europe, in R. Crompton (ed) *Restructuring gender relations and employment: the decline of the male breadwinner*, Oxford: Oxford University Press: 60–79.

Sibbald, B. and Young, R. (2001) *The general practitioner workforce 2000*, National Primary Care Research and Development Centre, Manchester: University of Manchester.

Sullivan, O. (2000) The division of domestic labour, *Sociology* 34 (3): 437–456.

Taylor, D. and Field, D. (1997) *Sociology of health and the health service*, Oxford: Blackwell.

Windebank, J. (2001) Dual-earner couples in Britain and France, *Work, Employment and Society* 15 (2): 269–290.

Witz, A. (1992) *Professions and patriarchy*, London: Routledge.

Young, R., Leese, B. and Sibbald, B. (2001) Imbalances in the GP labour market in the UK, *Work, Employment and Society* 15 (4): 699–719.

THE FEMINIZATION THESIS
Discourses on gender and medicine

Elianne Riska

Source: *NORA—Nordic Journal of Feminist and Gender Research*, 16:1 (2008), 3–18.

Abstract

This study examines the multiple meanings of the term *feminization*. The term is commonly used in the media and in research to indicate the increase of women in professions in which a majority of the practitioners previously have been men. This study examines three discourses on the "feminization of medicine"—the research discourse, the medical discourse, and the public discourse—in order to explore how the term is defined and used by different actors in different social contexts and the predictions these actors make about the future work conditions of the medical profession. In the medical and public discourses the term tends to identify the category of women as responsible for changes in medicine rather than the structural and cultural changes going on in medicine that require new skills in medical work.

Introduction

During the past decades the increasing number of women in medicine has given rise to the expression "feminization of medicine". The term feminization is often poorly defined and tends to carry multiple meanings. It is frequently used to indicate the numerical turn in the gender composition in medicine (Nordgren 2000), but the term also contains predictions about qualitative changes in the practice of medicine (e.g. Coventry 1999; Paik 2000; Adams 2005; Lindsay 2005). It is telling that a recent thematic issue on "Feminization of the professions" of an international sociology journal did not define the term (Giannini 2005). Similarly, a recent review article on women in medicine set out to explore "what is meant by the feminization of medicine and 'pink-collar medicine'" (Heru 2005: 20) but still left the term undefined.

There is a need to look more closely at the term *feminization* as a discourse on gender and medicine. The expression reflects and constructs the gendered organization of medicine in a number of ways. The term appears in the discourses of different social actors, and it is therefore important to analyse the meanings that these actors give the term. This study examines three discourses—the research discourse, the medical discourse, and the public discourse—in order to explore how the term is defined and used by different actors in different social contexts and the predictions these actors make about the gendered work conditions of the profession. The research discourse is an effort by sociologists to illuminate the implications of an increasing number of women on changes in medical work. The medical discourse is illustrated by how editorials in medical journals have used the term. This discourse tends to reconstruct medicine as a gender-neutral organization by signalling the gendered character of women. Finally, the public discourse is exemplified by an editorial on the topic in a leading Finnish newspaper which recaptures themes in the research and medical discourses.

The methodological approach is discourse analysis (Fairclough 1992) in an effort to locate the texts within a wider social context of discursive production. The aim is to examine the underlying beliefs and assumptions in discursive statements about feminization. Such statements often draw on binary thinking about gender and tend to reproduce the gendered organizational practices in medicine.

The research discourse

In the mid-1980s sociologists of the professions became interested in structural changes in the medical profession (Starr 1982). The debate concerned the status of the profession's authority and medical knowledge, and some saw the profession's previous power position as challenged. The terms "deprofessionalization" (Haug 1975) and "proletarianization" (McKinlay & Arches 1985) were used to describe the loss of power of the profession. The "restratification" thesis (Freidson 1984) was a way of describing the process whereby the knowledge elite of the profession would strive to maintain the knowledge monopoly of the doctors vis-à-vis other health professionals. Furthermore, it was envisioned that a new internal stratification within the profession would result in a reorganization of medical work and in a status quo of the profession's knowledge monopoly and organizational power. This scholarly discussion within mainstream sociology of professions did not recognize the changing gender composition of medicine or the new stratification of gender in these processes. In the 1970s and 1980s, the term feminization did not occur in the scholarly debate.

Instead, the research about women's influx into the labour market and its impact on existing work arrangements appeared later in the sociology of occupations and organizations. Three major types of interpretations of the impact of women's increasing numbers in male-dominated occupations or professions can be discerned in this genre of research. For example, Reskin and Roos (1990: 71) foresaw three outcomes: women's genuine integration in the profession, a resegregation of the profession, or a ghettoization of women within the profession. Researchers who have argued that there is or will be a genuine integration of women have noted women's increasing numbers and concluded that women will enjoy equal status at all levels of the profession. Others who have interpreted the changes as resegregation and ghettoization predict that structural and cultural barriers will prevent women's full integration.

The most frequent and general meaning of the term feminization implies a shift in the numerical gender composition of the practitioners: women will become a majority. For example, the proportion of the first-year women medical students has been used as a predictor of a future proportion of women in the profession (e.g. Paik 2000: 666; Adams 2005: 72; Heru 2005: 20). Accordingly, if the majority of the medical students are women, the medical profession will become female-dominated. The implication of this demographic fact has a soft and a strong version. The soft version notes that the profession will be resegregated: it will become "women's work". Another version of the resegregation argument adds a stronger qualitative dimension to the numerical shift. This version suggests that when women enter a high-status profession in increasing numbers, and specifically when women approach a majority, the authority and prestige of the whole profession will inevitably decline. Some proponents of this version of the term feminization further suggest that the inherent (male) ethos of the profession will disappear and the quality of medical work decline: a female majority in a profession will result in a deprofessionalization (Haug 1975), and the profession will become a regular (female) occupation. The feminization of a profession is here equated with femininity and powerlessness (Britton 2000: 420). A reference is often made to the fate of the Russian medical profession as a historical example of what may happen when a majority of practitioners are women, though the devalued status of Soviet medicine is related to other historic and economic circumstances than merely the influx of women into the profession (Field 1957).

The deprofessionalization version of the feminization thesis has been challenged by several scholars. A classic in the field of occupational gender segregation of work is the queuing theory presented by Reskin and Roos (1990). They contend that labour markets have strong vertical dynamics that are visible in men's domination of the best paying and most prestigious jobs. Reskin and Roos show that when an occupation's status declines, because of changed conditions in the labour or economic market, men leave the occupation. This situation creates an opportunity for women to enter the occupation in increasing numbers. This interpretation has been supported by a number of North American studies (Muzzin et al. 1994; Coventry 1999; Adams 2005; Lindsay 2005), but recent studies of the labour market in the Scandinavian countries have shown the process to be complex if sectors and occupational levels are controlled for (Nordgren 2000; Charles & Grusky 2004: 302–304).

In addition to the resegregation version of the feminization thesis, there is the ghettoization argument. It suggests that even though the number of women might increase in a profession, women will be channelled to work in highly segregated niches within the profession, while other more prestigious areas of medicine will remain in the hands of men. There are two types of dynamics that create extreme gender segregation (Charles & Grusky 2004: 7). Horizontal dynamics segregate men and women across different fields, while vertical dynamics result in the allocation of men to the most desirable occupations and positions. These dynamics are supported by two cultural trends that Charles and Grusky (2004: 15) call gender essentialism and male primacy. Horizontal gender segregation is rooted in gender essentialism that "defines women as more competent than men in service, nurturing, and social interaction". Vertical gender segregation is reproduced by male primacy, a view that "represents men as more status worthy than women and accordingly more appropriate for positions of authority and domination" (ibid.).

In the field of medicine, horizontal segregation means the clustering of female and male physicians in different specialties that are seen as embodying characteristics regarded as prototypically male or female, e.g. women in paediatrics and men in surgery. The female-dominated niches are characterized by low status and pay, while the high-status specialties and the organizational leadership of the profession tend to be dominated by men. Most studies on the gender composition of medicine and of various specialties have found that women have not achieved the same kind of status positions and income levels as men (Lorber 1984; Pringle 1998; More 1999; Cassell 2000; Riska 2001; Crompton & Le Feuvre 2003; Eriksson 2003; Heru 2005).

Feminist research on organizations has portrayed vertical gender segregation as an inherent or embedded feature of complex organizations. It has been argued that organizations (Acker 1990; Britton 2000) and professions (Witz 1992; Davies 1996) are inherently male-gendered: the workings of these institutions valorize the masculine and features associated with masculinity (e.g. scientific objectivity, efficiency, hierarchical structures, autonomy of the professions). It has been suggested that even if women enter a profession in increasing numbers, its values and organization of work will remain male-gendered, because men control the knowledge and power of the profession. More recently the term inequality regimes (Acker 2006) has been introduced as a way to understand the production of gender, race, and class in organizations and to shed light on why so many organizational equality projects have failed or have had minor impact.

In contrast to the foregoing view of the fixed and embedded male-gendered nature of professions and organizations, another more optimistic view suggests that a strategic increase in the number of women will substantially change the professional identity and practice of the profession. This is the argument presented by Kanter (1977). This "sociology of numbers" approach proposes that when the number of any group, for example women, reaches about a third in an organization, the organization will adapt to their views and behaviour. The optimists suggest, therefore, that a female majority will change the attitudes of physicians and give rise to more humane and empathic physicians (e.g. Ulstad 1993). Women are assumed to be more caring and empathic and to bring these skills with them to the practice of medicine. Although some research has documented that women physicians tend to be more empathic than their male colleagues towards patients, these gendered skills have not been shown to generate gender differences in the biomedical content of practice (Lorber 1984, 2000; Roter & Hall 2004; Heru 2005).

The medical discourse: editorial views

In the early 2000s the discourse on feminization of medicine began to appear in the editorials and articles in leading medical journals. By using the key words "feminization of the medical profession", "women and medicine" and "women physicians" in the search engine MEDLINE (Entrez PubMed, available at www.ncbi.nlm.gov/sites/entrez) a variety of articles appeared which dealt with the impact of women's recent increasing numbers in the medical profession. The initial search with the key word "feminization of the medical profession" (6 November 2006) yielded 16 articles on the topic, and through these articles a further set of articles on the topic was accessed. The articles selected here for analysis do not constitute a representative sample of all editorials on this topic in the 2000s, because MEDLINE does not provide a complete and hence reliable register of articles on the topic. Yet the medical discourse on the term feminization became evident after reading the texts on feminization listed in MEDLINE.

A concern about the possible effects of women physicians' increase in medicine was expressed in editorials in leading American and British medical journals in the early 2000s (e.g. Paik 2000; Heath 2004; *The Lancet* 2004). The editorials make an attempt to grapple with the structural changes taking place in medicine and use feminization as a discursive statement on the implications of the shift in the gender composition regarding the power and practice of the medical profession.

There is a tendency in editorials and articles in 2004 to predict that feminization of medicine will result in a downfall of the rationality inherent in organizations and the workings of the economy in general. An example of this kind of far-reaching consequence of women's increasing numbers in medicine is expressed in an editorial named "Women in Medicine" in the *British Medical Journal* in 2004:

> The worry is that the enduringly unequal status of women means that the feminization of professions may further diminish the independence, power and influence of civil society at a time when it is already under threat.
>
> (Heath 2004: 413)

A similar concern about the macro-level consequences of women's take-over of medicine is expressed in an editorial with the heading "Gender Quo Vadis: 21 the First Female Century?" in the *Journal of Men's Health and Gender*:

> Those in favour of a matriarchal society should however be warned. Women are suggested traditionally to be more compliant and less creative than men. Accordingly unless women change, any profession they dominate is in danger of stagnation, with reverberations for the economy.
>
> (Meryn 2004: 4)

Another set of editorials and articles in medical journals is concerned with intraprofessional consequences. The articles speculate about what kind of effects the increased proportion of women physicians will have on the status and the internal division of labour of the profession. This view is represented by an article in the *Annals of Internal Medicine*, which analyses the consequences when "the profession of medicine is becoming feminized". The underlying theme here is that an increase of women in medicine will imply a deprofessionalization.

> To the degree that compensation is correlated with social status, increasing the number of female physicians with less earning power may lead to reduced status of the medical profession and less generous compensation for the profession as a whole.
>
> (Levinson & Lurie 2004: 473)

The editorials cited above have not been read by sympathetic adherents of the feminization argument only. They have also been read by critics, and some sent critical responses to the journal. One letter to the *British Medical Journal* fumed:

> What is the logic in saying that a feminized profession loses status and influence? We cannot compare ourselves with totalitarian societies such as the Soviet Union.
>
> (Fabre 2004: 743)

And another letter contended that women doctors will help to humanize the profession:

The eroding social status of doctors should be viewed positively for professional vanity has divided the profession and alienated patients. The influx of people from lower social classes and of women has done much to break the old hierarchy and the destructive "status culture" over the past 30 years. . . . Finally, women have helped "humanize" the medical profession. We should strive to have a profession dominated by doctors who care and not encourage more self obsessed and status driven applicants.

(Spence 2004: 743)

Such views of critical readers have also been expressed in editorials in leading medical journals. For example, an editorial in *The Lancet*, entitled "Women in Medicine: Status Cannot Be the Driver", represents an optimistic stance:

The goal of the medical profession must be to provide the best care possible to patients, in a safe and appropriate working environment for doctors. If increasing numbers of women doctors drive change towards a more flexible working environment then that change should be welcomed and encouraged.

(*The Lancet* 2004: 556)

In conclusion, the discourse on feminization in medical journals portrays the organization of medicine as gender-neutral, and it is women as practitioners who bring in gender to an otherwise impartial and gender-neutral practice. This discourse constructs medicine as previously unmarked by gender although both medical education and practice have been shown to be male-gendered (e.g. Lorber 1984, 2000; Beagan 2000; Cassell 2000; Heru 2005).

The above editorials have appeared in medical journals of a country where about a fourth of the physicians are currently women. What is the situation in societies, like the Scandinavian, where women are already or soon approaching a majority? In 2007, women comprised 51% of the physicians in Finland, 43% in Sweden, and 40% in Norway (Finnish Medical Association 2007; Swedish Medical Association 2007; Norwegian Medical Association 2007). The next section will explore how the feminization thesis is dealt with in public media in these social contexts by examining an editorial on the topic in the Finnish daily newspaper *Helsingin Sanomat*.

The news media discourse

On 27 April 2005, the leading Finnish daily *Helsingin Sanomat* featured an editorial under the heading "An Increasing Number of Physicians Are Women" (in Finnish: "Yhä useampi lääkäri on nainen").[1] The article was an attempt to describe in a gender-sensitive way the increase of women in the medical profession. It will be used here as a case study, not only because it is a fair representation of the arguments and assumed implications of the feminization of medicine, but also because Finland has the highest proportion of women in the medical profession: 51% in 2007. The analysis, presented below, will proceed stepwise and examine each paragraph of the editorial from beginning to end (the whole editorial can be read in endnote 1).

The editorial starts off by presenting the facts: a majority of physicians are women, and among the younger physicians in Finland as many as 70% are women:

> An increasing number of physicians are women. Among physicians of working age, 53% are women, but among the young physicians who have recently graduated, the proportion of women already exceeds 70%. The proportion of women among healers is fast approaching the level of women teachers, which in primary schools is about 72% and in high schools 66%.

A critical reading of the quotation would suggest that the current majority of women in the medical profession in Finland—by 3%—is here presented as an indicator of the future feminized state of the profession rather than interpreted as a sign of a gender-balanced situation. Furthermore, the newly graduated physicians, a majority of whom are women, are used as evidence to project women's take-over of the profession in the future. A reference is made to another occupational group: teachers—an occupation that has changed from male-dominated to female-dominated. It is not evident what the analogy is here. There is one common denominator that unites the loss of autonomy and economic status of teachers and physicians in the Scandinavian countries: local government. Physicians, who work as employees at local health centres run by the county/city government, tend to have less autonomy than physicians in private practice. Yet, physicians are licensed and have a monopoly over their knowledge and tasks, which is the basis for the ranking of other professions in the health care system (Freidson 1984). Despite sociologists' prophecies of deprofessionalization (Haug 1975) and proletarianization (McKinlay & Arches 1985) of the medical profession, the licensure and the medical control of the profession have changed little (Freidson 1984) as compared to the social position of teachers in the local school system. Yet, teachers still enjoy a high status in Finland, as recently documented in international evaluations of the Finnish school system.

The next paragraph claims that women physicians have different values from men's: "Women are certainly as good physicians as men are, but their attitudes and life values are often different from those of the opposite sex". The above statement touches on a number of issues. First, most international studies on male and female physicians' values and behaviour have been done on primary care physicians. In primary care, women physicians tend to see different patients from men—medically complex patients and patients with psycho-social problems (Heru 2005: 22). In general, women physicians, more than men, are involved in patient-centred communication with their patients. This means that women generally provide more health-promoting information and services, but no gender differences among physicians have been found in the biomedical information provided to patients (Roter & Hall 2004; Heru 2005). Second, some studies have found patients more satisfied with female physicians (Bertakis et al. 1995), while more recent research has found no effect of the physician's gender on patient satisfaction with the care provided (Wolosin & Gesell 2006). While these issues have been explored in American and British research, they have so far not been examined in Finnish research. As Bergman (2002: 215) has shown, the Finnish gender equality policy has been built upon a gender-neutral discourse which has portrayed women's and men's position related to larger structural changes rather than merely to men's superordination. The notion of gender-neutral welfare-state professionalism, including the health care division of labour, has been part of the Finnish gender order (Wrede 2008).

The genre of studies on women physicians' empathic skills alludes to a change of medicine that is seldom explicated. Medical knowledge and the way medicine is practised are changing dramatically: For example, the Internet has challenged the knowledge monopoly of the medical profession. Nettleton and Burrows (2003: 10) point out that medical information on the Web has blurred the boundaries of users and producers of medicine. They argue that medical knowledge today is dispersed and has "e-scaped" and altered the relationships between patients and physicians. Similarly, Zetka (2003) documents how laparoscopic technology and endoscopy have changed the skills needed and the structure of work to team-work in general surgery. These new forms of medical work have created a need for new skills, and women physicians seem to have been drawn to the work in the new authority and knowledge structures in medicine.

Third, different views on the importance of family that, it is claimed, are held by men and women physicians (Heru 2005: 25–27) could be culture-specific. It seems that the belief that female physicians more often than male physicians cherish family values is based on studies in countries, like the United States, that do not have a publicly supported childcare system or maternity leave. In such societies women have to make hard choices if they want to combine work and motherhood (Hochschild 2000; Jacobs & Gerson 2004; Heru 2005: 25; Lindsay 2005). Finnish women tend to work full time, and public family policies have been developed to respond to the needs of working women, in order to improve the balance between the demands of work and family (Anttonen 2002; Crompton & Lyonette 2006a: 385).

The next paragraph in the editorial hints at the gender segregation of medical work; but the clustering of men and women in different organizational settings—e.g. women in health centres or in certain medical specialties; or, e.g., men in surgery—is presented as a result of women's own choice.

> Women often work in health centres, where 60% of the physicians are women, but they are reluctant to do hard on-duty work. That taxes their strength too much and may have bad consequences for family life and childcare. Therefore, on-duty fields, like surgery and anaesthesiology, are still quite male-dominated.

The excerpt is in line with the arguments of the "preference theory" (Hakim 2000, 2004) that suggest that women's employment pattern is an aggregate outcome of their choices. It is claimed that women prioritize work or family differently from men, and women's particular choices will therefore result in a gender difference in career patterns. Crompton and Lyonette (2006b) tested the assumptions of the preference theory in a study that included Britain, Finland, France, Norway, Portugal, and the United States and found little empirical support for the theory.

Surgery is often used, as in the editorial, to point to women's conflict between work and family demands. International research shows that surgery has a very low proportion of women, although there might be a high proportion of women in the profession or in other specialties (Pringle 1998; Riska 2001). For example, although women constituted 51% of the physicians in Finland in 2007, 20% of the surgeons were women. This contrasts with the field of paediatrics, where 61% were women, and with child psychiatry, where 85% were women (Finnish Medical Association 2007). In Lithuania, where women constituted 70% of the physicians in 2004, in surgery only 11% were women, but in paediatrics 93% were women (Riska & Novelskaite 2007).

Research has shown that surgery is a closed professional group (Fox 1992; Conley 1998; Lindgren 1999; Cassell 2000; Eriksson 2003; Zetka 2003). The surgical ethos is called a "masculinist" ethos, regardless of the gender of its practitioner (e.g. Conley 1998; Cassell 2000; Eriksson 2003). Studies have shown that women medical students are, by means of tracking, channelled to areas associated with traditional female skills (child psychiatry, geriatrics), while men medical students are picked by male mentors to be trained to become surgeons. Mentoring is a crucial part of learning the skills of surgery, and it has been argued that it is not female medical students' choice but rather the mentor's choice that decides who becomes a surgeon (e.g. Conley 1998; Cassell 2000; Eriksson 2003).

The beginning of the next paragraph of the editorial alludes to the historical fact that men have previously held the top positions because they have been in the majority in the profession. The second part of the paragraph suggests that the increasing number of women in the younger cohort will in the future change the gender composition of the top positions. It is assumed that women physicians' careers proceed in a linear fashion, and that women physicians will automatically move from lower levels of the profession to the top.

> Also, half of the senior physicians and junior physicians are men, but the situation will change when young women physicians advance in their career.

This prophecy does not take into account the vertical and horizontal gender segregation that serves as structural barriers for any automatic linear mobility in the organization of medicine. Vertical gender segregation has been called the glass-ceiling phenomenon, a thesis that suggests that it is difficult for women to advance in their career in hierarchical organizations (Baxter & Olin Wright 2000). This pattern was confirmed in a study of Norwegian female and male physicians, who tended to enter internships to the same extent, but women later changed specialty and type of practice more than men because of difficulties in advancing in the chosen specialty or practice, a pattern that resulted in a gender segregation in medical work (Gjerberg 2002).

There is also a pessimistic prediction that suggests that physicians' work conditions will get worse because women, it is assumed, are less committed to the profession and tend to take leave and/or work shorter hours than men do (Heru 2005). It is argued that in order to get the work done in health care, more physicians are needed (Denekens 2002). The "deviant" behaviour of women is constructed against the male behaviour as the norm.

> Even though there are no differences between the professional skills of women physicians and those of men physicians, the gendered structure of the medical profession, like that of other fields, influences many things. Because of maternity leave and childcare leave, for example, women often have a shorter career than men. Women are also more interested in part-time work and partial retirement. Therefore there is a need for more physicians in a female-dominated medical profession than in a male-dominated one, so that the work will get done.

The need for more physicians "to get the work done" has been redefined more recently in many health care systems. A Canadian study shows that the state has had an interest in rationalizing the division of labour in health care as a means of cutting costs and has supported the professional projects of nurse practitioners and midwives (Bourgeault 2005). The delegation of some of the physicians' work to other female-dominated health professions not only redefines the boundaries of medical work but also provides opportunities for professionalization of "women's work" in health care. There are several levels of "women's work" in health care, and the boundary work and professional projects concern many different female health professions in the Finnish health care system (Wrede 2007).

The next paragraph of the editorial regresses to the crude version of the feminization thesis: a female majority in a profession will result in a lower status of the profession and therefore in fewer male applicants.

> So far there are no signs that the feminization of the academic fields will stop. On the contrary, there are in general fewer male candidates when a field is changing to a female-dominated one.

The causality of feminization and the occupational decline argument has been contested in research on occupational gender segregation (e.g. Reskin & Roos 1990; Charles & Grusky 2004). Nordgren (2000) showed in her study of the Swedish medical profession that the features associated with the "feminization" of a profession were consequences of broader changes in the Swedish labour market—for example, an expansion of the public sector in health care, women's high rate of employment in this sector, and women's increase in higher education in general. These changes had affected the salaries of all high-education professions in the public sector in a direction that was in contrast to the improved economic position of occupations with vocational education and jobs in the private sector.

The last paragraph of the editorial identifies the gendered structure of medicine: the values and work arrangements are based on male values. The editorial takes a pro-feminist stance here and contends that the work commitment of men in professions can no longer serve as a guideline for women. Instead medical work has to be restructured so that more people (women) do the same work that was previously done chiefly by men.

> In the future, work arrangements will also have to be changed. If women physicians do not want to do the current hard on-duty work, it must be made easier by sharing it among more people.

The common theme in most of the foregoing paragraphs from the editorial, featured in the Finnish daily newspaper *Helsingin Sanomat*, is that feminization is a lens through which the larger cultural and structural changes in medicine can be interpreted and understood. Structural changes in work and concomitant altered attitudes towards work and leisure are interpreted to be a result of women's increasing numbers in medicine rather than a product of broad transformations affecting all sectors and genders. The reason for and the essence of the changes are attributed to the traditional gender-specific characteristics of women as a category. The feminization thesis not only homogenizes women as a social category but also confirms the traditional attributes of men.

The discourses on feminization of medicine constitute attempts to capture the changes of medical work. The emphasis has been on medical work becoming "feminized" or "women's work" rather than asking the important question: What is there in current medical work that requires new skills, and why is it that mainly women are drawn to this new content? This inquiry captures the Parsonsian legacy (Parsons 1951) of using the medical profession as a prototype that allows an understanding of the impact of broader structural changes in society on social relationships.

Conclusion

The term feminization of medicine is used in research, medicine, and newspapers as a discourse on gender and medicine. The feminization thesis is physician-focused and does not address the fact that the health care labour force has for a long time been "feminized" because of the existence of a number of subordinated female health professions. Furthermore, the discourse on feminization reproduces notions of the organization of health care, medical knowledge, and medical practice as being gender-neutral in the past, whereas in the present it is women as a category that bring in gender to the previously unmarked character of medicine.

The statements about the "feminization of medicine" contain three types of predictions. The first one is a nominal definition: a numerical increase of women in the medical profession will lead to a numerical shift of the practitioners and change the profession from having a male majority to a female majority. This means a resegregation of the gender composition of the profession.

The second prediction has attached a qualitative meaning to the increase of women in a profession. It suggests that the influx of women into a profession is linked to professional decline. A profession's golden age tends thus to be defined in masculine terms, and the authority and practice of the profession are directly or indirectly portrayed as male-gendered. This connotation of the term feminization equals the deprofessionalization argument.

The third prediction maintains that, regardless of the proportion of women, the profession will continue to reflect the rest of the gender order, in which men's superordination governs women's subordination. In more general terms this means that female and male physicians will work in gender-segregated niches and in a profession where male gender is embedded. This connotation equals the ghettoization argument.

All three arguments and predictions were found in the three discourses on the feminization of medicine—the research discourse, the medical discourse, and the public media discourse. The analysis pointed to three types of arguments concerning the impact of women's increase in the profession, which appeared particularly in the medical discourse and the public discourse.

First, structural changes in medicine were primarily identified as caused by the influx of women into the profession. It was women's values and behaviour that caused changes in a profession that could have gone on pursuing its previous mandate if a male majority had been maintained. The assumption seems to be that men have remained unchanged and they have nothing to do with the current changes in medicine.

Second, there is a vision that nothing can stop women. They are taking over medicine, and their careers are proceeding in a linear fashion. They are in the future going to take over the top-level positions in the knowledge and administrative leadership positions in medicine.

Third, there is also a positive component to the predictions. Some envision that women's values will be good for medicine and restore the culture of doctoring from back when the old-time family doctor knew and was skilful in communicating with his patient. It is assumed that the humane tradition of medicine will be revived with the aid of women.

As the analysis of the editorials shows, a number of the arguments are based on a direction of causality which could in fact be the reverse—for example, the link between feminization and professional decline (Reskin & Roos 1990; Nordgren 2000). Some arguments rest on gender essentialism without taking into account the gender segregation—both vertical and horizontal—that characterizes medicine. Others explain the gender-segregated pattern of medicine as the aggregated sum of choices made by individual women, who have to balance family and work demands. This "preference theory" has found little empirical support in studies on working women in various countries (Crompton & Lyonette 2006b).

The term feminization should be used with some caution in social science vocabulary. Instead of feminization a compound term could be used to capture the character of women's increase in and impact on professions. The term *female-majority profession* could be used to indicate the quantitative dimension—a clear numerical majority of women (over 60%). The term *gendered profession* should be used to indicate the gender-related values of the profession. The latter term suggests that masculine values or feminine values are embedded in the practice and organization of the profession.

Externally induced changes in medicine today pose new demands and needs in medical practice. Some changes are state-initiated—for example, new governance structures in health care; other changes are market-driven—for example, Web-based medicine and drug advertising in public media which have changed the relationships between the patients and the physicians. These changes require new skills of physicians—for example, in primary care (e.g. Nettleton & Burrows 2003; Jones & Green 2006; Wolosin & Gesell 2006: 102) and in surgery (e.g. Zetka 2003). The discourses on feminization of medicine have raised an important issue: the existence of different styles of doctoring. The challenge is to utilize fully the potential of different styles of practice, but to degender them, to meet the demands for new skills in medicine.

Acknowledgements

I wish to thank Judith Lorber, Sirpa Wrede, Stina Johansson, Katherine McCracken, and the anonymous reviewers for their insightful comments on earlier versions of this article.

Note

1 Editorial in *Helsingin Sanomat*, 27 April 2005 (translated from Finnish to English by E.R.):

"An Increasing Number of Physicians Are Women"
An increasing number of physicians are women. Among physicians of working age, 53% are women, but among the young physicians, who have recently graduated, the proportion of women already exceeds 70%. The proportion of women among healers is fast approaching the level of women teachers, which in primary schools is about 72% and in high schools 66%.

Women are certainly as good physicians as men are, but their attitudes and life values are often different from those of the opposite sex.

Women work often in health centres, where 60% of the physicians are women, but they are reluctant to do hard on-duty work. That taxes their strength too much and may have bad consequences for family life and childcare. Therefore, on-duty fields, like surgery and anaesthesiology, are still quite male-dominated.

Also, half of the senior physicians and junior physicians are men, but the situation will change when young women physicians advance in their career.

Even though there are no differences between the professional skills of women physicians and those of men physicians, the gendered structure of the medical profession, like that of other fields, influences many things. Because of maternity leave and childcare leave, for example, women often have a shorter career than men. Women are also more interested in part-time work and partial retirement. Therefore there is a need for more physicians in a female-dominated medical profession than in a male-dominated one, so that the work will get done. So far there are no signs that the feminization of the academic fields will stop. On the contrary, there are in general fewer male candidates when a field is changing to a female-dominated one. In the future, work arrangements will also have to be changed. If women physicians do not want to do the current hard on-duty work, it must be made easier by sharing it among more people.

References

Acker, Joan (1990) Hierarchies, jobs, bodies: A theory of gendered organizations, *Gender and Society*, 4(2), pp. 139–158.

Acker, Joan (2006) Inequality regimes: Gender, class, and race in organizations, *Gender and Society*, 20(4), pp. 441–464.

Adams, Tracey L. (2005) Feminization of professions: The case of women in dentistry, *Canadian Journal of Sociology*, 30(1), pp. 71–94.

Anttonen, Anneli (2002) Universalism and social policy: A Nordic-feminist revaluation, *NORA—Nordic Journal of Women's Studies*, 10(2), pp. 71–80.

Baxter, Janeen & Olin Wright, Erik (2000) The glass-ceiling hypothesis: A comparative study of the United States, Sweden, and Australia, *Gender and Society*, 14(4), pp. 275–294.

Beagan, Brenda L. (2000) Neutralizing differences: Producing neutral doctors for (almost) neutral patients, *Social Science & Medicine*, 51(8), pp. 1253–1265.

Bergman, Solveig (2002) *The Politics of Feminism: Autonomous Feminist Movements in Finland and West Germany from the 1960s to the 1980s* (Åbo: Åbo Akademi University Press).

Bertakis, Klea D.; Helms, Jay L.; Callahan, Edward J.; Azari, Rahman & Robbins, John A. (1995) The influence of gender on physician practice style, *Medical Care*, 33(4), pp. 407–116.

Bourgeault, Ivy Lynn (2005) Rationalization of health care and female professional projects: Reconceptualizing the role of medicine, the state and health care institutions from a gendered perspective, *Knowledge, Work & Society*, 3(1), pp. 25–52.

Britton, Dana M. (2000) The epistemology of the gendered organization, *Gender and Society*, 14(3), pp. 418–134.

Cassell, Joan (2000) *The Woman in the Surgeon's Body* (Cambridge, MA: Harvard University Press).

Charles, Maria & Grusky, David B. (2004) *Occupational Ghettos: The Worldwide Segregation of Women and Men* (Stanford: Stanford University Press).

Conley, Frances K. (1998) *Walking Out on the Boys* (New York: Farrar, Straus & Giroux).

Coventry, Barbara Thomas (1999) Do men leave feminizing occupations?, *Social Science Journal*, 36(1), pp. 47–64.

Crompton, Rosemary & Le Feuvre, Nicky (2003) Continuity and change in the gender segregation of the medical profession in Britain and France, *International Journal of Sociology and Social Policy*, 23(4/5), pp. 36–58.

Crompton, Rosemary & Lyonette, Clare (2006a) Work-life balance in Europe, *Acta Sociologica*, 49(4), pp. 379–393.

Crompton, Rosemary & Lyonette, Clare (2006b) The new gender essentialism—Domestic and family "choices" and their relation to attitudes, *British Journal of Sociology*, 56(4), pp. 601–620.

Davies, Celia (1996) The sociology of professions and the profession of gender, *Sociology*, 30(4), pp. 661–678.

Denekens, J. P. (2002) The impact of feminization on general practice, *Acta Clinica Belgica*, 57(1), pp. 5–10.

Eriksson, Kristina (2003) *Manligt läkarskap, kvinnliga läkare och normala kvinnor. Köns- och läkarskapande symbolik, metaforik och praktik* [Physicianship, female physicians and normal women. The symbolical, metaphorical and practical doing(s) of gender and physicians] (Stehag: Förlags AB Gondolin).

Fabre, Clarissa (2004) Women in medicine: Women do not have to choose, *British Medical Journal*, 329(7468), p. 743.

Fairclough, Norman (1992) *Discourse and Social Change* (Cambridge: Polity Press).

Field, Mark (1957) *Doctor and Patient in Soviet Russia* (Cambridge, MA: Harvard University Press).

Finnish Medical Association (FMA) (2007) *Statistics on Physicians 2007*. Available at: www.laakariliitto.fi/tilastot/laakaritilastot/erikoislaakarit.html (accessed 27 December 2007).

Fox, Nicolas J. (1992) *The Social Meaning of Surgery* (Milton Keynes: Open University Press).

Freidson, Eliot (1984) The changing nature of professional control, *Annual Review of Sociology*, 10(1), pp. 1–20.

Giannini, Mirella (Ed.) (2005) The feminization of the professions. Thematic issue of *Knowledge, Work & Society*, 3(1).

Gjerberg, Elisabeth (2002) *Kvinner i norsk medisin—mot full integrering: En studie av kjønnsdifferensieringen i legers spesialitetsvalg* [Women in Norwegian medicine—Towards full integration: A study of gender differentiation in physicians' choice of specialty] The Work Research Institute's Publication Series 10 (Oslo: Arbeidsforskningsinstituttet).

Hakim, Catherine (2000) *Work-lifestyle Choices in the 21st Century: Preference Theory* (Oxford: Oxford University Press).

Hakim, Catherine (2004) *Key Issues in Women's Work* (London: Glass House Press).

Haug, Marie R. (1975) The deprofessionalization of everyone, *Sociological Focus*, 8(3), pp. 197–213.

Heath, Iona (2004) Women in medicine (Editorial), *British Medical Journal*, 329(7463), pp. 412–413.

Helsingin Sanomat (2005) Yhä useampi lääkäri on nainen [An increasing number of physicians are women] (Editorial) 27 April 2005.

Heru, Alison M. (2005) Pink-collar medicine: Women and the future of medicine, *Gender Issues*, 22(1), pp. 20–34.

Hochschild, Arlie R. (2000) *The Time Bind: When Work Becomes Home and Home Becomes Work* (New York: Henry Holt).

Jacobs, Jerry A. & Gerson, Kathleen (2004) *The Time Divide: Work, Family and Gender Inequality* (Cambridge, MA: Harvard University Press).

Jones, Lorelei & Green, Judith (2006) Shifting discourses of professionalism: A case study of general practitioners in the United Kingdom, *Sociology of Health and Illness*, 28(7), pp. 927–950.

Kanter, Rosabeth Moss (1977) *Men and Women of the Corporation* (New York: Basic Books).

The Lancet (2004) More doctors needed, without discrimination (Editorial), *The Lancet*, 364(9434), pp. 555–556.

Levinson, Wendy & Lurie, Nicole (2004) When most doctors are women: What lies ahead? *Annals of Internal Medicine*, 141(6), pp. 471–474.

Lindgren, Gerd (1999) *Klass, kön och kirurgi* [Class, gender and surgery] (Malmö: Liber).

Lindsay, Sally (2005) The feminization of the physician assistant profession, *Women & Health*, 41(4), pp. 37–61.

Lorber, Judith (1984) *Women Physicians: Careers, Status, and Power* (London: Tavistock).

Lorber, Judith (2000) What impact have women physicians had on women's health, *Journal of the American Medical Women's Association*, 55(1), pp. 13–15.

McKinlay, John B. & Arches, Joan (1985) Towards the proletarianization of physicians, *International Journal of Health Services*, 15(2), pp. 161–195.

Meryn, Siegfried (2004) Gender Quo Vadis: 21 the first female century? (Editorial), *The Journal of Men's Health & Gender*, 1(1), pp. 3–7.

More, Ellen S. (1999) *Restoring the Balance: Women Physicians in the Profession of Medicine, 1850–1995* (Cambridge, MA: Harvard University Press).

Muzzin, L. J.; Brown, G. P. & Homosty, R. W. (1994) Consequences of feminization of a profession: The case of Canadian pharmacy, *Women & Health*, 21(2/3), pp. 39–56.

Nettleton, Sarah & Burrows, Roger (2003) E-scaped medicine? Information, reflexivity and health, *Critical Social Policy*, 23(2), pp. 165–185.

Nordgren, Margreth (2000) *Läkarprofessionens feminisering: ett köns- och maktperspektiv* [The feminization of the medical profession: a gender and power perspective] (Stockholm: Department of Political Science, Stockholm University).

Norwegian Medical Association (2007) *Historisk legestatistikk 1920–2007* [Historical Statistics on Physicians 1920–2007]. Available at: www.legeforeningen.no (accessed 27 December 2007).

Paik, Jodi Elgart (2000) The feminization of medicine (Editorial), *Journal of the American Medical Association*, 283(5), p. 666.

Parsons, Talcott (1951) *The Social System* (New York: Free Press).

Pringle, Rosemary (1998) *Sex and Medicine: Gender, Power, and Authority in the Medical Profession* (Cambridge: Cambridge University Press).

Reskin, Barbara F. & Roos, Patricia A. (1990) *Job Queues, Gender Queues: Explaining Women's Inroads into Male Occupations* (Philadelphia: Temple University Press).

Riska, Elianne (2001) *Medical Careers and Feminist Agendas: American, Scandinavian, and Russian Women Physicians* (New York: Aldine de Gruyter).

Riska, Elianne & Novelskaite, Aurelija (2007) Professionals in transition: Physicians' careers, migration and gender in Lithuania, in: Ellen Kuhlmann & Mike Saks (Eds) *Rethinking Governance, Remaking Professions: International Directions in Health Care*, pp. 217–230 (Bristol: Policy Press).

Roter, Debra L. & Hall, Judith A. (2004) Physician gender and patient-centered communication: A critical review of empirical research, *Annual Review of Public Health*, 25(1), pp. 497–519.

Spence, Des (2004) Women in medicine: Status cannot be the driver, *British Medical Journal*, 329(7468), p. 743.

Starr, Paul (1982) *The Social Transformation of American Medicine* (New York: Basic Books).

Swedish Medical Association (2007) *Läkarfakta 2007* [Statistics on Physicians 2007], Available at: www.lakarforbundet.se (accessed 27 December 2007).

Ulstad, Valerie K. (1993) How women are changing medicine, *Journal of the American Medical Women's Association*, 48(3), pp. 75–78.

Witz, Anne (1992) *Professions and Patriarchy* (London: Routledge).

Wolosin, Robert J. & Gesell, Sabina B. (2006) Physician gender and primary care satisfaction: No evidence of "feminization", *Quality Management in Health Care*, 15(2), pp. 96–103.

Wrede, Sirpa (2007) Educating generalists: The flexibilisation of Finnish auxiliary nursing and the dilemma of professional identity, in: Ellen Kuhlmann & Mike Saks (Eds) *Rethinking Governance, Remaking Professions: International Directions in Health Care*, pp. 127–140 (Bristol: Policy Press).

Wrede, Sirpa (2008) Unpacking gendered professional power in the welfare state, *Equal Opportunities International*, 27(1), pp. 19–33.

Zetka Jr., James R. (2003) *Surgeons and the Scope* (Ithaca, NY: Cornell University Press).

Part 12

ACCESSING AND EXPERIENCING HEALTHCARE

56

HELP SEEKING FOR CARDIAC SYMPTOMS
Beyond the masculine–feminine binary

*Paul M. Galdas, Joy L. Johnson,
Myra E. Percy and Pamela A. Ratner*

Source: *Social Science & Medicine*, 71 (2010), 18–24.

Abstract

Empirical and theoretical literature suggests that stereotypical gender roles shape men's and women's health help-seeking behavior, and plays an important role in the treatment seeking delays of cardiac patients. We were interested in exploring the ways in which gender informs the experiences and help-seeking behavior of men and women who experienced the symptoms associated with acute cardiac events. We undertook 20 in-depth interviews between October 2007 and July 2008 with 11 men and 9 women recently diagnosed with an acute coronary syndrome in British Columbia, Canada. Participants were encouraged to tell their 'story' of the event that led to hospitalization and diagnosis, with a focus on the symptoms and decision making processes that occurred before and during the activation of health services: seeking the advice of others including colleagues, family members and healthcare professionals; calling 911; and attending an emergency department. Although we anticipated that distinctive patterns of help-seeking behavior aligned with stereotypical masculine and feminine ideals might emerge from our data, this was not always the case. We found some evidence of the influence of gender role ideology on the help-seeking behavior of both male and female participants. However, men's and women's experiences of seeking health care were not easily parsed into distinct binary gender patterns. Behavior that might stereotypically be considered to be 'masculine' or 'feminine' gender practice was shared by both male and female participants. Our findings undermine simple binary distinctions about gendered help-seeking prevalent in the literature, and contribute towards setting the direction of the future health policy and research agenda addressing the issue of gender and health help-seeking behavior.

© 2010 Elsevier Ltd. All rights reserved.

Introduction

Women's and men's health-seeking behavior are purported to be closely tied to stereotypical/traditional ideals of femininity and masculinity. Within Western culture, the predominant stereotype of women has placed a heavy emphasis on beauty, youth, and physical attractiveness (Avsec, 2006; Baker-Sperry & Grauerholz, 2003; Beben, 2002; Cole & Zucker, 2007; Stankiewicz & Rosselli, 2008; Wu, Rose, & Bancroft, 2006). This stereotype is accompanied by the traditional gender role ideology of women as primary care givers and the perception that women are gentle, emotionally expressive, reluctant to bother others with their problems, sensitive and sociable (Prentice & Carranza, 2002). Accordingly, women are typically viewed as possessing a desire to have and raise children, as nurturers who have domestic skills, take care of their own and others' health, and have a need for intimacy, connectedness, and self-disclosure (Barnett, 2006; Cole & Zucker, 2007; Emslie & Hunt, 2008; Kristofferzon, Löfmark, & Carlsson, 2003; Wood, Conway, Pushkar, & Dugas, 2005). Thus, in Western cultures, feminine 'ideals' (in the context of health help-seeking behavior) are typically seen as asking for help, caring about health, nurturing and monitoring partners' and children's health and well being, and pressuring male partners to see a physician if they are reluctant (Courtenay, 2000b; O'Brien, Hunt, & Hart, 2005).

By contrast, the espoused masculine ideal in Western culture emphasizes toughness, controlled emotions, decisiveness, heroism, and independence (Seem & Clark, 2006). Men are typically viewed as risk takers who possess a high threshold for pain or discomfort, enjoy challenges, are self-reliant, and are responsible for the family's economic protection. Rather than emotional, 'real' men are considered to be stoic and rational, and typically suppress the need for self disclosure, intimacy, and connectedness (Connell, 1995; Courtenay, 2000a; Emslie, Ridge, Ziebland, & Hunt, 2006; Mahalik, Levi-Minzi, & Walker, 2007; Wu et al., 2006). Although recent work has identified differences and diversity among men and masculinities in the context of health and help seeking (Galdas, Cheater, & Marshall, 2007; O'Brien et al., 2005; Robertson, 2006), these culturally-dominant masculine ideals have been implicated to play out in some men's reluctance to seek health care promptly (Galdas, 2009). Indeed, despite variations in how gender has been understood and conceptualized by social scientists and health researchers, the aforementioned (Western) gender roles and stereotypical ideals of masculinity and femininity have been widely used to inform a variety of studies of health behavior.

Mahalik, Lagan, and Morrison (2006) found that men who reported greater conformity to the 'masculine norms' of sexual promiscuity, self-reliance, and violence were less likely to engage in health-promoting behavior, and were more likely to engage in health risk behavior. Regardless of nationality, conformity to traditional norms was associated with unhealthy alcohol use, neglect of preventive health care, such as health screenings and skin cancer protection, entering into fights, and taking general as well as specific risks related to sexual behavior and the use of cars. Parslow, Jorm, Christensen, Jacomb, and Rodgers (2004) reported that being married or in a relationship was positively associated with men making an initial family physician visit, and also with making further visits, indicating that, for married heterosexual men, women were monitoring and successfully ensuring that their male partners sought health care. However, men are less likely to discuss mental and emotional problems with their primary care providers, and spend less time in office visits than do women (Smith, Braunack-Mayer, & Wittert, 2006). When the use of reproductive services have been accounted for, Western men use health services less often than do women, especially after the age of 16 years, and are twice as likely to have gaps of two or more years between physician visits (Mansfield, Addis, & Mahalik, 2003; Mason & Strauss, 2004; Smith et al., 2006). The reasons for these differences may include perceptions of invulnerability and espousing the masculine 'ideals' of independence, self-reliance, stoicism, and fear of discrimination for mental or physical health problems (George & Fleming, 2004; Smith et al., 2006; White, Fawkner, & Holmes, 2006). Mahalik, Burns, and Syzdek (2007) found that men who rated themselves as having higher 'traditional masculinity' scores reported more health risk behavior and less health promotion behavior, and were less likely to consult a mental health professional if feeling sad or depressed for longer than a month, or to consult with a health care provider when having unfamiliar symptoms.

According to the popular press, women are seen as experts in terms of diet and health (Gough, 2007), which is framed as women's work, with a caretaking role expected of them (Barnett, 2006). Similarly, compared with men, women have been found to have more positive overall attitudes toward professional help-seeking, a greater willingness to recognize the need for help, and a greater tolerance for any societal stigma associated with help seeking (Ang, Lim, Tan, & Yau, 2004; Krogh, 2007). Hunt, Lewars, Emslie, and Batty (2007) reported that higher 'femininity' scores in men were associated with a lower risk of coronary heart disease death, while no such relationship was observed with the women in their study. Thus it would seem that traditional gender roles and stereotypes exist and influence the health behavior of men and women. Moreover, researchers continue to rely on these notions to explain health behavior.

The literature concerning help seeking and cardiac care is conflicting in that some researchers have reported that women delay seeking help, compared with men's responses (Ottesen, Dixen, Torp-Pedersen, & Køber, 2004; Ting et al., 2008), and others have reported that there is no sex/gender difference in the interval between the onset of cardiac symptoms and seeking care (Løvlien, Schei, & Hole, 2007; Moser, McKinley, Dracup, & Chung, 2005). Those who have reported that there is a sex-based difference (anatomical or physiological in nature) have postulated that women do not recognize their cardiac symptoms because health educators' characterizations are based on men's experiences when women's symptoms are different from the "hallmark" symptoms – they are "atypical" and consequently not recognized as serious (O'Keefe-McCarthy, 2008). Canto et al. (2007) however hypothesized that this apparent difference is more likely the result of differences in age at the time of a cardiac event, rather than being a sex difference (women are generally older than men when they first experience an acute coronary syndrome and age influences the symptom experience). Others have suggested that there are gender differences in help-seeking behavior and they are social in nature. For example, Moser et al. (2005) reported that being concerned about troubling others led to delay for women but not for men. They argued that the importance placed on their numerous social demands may cause women to ignore their own health needs. Galdas et al. (2007) reported that some men need to portray high tolerance for pain and to avoid appearing weak or hypochondriacal, which influences their help seeking.

Whether there is a difference in the timing of help-seeking, much of the empirical literature suggests that stereotypical (or "traditional") gender roles and norms – culturally dominant behavior considered to be essentially "masculine" and "feminine" – are an important factor that shapes both men's and women's health help-seeking behavior. Indeed, these masculine and feminine gender roles are purported to play an important role in treatment seeking delays in cardiac patients. We were interested in exploring the ways in which gender informs the experiences and help-seeking behavior of men and women who have symptoms of an acute cardiac event.

Methods

Sampling and data collection

We used purposive sampling to recruit a heterogeneous sample in terms of gender, age, socio-economic status and health status. Participants were invited to be interviewed based on the following criteria: an admitting diagnosis of chest pain suspected to be of cardiac origin or confirmed Acute Coronary Syndrome (ACS); completion of a survey questionnaire while in an acute care facility for ACS; an expressed interest in participating in a qualitative interview once discharged home and medically stable; and the ability to communicate in English. Ethics approval was obtained from relevant ethics committees, and written informed consent was obtained from all participants. Participants continued to be recruited and interviewed until nothing new emerged from the data about the themes being explored, and 'conceptual density' was deemed to have been achieved (Strauss & Corbin, 1998). Twenty interviews were completed in British Columbia, Canada (see Table 1).

An interviewer's and participant's gender likely affects the dynamic and information shared in a qualitative interview: participants tend to gauge interviewers' orientations and opinions and consequently develop their responses within a gendered context (Schwalbe & Wolkomir, 2001; Williams & Heikes, 1993). To ensure consistency, one (female) researcher conducted all 20 interviews and ensured the accuracy of all the transcriptions.

Data were collected between October 2007 and July 2008 using in-depth semi-structured interviews that took place at a time and location convenient to the participant. Each participant was provided with a $25 honorarium. Interviews were digitally audio-recorded and transcribed verbatim. The initial interview guide consisted of open-ended questions that encouraged participants to tell their 'story' of the event that led to their hospitalization

Table 1 Demographic information.

Participant number	Age/sex	Marital status	Admission diagnosis	Discharge diagnosis	Relevant past medical history
1	80/male	Married	Chest pain	AMI	Chest pain
2	89/female	Widowed	ACS	Pulmonary edema	Hypertension, atrial fibrillation/ pacemaker insertion
3	58/female	Divorced	Chest pain	AMI	Hypertension
4	59/male	Married	ACS	AMI	None relevant
5	54/male	Married	Chest pain	AMI	Hypertension, chest pain
6	48/female	Married	Chest pain	AMI	Diabetes
7	69/female	Married	Chest pain	AMI	None relevant
8	80/male	Married	ACS	AMI	Coronary artery bypass grafts, angina
9	61/male	Married	AMI	AMI	Hypertension
10	52/male	Single	Chest pain	AMI	None relevant
11	68/male	Married	ACS	AMI	ACS
12	58/female	Married	AMI	AMI	None relevant
13	69/female	Married	Chest pain	AMI	AMI
14	60/female	Married	Chest pain	AMI	AMI, diabetes
15	54/male	Married	Chest pain	AMI	Hypertension
16	66/female	Married	AMI	Unstable angina	None relevant
17	73/male	Single	ACS	Unstable angina	ACS
18	67/female	Widowed	AMI	AMI	None relevant
19	54/male	Married	Chest pain	AMI	Hypertension
20	78/male	Married	AMI	AMI	AMI

and diagnosis of ACS, with a focus on the symptoms and decision making processes that took place before and during the activation of health care services: seeking the advice of others, including colleagues, family members and healthcare professionals; calling emergency services; and attending an emergency department. When participants discussed or alluded to delays in their help seeking, the interviewer sought clarification and a deeper understanding of the context and influencing factors surrounding such delays. Further, the interviewer sought to understand the influences of being male or female, married or single, location of the event(s), and the role of previous cardiac events or co-morbidity on the actions taken. The interview guide underwent several revisions based on insights that emerged from the analysis of completed interviews.

Sample characteristics

The sample was composed of 20 people (11 men and 9 women; see Table 1). These participants ranged in age from 48 to 89 years; 15 were married and 5 were either divorced, widowed, or never married, and hence lived alone at the time of the event. Sixteen participants were either retired or worked part-time; 2 participants worked full-time, and 2 participants were on long-term disability leave owing to non-cardiac health issues. One participant reported no previous health problems of any kind. For those 8 participants with a previous cardiac history, the problems reported were: one or more previous myocardial infarctions; a pacemaker insertion; hypertension; angina; and angioplasty. The remaining 11 participants reported various non-cardiac chronic conditions, such as asthma, arthritis, trigeminal neuralgia, cerebral aneurysm, diabetes, *Helicobacter pylori*, and end-stage renal failure. All 20 participants communicated in English.

Data analysis

The data were analysed using an inductive thematic approach that occurred concurrently with data collection. The analytical process involved grounded theory methods of coding and constant comparative analysis as described by Strauss and Corbin (1998); 'tools' which have been widely used in exploratory qualitative research studies seeking to explore and describe social situations and to understand social phenomena (Charmaz, 2000). Transcripts were entered into the qualitative data management software *NVivo* (version 8.0) and initially subjected to a line-by-line analysis. First-level coding involved making comparisons between transcripts, searching for similarities and differences, and then labelling similar phenomena as open codes. Second-level coding involved making propositions about connections between open codes and reassembling them into 'tentative themes' to form a more precise and complete explanation of the phenomena (Strauss & Corbin, 1998). The 'tentative themes' were discussed by the entire research team on several occasions until a consensus on the interpretation of patterns in the data was reached. A key feature of this process involved each member of the research team testing themes against individual transcripts and the entire data set, and reformulating them where necessary, in an iterative process of constant comparative analysis that led to the generation of the final themes (Strauss & Corbin, 1998). The final themes were considered to represent a level of patterned response or meaning in the data that described the phenomena taking place in the participants' experiences of seeking help for cardiac symptoms (Attride-Stirling, 2001; Braun & Clarke, 2006).

Findings and discussion

Although we anticipated that distinctive patterns of help-seeking behavior aligned with stereotypical masculine and feminine gender roles might emerge from our data, we found that this was not always the case. Indeed, our findings reveal that men's and women's behavior is not easily parsed into distinct binary gender patterns. Behavior that might stereotypically be thought of as "masculine" or "feminine" was shared by both men and women. We begin by discussing the responses of men and women that tended to fit the stereotypical gender-role pattern of help-seeking behavior, themes we conceptualized as "stoic men" and "vulnerable or accommodating women"; before going on to address those participants whose narratives were not reflective of stereotypical gender ideology: a theme we conceptualized as "beyond the masculine–feminine binary".

Stoic men

For several of the men we interviewed, from the onset of their symptoms to their decision to seek help they described what could be considered to be 'stereotypical' masculine help-seeking behavior: being extremely reluctant to relinquish control of their situation to a health care professional, and attempting to manage their condition independently. For some, retaining control and independence meant continuing with a planned schedule involving work or leisure activities. For instance, one 54-year-old male participant experienced recurrent exercise-induced chest tightness and arm weakness over a period of two days, which prompted him to research his condition on the internet. Despite suspecting he had angina, he decided to delay visiting a physician so that he could continue with his planned work schedule. An additional striking feature of his account was his great reluctance to admit to colleagues that an appointment with a physician was the reason he could not attend a pre-planned game of golf. Instead, he offered a work-related excuse to avoid being seen to be 'bailing out'. He was later diagnosed with an acute myocardial infarction (AMI).

> I felt brief spells when I was walking, exerting myself, of this sensation. So, during the weekend, I poked around on the internet to see, 'What is this that's going on?' I suspected it was angina.... I had meetings all day Monday ... so I didn't have an opportunity to go to the doctor.... So, the next day, I was actually supposed to play a game of golf with some of my colleagues ... and I was looking for an excuse not to do that because I was thinking, 'I better go see the doctor and see what this is about.' As it turned out, I got a phone call from the office ... saying, 'We need you here to meet with some people at 3 o'clock on Thursday afternoon.' So, ha! My perfect excuse, I didn't have to bail out totally. I had an excuse to leave on Thursday morning, which I did.
> [P#19, 54-year-old man, first time AMI]

Similar stories were told by several other male participants who recounted their reluctance to accept the potential severity of their condition. These men's accounts of stoicism and self-reliance clearly align with the assumed stereotypical pattern of male help-seeking and masculine gender role ideology (Seem & Clark, 2006), and echo the findings of other qualitative studies of men's cardiac disease related help-seeking behavior (Galdas et al., 2007; White & Johnson, 2000). Consistent with this pattern, several men in the study also frequently spoke of having 'played down' or denied their symptoms to continue with their daily activities. One participant was skiing at the time of his symptom onset and minimized the suggestions of his friends that his symptoms might be indicative of a 'heart attack.' He vowed to continue with his ski trip. Even though some of these men had been informed by their family physicians that their condition was serious and required immediate emergency care, many admitted that they remained extremely reluctant to forgo their independence and self-determination. For instance, one participant with a history of previous AMI described his determination to view the end of a theatre show he was attending during the onset of his symptoms – despite suspecting he was having a 'heart attack' at the time. It was clear from these men's accounts that they were determined to engage with health care services on their own terms.

> I had gone a thousand miles to see two operas and, by God, saw them.... I was not going to allow myself to be sick. Even though, in retrospect, I realize I was a having a heart attack during Samson and Delilah.
> [P#11, 68-year-old man, fourth AMI]

Vulnerable or accommodating women

Along the same lines as the 'stoic men' theme, several of the women we interviewed recounted stories that could be considered to be a 'stereotypical' health help-seeking pattern that was consistent with female gender role ideology (Prentice & Carranza, 2002). The key aspects of these women's accounts were associated with self-disclosure and asking for help promptly, caring about health matters, monitoring partners' and children's health and well being, and nurturing the family. The features of the participants' stories cohere with previous literature that has highlighted the often deleterious impact of 'femininity' and feminine gender roles on help-seeking for the symptoms of an acute cardiac event (Lockyer, 2005; Rosenfeld, Lindauer, & Darney, 2005; Turris & Finamore, 2008). For instance, one woman in our study, who had realized she was having a heart attack at home, talked of her fear that she might die with an unkempt appearance and be found by her sister.

> [I had] no makeup on, nothing, I think my hair was brushed. My hands were washed and my face was washed, but still.... You just feel like ... ugh ... I hadn't brushed my teeth either, that was the thing that really bothered me.
> [P#18, 67-year-old woman, first time AMI]

A 59-year-old woman spoke of her relief when paramedics arrived at her home. In her narrative, she indicated her willingness to surrender control of the situation and let others 'take charge' and take her to hospital, despite thinking throughout the process that her condition was not serious. Another female participant, a 69-year-old married woman with two children and with a history of previous AMI, clearly positioned herself as a mother and care giver in her narrative. She described being preoccupied with caring for her husband and children before tending to her own needs despite experiencing several days of 'typical', often severe, AMI symptoms. Later in her interview, she described how she felt the need to straighten up the house before going to seek help:

> I got up and walked around and thought, 'Oh, I feel just awful.' And I didn't want to bother K., my youngest, because she's got two babies and you know, she didn't need that, and C. and J. [the participant's other children] were away somewhere that weekend, or they had something else on ... [later in interview] ... I guess I thought I had to make the bed, I had to make the place tidy, loading the dishwasher and stuff like that.
> [P#13, 69-year-old woman, second AMI]

Beyond the masculine–feminine binary

Although many aspects of our participants' stories fit with the stereotypical pattern of masculine and feminine gender roles in the context of help-seeking behavior, several participants reported responses that were *not* reflective of their respective gender roles. Indeed, several participants explicitly positioned some of their behavior during their cardiac event as atypical of their gender. For female participants, this was most often displayed through accounts of behavior that would more commonly be aligned with masculine ideals embodied by stoicism, control, the denial of weakness, and endurance. For instance, in describing her symptoms, one woman explained,

> I was playing badminton. I had no idea, and everyone was extremely shocked, because I've always been active, that I would have a heart attack. I was playing badminton, and had the pain in my chest. Fortunately, it was the crushing pain, the deep pain, so I knew what it was, not like a lot of women who really, their sense is so different.
> [P#7, 69-year-old woman, first time AMI]

It was also apparent that a large proportion of the men's responses contrasted with stereotypical, stoic masculine ideology. For these men, 'atypical' responses were often characterized by accounts of explicit concern for their health, relinquishing their control to healthcare professionals, and overt displays of vulnerability during their cardiac event. For example, one man took pride in facing his symptoms 'head on', rather than trying to 'wait it out', he took immediate action.

> This was a little more serious, and then I started thinking to myself, "Am I going to let this go because it seems to be passing already?" And, I thought to myself, "No, this has been, this is probably the most pronounced thing I've ever felt, so I'm doing to do something about this." And, I turned around behind me, two steps away was the foreman's doorway to his office, and I backed into his office, sat down on a chair and I said, "I have to go to the hospital now, I'm not feeling good." They know me at work, that I have a heart problem; have been on some medications, and have had ups and downs at times . . . been going over the last couple of years. I think that's kind of been good for me, in the fact that I've never run from this, I've always faced it face on. I'm not going to hide; I want to try and be around as long as I can, to put it that way. Nobody wants to die or anything like that. But I have a positive outlook too, from my own personal experience.
> [P#15, 54-year-old man, first time AMI]

The above accounts serve to illustrate that many men's and women's responses to their acute cardiac symptoms were not simply a reflection of assigned gender roles and expectations. It was clear in the data that contextual factors (most notably the time and location of the event, and the people present) frequently influenced the participants' behavior and responses to their symptoms. The circumstances persons found themselves in when they first experienced their symptoms were powerful moderators, as were the nature and severity of their symptoms.

The reticence of some participants to relinquish control to healthcare professionals was often compounded by a sense of ambiguity about the seriousness of their condition. The transient nature of their symptoms, including chest pain, was frequently confusing for the participants. These findings accord with those of a previous investigation that showed the help-seeking decision-making process of people admitted to hospital with an AMI to be a complex interaction of knowledge and experience, beliefs, emotions, and the context of the event (Pattenden, Watt, Lewin, & Stanford, 2002). Pattenden et al. (2002) found that patients experiencing the symptoms of AMI were often reluctant to relinquish control to healthcare professionals, and frequently attributed their symptoms to a benign, non-cardiac cause. As other researchers have described (Clark, 2001; Dracup et al., 1995; Galdas et al., 2007; Pattenden et al., 2002), several participants in our study had waited until their attempts at self-treatment had failed, or their symptoms were viewed as being persistent or more severe, until they decided that their condition was serious and they required health care. This observed pattern of behavior is consistent with Clark's (2001) analysis of the role of the body and self as an important part of the interpretive frames used to understand the meaning of AMI symptoms and the action to take thereon. Clark (2001) drew a distinction between individuals' interpretations of the body (symptoms, including chest pain) and self (perception of level of risk to health) in the context of experiencing an AMI; with the latter seen as more influential in prompting help seeking. He also found that it was only when numerous and often lengthy attempts to alleviate symptoms failed and symptoms appeared to be more severe that participants saw the self as being at "high risk" and sought help. Akin to the participants in our study, it was the view of the self at risk as opposed to the body in great pain that appeared to prompt individuals' decisions to seek medical help.

> I waited to see if the pain would go. You always try to ignore things, you know? But even though I sort of knew what it was, I just waited about 15 min or so, and the pain didn't go. That's when I phoned him.
> [P#7, 69-years-old woman, first time AMI]

The narratives in our study show that gender is not simply a matter of identity and role, but that it is constructed and lived in a social and cultural context. The men and women we interviewed were responding to the gendered expectations that were subtly and not so subtly cuing them to respond in certain ways depending on the context of their event. Simply put, their construction of health and gender did not occur in isolation from other forms of social action (Courtenay, 2000b); a perspective in keeping with the insights of gender-relations theory, which positions gender as a socially produced practice with attention to how it is accomplished vis-à-vis "norms" of femininity and masculinity (Connell, 1995). This is important to note because it highlights gender as being both fluid and reciprocal. The findings presented in this final theme serve to illustrate the fluidity of gender, refuting much of the recent work that has explored men, women, and heart disease (Emslie, 2005), which has suggested that women predominantly respond one way and men another when experiencing the symptoms of an acute cardiac event. The discourses of several men we interviewed exemplified what could more commonly be considered to be 'feminine' gender roles/behavior, and several women spoke of 'masculine' gender roles/behavior. Furthermore, several participants recounted behavior that could be aligned with both 'masculine' (stoical) and 'feminine' (vulnerable/accommodating) gender ideals in the context of seeking health care, as seen in this excerpt:

> I made a doctor's appointment, and at the beginning of March, my son, he had a stroke. But it turned out to be, he got over it in a couple of weeks ... anyway, so I thought, "I'm not going to say anything to anybody [about cardiac symptoms] because I don't want ... Let's let him get over his problem first and then I'll deal with this." There's always family things that seem to, and I'm not one to complain about everything like that ... I think my symptoms, I tended to put onto other stuff. I'm pretty sure, somewhere back there, I knew there was a problem long before that, that I didn't acknowledge until late February [her first symptoms developed in December].
> [P#16, 68-year-old woman, first time AMI]

Clearly, men and women can and do behave in ways that both cohere with and contradict their respective gender role ideologies and 'normative' gender behavior when seeking health care for the symptoms of an acute cardiac event. The participants' stories illustrated that gender was not a 'stand alone' variable that determined their help-seeking decision making and behavioral patterns. Yet, the complex, fluid, and often contradictory nature of gender evident in the narratives of our study participants does not necessarily mean that gender is not an important and useful construct in exploring help-seeking behavior. Rather, we argue that the way in which gender interplays with men's and women's health behavior is highly complex and our treatment of it in empirical work – and in the study of health help-seeking behavior in particular – has often lacked the sophisticated approaches it deserves. Much of the work in this field has built on an oppositional, binaried approach. As a result, the key practices of masculinity and femininity in the context of seeking health services have been somewhat essentialized as either a masculine or feminine gender role or trait. A more nuanced investigation of the intersection of gender and help-seeking behavior is required to develop a progressive and more diversified conceptual lens that disrupts the ontological assumption of binaried categories.

The call to move beyond a binary conceptualization of gender is not a recent or novel insight. In the mid 1990s, authors such as Lorber (1996) called for a reconsideration of traditional gender categories. Lorber (1996) commented that in research "variations in gender displays are often ignored: A woman is assumed to be a feminine female; a man masculine male" (p. 144). Furthermore, a questioning of binary conceptions of gender is influencing other areas of health research such as HIV/AIDS (Dworkin, 2005). What is interesting to consider is why those working in the field of cardiac sciences have continued to reify these stereotypical typologies. Perhaps part of the problem is that there has been little opportunity to ask whether there are similar expressions of reluctance or willingness to seek health care amongst women and men because most recent insights from research on gender and health have arisen from empirical studies of single sex samples (Hunt, Adamson, & Galdas, 2010). Because of an often (perhaps unconsciously) tendency to highlight distinctions rather than similarities between male and female 'gendered' behavior, it is often presumed, for instance, that because some men adhere to the masculine ideals of stoicism and self-reliance in certain help-seeking contexts, women do not; or, that because some women may prioritize their domestic and family responsibilities over their own health, men do not. Our study clearly undermines these binary gender distinctions and suggests that, consistent with relational theoretical perspectives (Connell, 1995), masculinity and femininity are not polar opposites on a single gender continuum. As has been discussed elsewhere (Courtenay, 2000b; Robertson, 2007), a key feature of gender-relations theory concerns the understanding of gender as neither a character typology nor an isolated act, but as a configuration of social practice that is generated in particular situations in a changing structure of relationships. In this way, gender practices, such as those manifested by the participants of our study, can be understood as being historically and culturally contingent, but also open to change and not essentially determined by biology or processes of socialization (Robertson, 2007). Our findings suggest that this relational concept of gender fluidity may be a useful starting point in re-examining current binary assumptions about gender and help seeking. Further research using samples of both men and women will be crucial to avoid overly simplistic and binary assumptions about gendered behavior.

Conclusion

Our findings contribute towards setting the direction of the future health policy and research agenda addressing the issue of gender and health help-seeking behavior. Previous research has largely focused on single sex samples and emphasized the differences between men's and women's help-seeking behavior for acute cardiac symptoms, when it is apparent that there are many important similarities. Our findings illustrate that men's and women's decisions to seek or delay seeking treatment for acute cardiac symptoms cannot be easily parsed or categorized into distinct, gendered patterns. In terms of the cardiac literature and our understanding of help-seeking behavior, our findings suggest that attempts to tailor 'gender sensitive' health promotion messages based on culturally-dominant gender ideals to men or women might be misguided. Instead, a range of messages may be required that are sensitive to the complex nature of our gendered lives.

Acknowledgements

This research was supported by a Canadian Institutes of Health Research (CIHR) operating grant (MOP 145706). Dr. Ratner is supported by the Michael Smith Foundation for Health Research.

References

Ang, R. P., Lim, K. M., Tan, A., & Yau, T. Y. (2004). Effects of gender and sex role orientation on help-seeking attitudes. *Current Psychology, 23,* 203–214.

Attride-Stirling, J. (2001). Thematic networks: an analytic tool for qualitative research. *Qualitative Research, 1,* 385–405.

Avsec, A. (2006). Gender differences in the structure of self-concept: are the self-conceptions about physical attractiveness really more important for women's self-esteem? *Studia Psychologica, 48,* 31–43.

Baker-Sperry, L., & Grauerholz, L. (2003). The pervasiveness and persistence of the feminine beauty ideal in children's fairy tales. *Gender & Society, 17,* 711–726.

Barnett, B. (2006). Health as women's work: a pilot study on how women's magazines frame medical news and femininity. *Women & Language, 29,* 1–12.

Beben, A. A. (2002). *A Barbie who puts out: Adolescent cheerleaders contend with standards of femininity in high school and in sport* (Master's thesis). Available from ProQuest Dissertations & Theses database. (Publication No. AAT MQ71566)

Braun, V., & Clarke, V. (2006). Using thematic analysis in psychology. *Qualitative Research in Psychology, 3,* 77–101.

Canto, J. G., Goldberg, R. J., Hand, M. M., Bonow, R. O., Sopko, G., Pepine, C. J., et al. (2007). Symptom presentation of women with acute coronary syndromes: myth vs reality. *Archives of Internal Medicine, 167,* 2405–2413.

Charmaz, K. (2000). Grounded theory: objectivist and constructivist methods. In N. K. Denzin, & Y. S. Lincoln (Eds.), *Handbook of qualitative research* (2nd ed.). (pp. 509–535) London: Sage.

Clark, A. M. (2001). Treatment decision-making during the early stages of heart attack: a case for the role of body and self in influencing delays. *Sociology of Health & Illness, 23,* 425–446.

Cole, E. R., & Zucker, A. N. (2007). Black and white women's perspectives on femininity. *Cultural Diversity & Ethnic Minority Psychology, 13*, 1–9.

Connell, R. W. (1995). *Masculinities*. Oxford: Polity Press.

Courtenay, W. H. (2000a). Behavioral factors associated with disease, injury, and death among men: evidence and implications for prevention. *Journal of Men's Studies, 9*, 81–142.

Courtenay, W. H. (2000b). Engendering health: a social constructionist examination of men's health beliefs and behaviors. *Psychology of Men and Masculinity, 1*, 4–15. doi:10.1037//1524-9220.1.1.4.

Dracup, K., Moser, D. K., Eisenberg, M., Meischke, H., Alonzo, A. A., & Braslow, A. (1995). Causes of delay in seeking treatment for heart attack symptoms. *Social Science & Medicine, 40*, 379–392. doi:10.1016/0277-9536(94)00278-2.

Dworkin, S. L. (2005). Who is epidemiologically fathomable in the HIV/AIDS epidemic? Gender, sexuality, and intersectionality in public health. *Culture, Health & Sexuality, 7*, 615–623. doi:10.1080/13691050500100385.

Emslie, C. (2005). Women, men and coronary heart disease: a review of the qualitative literature. *Journal of Advanced Nursing, 51*, 382–395.

Emslie, C., & Hunt, K. (2008). The weaker sex? Exploring lay understandings of gender differences in life expectancy: a qualitative study. *Social Science & Medicine, 67*, 808–816. doi:10.1016/j.socscimed.2008.05.009.

Emslie, C., Ridge, D., Ziebland, S., & Hunt, K. (2006). Men's accounts of depression: reconstructing or resisting hegemonic masculinity? *Social Science & Medicine, 62*, 2246–2257. doi:10.1016/j.socscimed.2005.10.017.

Galdas, P., Cheater, F., & Marshall, P. (2007). What is the role of masculinity in white and South Asian men's decisions to seek medical help for cardiac chest pain? *Journal of Health Services Research & Policy, 12*, 223–229. doi:10.1258/135581907782101552.

Galdas, P. M. (2009). Men, masculinity and help-seeking. In A. Broom, & P. Tovey (Eds.), *Men's health: Body, identity and social context* (pp. 63–82). London: John Wiley & Sons.

George, A., & Fleming, P. (2004). Factors affecting men's help-seeking in the early detection of prostate cancer: implications for health promotion. *Journal of Men's Health & Gender, 1*, 345–352. doi:10.1016/j.jmhg.2004.10.009.

Gough, B. (2007). 'Real men don't diet': an analysis of contemporary newspaper representations of men, food and health. *Sociol Science & Medicine, 64*, 326–337. doi:10.1016/j.socscimed.2006.09.011.

Hunt, K., Adamson, J., & Galdas, P. (2010). Gender and help-seeking: toward gender-comparative studies. In E. Kuhlmann, & E. Annandale (Eds.), *Palgrave handbook of gender and healthcare*. London: Palgrave. pp. 207–221.

Hunt, K., Lewars, H., Emslie, C., & Batty, G. D. (2007). Decreased risk of death from coronary heart disease amongst men with higher 'femininity' scores: a general population cohort study. *International Journal of Epidemiology, 36*, 612–620. doi:10.1093/ije/dym022.

Kristofferzon, M., Löfmark, R., & Carlsson, M. (2003). Myocardial infarction: gender differences in coping and social support. *Journal of Advanced Nursing, 44*, 360–374. doi:10.1046/j.0309-2402.2003.02815.x.

Krogh, J. H. (2007). Personal and social influences: internal and external factors in predicting intentions to seek professional psychological help (Doctoral dissertation). Available from Dissertations and Theses database (Publication No. AAT 3256823).

Lockyer, L. (2005). Women's interpretation of their coronary heart disease symptoms. *European Journal of Cardiovascular Nursing, 4,* 29–35. doi:10.1016/j.ejcnurse.2004.09.003.

Lorber, J. (1996). Beyond the binaries: depolarizing the categories of sex. sexuality, and gender. *Sociological Inquiry, 66,* 143–159.

Løvlien, M., Schei, B., & Hole, T. (2007). Prehospital delay, contributing aspects and responses to symptoms among Norwegian women and men with first time acute myocardial infarction. *European Journal of Cardiovascular Nursing, 6,* 308–313. doi:10.1016/j.ejcnurse.2007.03.002.

Mahalik, J. R., Burns, S. M., & Syzdek, M. (2007). Masculinity and perceived normative health behaviors as predictors of men's health behaviors. *Social Science & Medicine, 64,* 2201–2209. doi:10.1016/j.socscimed.2007.02.035.

Mahalik, J. R., Lagan, H. D., & Morrison, J. A. (2006). Health behaviors and masculinity in Kenyan and U.S. male college students. *Psychology of Men & Masculinity, 7,* 191–202. doi:10.1037/1524-9220.7.4.191.

Mahalik, J. R., Levi-Minzi, M., & Walker, G. (2007). Masculinity and health behaviors in Australian men. *Psychology of Men & Masculinity, 8,* 240–249. doi:10.1037/1524-9220.8.4.240.

Mason, O. J., & Strauss, K. (2004). Testicular cancer: passage through the help-seeking process for a cohort of U.K. men (part 1). *International Journal of Men's Health, 3,* 93–110.

Mansfield, A. K., Addis, M. E., & Mahalik, J. R. (2003). 'Why won't he go to the doctor?': the psychology of men's help seeking. *International Journal of Men's Health, 2,* 93–109.

Moser, D. K., McKinley, S., Dracup, K., & Chung, M. L. (2005). Gender differences in reasons patients delay in seeking treatment for acute myocardial infarction symptoms. *Patient Education & Counseling, 56,* 45–54. doi:10.1016/j.pec.2003.11.011.

O'Brien, R., Hunt, K., & Hart, C. (2005). 'It's caveman stuff, but that is to a certain extent how guys still operate': men's accounts of masculinity and help seeking. *Social Science & Medicine, 61,* 503–516. doi:10.1016/j.socscimed.2004.12.008.

O'Keefe-McCarthy, S. (2008). Women's experiences of cardiac pain: a review of the literature. *Canadian Journal of Cardiovascular Nursing, 18*(3), 18–25.

Ottesen, M. M., Dixen, U., Torp-Pedersen, C., & Køber, L. (2004). Prehospital delay in acute coronary syndrome – an analysis of the components of delay. *International Journal of Cardiology, 96,* 97–103, doi:10.1016/j.ijcard.2003.04.059.

Parslow, R., Jorm, A., Christensen, H., Jacomb, P., & Rodgers, B. (2004). Gender differences in factors affecting use of health services: an analysis of a community study of middle-aged and older Australians. *Social Science & Medicine, 59,* 2121–2129. doi:10.1016/j.socscimed.2004.03.018.

Pattenden, J., Watt, I., Lewin, R. J. P., & Stanford, N. (2002). Decision making processes in people with symptoms of acute myocardial infarction: qualitative study. *British Medical Journal, 324,* 1006–1009.

Prentice, D. A., & Carranza, E. (2002). What women should be, shouldn't be, are allowed to be, and don't have to be: the contents of prescriptive gender stereotypes. *Psychology of Women Quarterly, 26,* 269–281.

Robertson, S. (2006). 'Not living life in too much of an excess': lay men understanding health and well-being. *Health, 10,* 175–189. doi:10.1177/1363459306061787.

Robertson, S. (2007). *Understanding men and health: Masculinities, identity and wellbeing.* Maidenhead, England: McGraw Hill/Open University Press.

Rosenfeld, A. G., Lindauer, A., & Darney, B. G. (2005). Understanding treatment-seeking delay in women with acute myocardial infarction: descriptions of decision-making patterns. *American Journal of Critical Care, 14,* 285–293.

Schwalbe, M., & Wolkomir, M. (2001). The masculine self as problem and resource in interview studies of men. *Men & Masculinities, 4,* 90–103. doi:10.1177/1097184 X01004001005.

Seem, S. R., & Clark, M. D. (2006). Healthy women, healthy men, and healthy adults: an evaluation of gender role stereotypes in the twenty-first century. *Sex Roles, 55,* 247–258. doi:10.1007/s11199-006-9077-0.

Smith, J. A., Braunack-Mayer, A., & Wittert, G. (2006). What do we know about men's help-seeking and health service use? *Medical Journal of Australia, 184,* 81–83.

Stankiewicz, J. M., & Rosselli, F. (2008). Women as sex objects and victims in print advertisements. *Sex Roles, 58,* 579–589. doi:10.1007/s11199-007-9359-1.

Strauss, A. L., & Corbin, J. M. (1998). *Basics of qualitative research: Techniques and procedures for developing grounded theory* (2nd ed.). Thousand Oaks, CA: Sage.

Ting, H. H., Bradley, E. H., Wang, Y., Lichtman, J. H., Nallamothu, B. K., Sullivan, M. D., et al. (2008). Factors associated with longer time from symptom onset to hospital presentation for patients with ST-elevation myocardial infarction. *Archives of Internal Medicine, 168,* 959–968.

Turris, S. A., & Finamore, S. (2008). Reducing delay for women seeking treatment in the emergency department for symptoms of potential cardiac illness. *Journal of Emergency Nursing, 34,* 509–515. doi:10.1016/j.jen.2007.09.016.

White, A., Fawkner, H. J., & Holmes, M. (2006). Is there a case for differential treatment of young men and women? *Medical Journal of Australia, 185,* 454–455.

White, A. K., & Johnson, M. (2000). Men making sense of their chest pain – niggles, doubts and denials. *Journal of Clinical Nursing, 9,* 534–541.

Williams, C. L., & Heikes, E. J. (1993). The importance of researcher's gender in the in-depth interview: evidence from two case studies of male nurses. *Gender & Society, 7,* 280–291.

Wood, W., Conway, M., Pushkar, D., & Dugas, M. J. (2005). People's perceptions of women's and men's worry about life issues: worrying about love, accomplishment, or money? *Sex Roles, 53,* 545–551. doi:10.1007/s11199-005-7141-9.

Wu, T., Rose, S. E., & Bancroft, J. M. (2006). Gender differences in health risk behaviors and physical activity among middle school students. *Journal of School Nursing, 22*(1), 25–31.

57

GENDER AND HELP-SEEKING
Towards gender-comparative studies

Kate Hunt, Joy Adamson and Paul Galdas

Source: E. Kuhlmann and E. Annandale (eds), *The Palgrave Handbook of Gender and Healthcare*, London: Palgrave, 2010, pp. 207–21.

Introduction

The question of whether there are differences in the use that men and women make of healthcare services has occupied researchers for many decades (see, for example, Cleary et al., 1982; Mechanic, 1976; Nathanson, 1977). It is often taken as a given that men make lesser use of healthcare services than women (see, for example, White and Witty, 2009). Statements such as that 'men are less likely than women to actively seek medical care when they are ill, choosing instead to "tough it out" ' (Tudiver and Talbot, 1999: 47) are common. Men's supposed 'underuse' or delayed use of healthcare is often taken to be a key part of the explanation for men's shorter life expectancy in comparison with women (White and Witty, 2009). Their underuse of the healthcare system is constructed as a social problem (O'Brien et al., 2005: 503) and has moved up the policy agenda in countries such as the UK, the USA, Australia and Canada in recent years (see also Chapter 14 by Schofield).

Such definitive statements have contributed to a 'strong public narrative' which emphasizes 'expectations that rather than seek help, men will be strong, stoical and often silent in matters relating to health and well-being' (Robertson, 2003: 112). However, this creates problems for how women's help-seeking behaviour is interpreted. An unfortunate implication of this public narrative is that, in presumed contrast to men, women will go to the doctor more readily and will consult with less serious complaints. Such assumptions can lead to women's problems being trivialized when presented to doctors.

In this chapter we outline the origins of these widely held beliefs about gender and help-seeking, and how these have been translated into a binary assumption that, given the same health problems, men will delay seeking help for longer than women. We highlight studies which have shown that the way that men talk about their help-seeking behaviour is linked to their presentations of masculinity, or how they 'do' gender (Saltonstall, 1993; West and Zimmerman, 1986). We then consider exceptions to this dominant portrayal of the relationship between hegemonic masculinity and men's help-seeking behaviour (Connell and Messerschmidt, 2005) and present examples of gender-comparative research on help-seeking. Throughout the chapter we focus on research from Anglo-American countries. We conclude by agreeing, with others, that the 'research base in relation to the link between gender and use of health services is surprisingly poor' (Wilkins et al., 2009: 4) and outlining the reasons why it is important to conduct more gender-comparative studies if we are to better understand the links between gender and help-seeking.

Evidence for men's reluctance to seek help and some important exceptions

In the UK and other western countries, most data show that, *on average*, women consult their general practitioner (GP) more than men (McCormick et al., 1995). Gender differences in GP consultation rates overall are particularly marked in the reproductive years. For example, in Scotland in the 15 to 24 and 25 to 44 age groups women are twice as likely to visit a GP compared to men (ISD, 2000). This partly reflects the medicalization of childbirth, which means that most pregnant women see their GP several times for ante-natal and post-natal care, and many women rely on methods of contraception which are provided within primary care.

In the past two decades or so, following a period when interest in the links between gender and health was largely confined to issues with women's health, there has been increased interest in the links between men's health and their enactment of gender. The ways in which men adopt various expressions, or practices, of masculinity and how this is related to their health and health behaviours has been the focus of many fascinating studies. These have drawn on theoretical insights which have suggested that, although there are numerous expressions of masculinity and masculine identity, there is often a dominant form or hegemonic practice of masculinity in any given context which is recognized as being the most culturally valued (see, for example, Connell and Messerschmidt, 2005; Chapter 14 by Schofield).

Courtenay is one of the many scholars who has drawn a direct link between denial of weakness and the rejection of help as key practices of hegemonic masculinity. He has argued:

> The most powerful men among men are those for whom health and safety are irrelevant ... By dismissing their health care needs, men are constructing gender. When a man brags, 'I haven't been to a

doctor in years', he is simultaneously describing a health practice and situating himself in a masculine arena.

(Courtenay, 2000: 1389)

The observations of women's greater average use of primary care services *overall* – for all health problems and services combined – in interaction with studies of men which have examined the way that masculinities and health are linked, have led to a very widespread belief that men will delay seeking care longer than women whatever their underlying health problem. Galdas (2009) has recently reviewed a number of studies which demonstrate how notions of masculinity and help-seeking behaviours are intricately linked. Most of these are studies of men with male-specific illnesses (prostate or testicular cancer) or with coronary heart disease (CHD) which has often, erroneously, been characterized in the popular and medical imagination as a disease that is more common amongst men (Emslie et al., 2001; see also Chapter 9 by Riska on coronary heart disease).

It is not unusual for studies which have investigated the views of men with a particular condition, such as prostate cancer, to generalize their findings to how men will deal with all conditions. As one example, George and Fleming (2004) studied the factors affecting men's help-seeking in relation to the early detection of prostate cancer. From interviews with 12 men who had attended a charity-based service for the early detection of prostate cancer in Northern Ireland they came to the common conclusion that 'men experience social, psychological and structural barriers to help-seeking including a threat to masculinity, embarrassment, fear and guilt at using an under-resourced health service' (George and Fleming, 2004: 345). They go on to make the more sweeping assertion that 'men delay help-seeking when they are ill and under-use primary health care services' (2004: 346). Others have been a little more tentative in their conclusions. For example, Addis and Mahalik have argued that:

> Men may experience barriers to seeking help from health professionals when they perceive other men in their social networks as disparaging the process. This is especially so if a) other men are perceived as unanimous in their attitudes, b) a large number of men express similar attitudes, c) men see themselves as quite similar to the members of the reference groups, and d) the members of the men's reference groups are important to them.
>
> (2003: 11)

Undoubtedly, many well-conducted qualitative studies of men in a range of countries (including the UK, the USA, Canada and Australia) have found that men often express a reluctance to seek care and have taken this to be an important, if not emblematic, expression of their masculinity. We turn next, however, to consider a few studies which have argued not that masculinity and help-seeking are unrelated, but that the ways in which masculinities and help-seeking are linked are more multi-faceted and complex.

Examples of studies challenging the universality of men's reluctance to seek help

O'Brien and colleagues (2005) studied the links between masculinity and health, and specifically examined how men spoke about help-seeking behaviours. A total of 59 men participated in 15 focus groups. The sample was diverse by age (range 15 to 72 years), occupational status, socio-economic background and health status. Some groups of men were expected to have had unremarkable experiences of masculinity and health; these were largely occupationally based groups, such as gas workers, fire-fighters and students. Other groups were recruited because they were known to have had health problems which might have prompted greater reflection on masculinity and health, for example, groups with men who had prostate cancer, coronary heart disease or mental health problems. The majority of the men lived in central Scotland, and just one focus group was conducted with men of Asian origin, reflecting the limited ethnic diversity in this part of Britain.

These focus group discussions suggested a 'widespread endorsement of a "hegemonic" view that men "should" be reluctant to seek help, particularly amongst younger men' (O'Brien et al., 2005: 503). For example, one member of a focus group, made up of students, said:

> ... the only time I have (gone) to hospital or seen a doctor ... was when I had been punched in the face (and) ... I needed stitches ... or a relative tells you that you've got to go.... even then I've been reluctant to go.
>
> (O'Brien et al., 2005: 507)

This man related his reluctance to consult to 'the whole idea about what constitutes a man. A real man puts up with pain and doesn't complain' (O'Brien et al., 2003: 507–8). However, whilst similar sentiments were very commonly expressed in the groups, some men clearly distanced themselves from this dominant portrayal. A fire-fighter, for example, challenged the hegemonic view of men who trivialized symptoms and dismissed the need for help as 'naïve, I wouldn't say that's masculine' (O'Brien et al., 2005: 513), and his colleague described a reluctance to consult amongst men as 'completely moronic, I mean, it's caveman stuff, but that is to a certain extent how guys still operate'. Indeed, the men in the fire-fighters' group agreed that seeking help at the first sign of symptoms and asking for preventative health checks were important to their continuing ability to work effectively.

O'Brien and colleagues argued such exceptions rarely get considered, although they noted that Robertson (2003: 112) has commented that men struggle with balancing 'a dilemma between "don't care" and "should care"'. However, O'Brien and colleagues noted that these exceptions were not unrelated to men's constructions of their masculinity. They argued that, for the fire-fighters, help-seeking was a way of *preserving* the strongly valued sense of masculinity that they gained through their occupational status. In their working environment at least, the fire-fighters felt able to critique the constraints of an 'old school mentality', and to reject it without consequence for their sense of masculinity.

Other exceptions to men's reluctance to consult could also be understood by reference to a 'hierarchy of threats' to masculinity. O'Brien and colleagues (2005) interpreted some men's discussion of their apparent readiness to consult with putative problems with their sexual performance as indicating that they would rather 'risk' their masculine status by consulting for a sexual health problem than put it in greater jeopardy by not being able to have sex. For some men (such as those with myalgic encephalomyelitis), they argued that consultation – and through it, a diagnosis which to some extent legitimated being unable to fulfil certain roles, like working, 'providing' for the family, which the men felt they were expected to meet as men – presented a potential means to *restore* a masculine identity that had been undermined by the nature of their illness. Finally, men who had survived episodes of illness which they perceived to be life-threatening (cardiac problems, prostate cancer) were more reflective and sometimes critical about men's general reluctance to seek help and appeared to have accepted that preserving their future health assumed a higher priority than preserving their masculinity.

O'Brien and colleagues acknowledged that these men's accounts of their attitudes to help-seeking may not reflect their actual past actions, but

> they poignantly describe a culture, a 'practice of masculinity', which most men felt they were expected to conform to and reproduce, or to justify their rejection of such practices.
>
> (O'Brien et al., 2005: 515)

Another qualitative study which also explicitly challenged the universality of men's reluctance to consult contrasted accounts of the decision to seek medical help for cardiac chest pain by 36 men of 'white' ethnicity and UK ancestry and 20 South Asian men (English-speaking men of Indian or Pakistani ancestry) living in the northeast of England (Galdas et al., 2007). The men were recruited from two coronary care units and six cardiology wards in two teaching hospitals. All participants had been admitted after experiencing chest pain which was subsequently confirmed as a first acute myocardial infarction or newly diagnosed angina pectoris. Participants were interviewed at their hospital bedside, and were asked to give their own account of the 'events and actions relating to their experience from the outset of pain to hospital admission', before being asked further questions on their 'views, common behaviours and premises about seeking medical help "as a man" that aimed to elicit information on how constructions of masculinity were associated with a participant's experience of seeking help'; this approach was taken to limit the effect of 'masculine "impression management"' (Galdas et al., 2007: 224).

In this study, the majority of 'white' men were noted to perceive a need to demonstrate that they had endured a high level of pain before seeking help for chest pain symptoms (as in earlier studies, for example, White and Johnson, 2000). However, the accounts provided by most of the South Asian participants were quite different. These men described how they had consulted quickly when they experienced persistent or recurrent chest pain. They considered pain to be a legitimate reason to seek medical help and none appeared to think that seeking help for their chest pain was either 'unmanly' or a sign of weakness. What is more, they placed great emphasis on their responsibilities for their families, which they felt they could not fulfil if they were seriously ill (or if they died). The majority of Indian and Pakistani men had discussed their symptoms with their family, in contrast to the majority of white men who suggested that they only disclosed their chest pain to others as a last resort, when they could no longer tolerate the pain or when they felt confident it was a sign that they had a 'legitimate' illness that they should be worried about.

Many of the white men talked with pride about the lengthy periods since their last visit to the GP and only one had consulted a GP before being admitted to hospital with his chest pain symptoms. In stark contrast, all but one of the 20 Indian and Pakistani men had visited their GP before being admitted to hospital. Thus, it was apparent in this study that seeking medical help was portrayed as a 'last resort' by the white men and avoiding 'being perceived as a hypochondriac or weak by others played a part in many white men's decisions to delay seeking help from a healthcare professional until they became certain their pain could not be coped with alone', whereas the willingness to seek medical help observed amongst most Indian and Pakistani men can be seen to 'signify men's retention of a culturally distinct (non-dominant) form of masculinity' (Galdas et al., 2007: 227–8).

These interesting exceptions to the prevailing orthodoxy that men are always reluctant to present themselves as being willing to seek help for health problems are likely to be reflected in other studies. As Galdas has concluded:

> the simplistic notion of 'men' being consistently averse to seeking medical help in a timely manner is not wholly supported by the empirical evidence ... In developing an empirical basis from which to inform interventions to effectively engage men with health services, it is important to ... avoid universalising assumptions about hegemonic

> masculinity that propagate an essentialist discourse about the damaging affect of 'masculinity' on men's help-seeking behaviour.
>
> (2009, 77-8)

We would argue that two steps are essential to developing this empirical basis. The first is for researchers to critically investigate the particular circumstances in which men articulate or reject a link between reluctance and prevailing notions of appropriate demonstrations of their masculinity. Second, and perhaps most crucially, there is a need for many more studies to adopt a gender-comparative approach. These need to be of at least two kinds: 1) quantitative studies which compare patterns of help-seeking behaviours amongst men and women with similar underlying morbidity; and 2) qualitative research which critically explores the similarities and differences in the ways that women and men talk about their decisions to consult (or not) when faced with novel or ongoing symptoms. Such research is rare: most empirical investigations of gender and help-seeking have used single-sex samples and addressed problems that are either specific to men or specific to women (Annandale et al., 2007). In the next section we consider a few exceptions to this generalization.

Comparing patterns of healthcare use in men and women with similar conditions

Given the widespread and entrenched nature of the assumption that women consult more frequently, and more readily, than men, it is surprising how few studies have sought to systematically compare patterns of consultation amongst men and women with similar morbidity. We consider here a few exceptions. The first is a systematic review of two common symptoms, namely back pain and headache. Although these are often not indicative of serious underlying disease, they nonetheless can be troubling and disruptive and both symptoms contribute substantially to absence from work and to the burden of ill-health presented to primary care. The second is an empirical study which considers whether women are more likely to consult than men for particular groups of chronic conditions. The third considers gender and consultation prior to the diagnosis of one of the most common forms of malignancy, colorectal cancer, which is a major cause of death in most countries.

Gender and consultation for headache and back pain

Hunt and colleagues (2010) have recently undertaken a systematic review of consultation for headache or back pain in order to question the strength and consistency of evidence that women consult more frequently. To be eligible for inclusion, studies had to include both users and non-users of healthcare, have gender as an explanatory variable, and be based on epidemiological methods. The review was restricted to studies which were conducted in more developed countries and published in English. An extensive and systematic search identified just 14 publications (mostly reporting studies conducted in northern European countries, although four were from the USA, and one each from Australia and Greece) which reported data on consultation amongst men and women with symptoms of back pain. Overall, evidence for greater consultation by women with back pain in comparison with men was weak and inconsistent. Amongst those who reported symptoms of back pain, the odds ratios for women seeking help, in comparison with men ranged from 0.6 (95 per cent confidence intervals 0.3, 1.2, adjusted only for age) to 2.17 (95 per cent confidence intervals 1.35, 3.57, unadjusted for other factors), although none of the studies with an odds ratio of less than 1.00 (which would indicate that men were more likely to consult than women) were statistically significant. Three of the four studies which reported a statistically elevated odds ratio (which would suggest that women were consulting more than men) examined recent consultation (within the last six months).

The evidence for women being more likely to consult for headache than men was a little stronger. Five of the 11 studies reporting on gender and consultation for headache showed a statistically elevated odds ratio (indicating that women were more likely to have consulted than men), and none suggested that men were more likely to consult than women for headache.

However, this review highlights the paucity of evidence on gender and consultation *for specific conditions and symptoms*. First, few studies had the question of whether consultation patterns differ for men and women as the main focus of their analysis. Mostly gender was included as one of a number of socio-demographic variables, and often the numbers of men and women in the study, or the sex-specific prevalence of symptoms or of consulting, were difficult to extract from the papers. Second, the studies varied greatly in their definitions of the symptom (including its severity and duration) and of help-seeking. Some included consultation over a relatively short period – for example, the last month – whereas others used 'ever consulted' as their outcome. Some confined themselves to consultation with a general practitioner whilst others included other healthcare professionals or alternative practitioners. Third, the studies were conducted in countries with very different healthcare systems (including those which rely heavily on private healthcare insurance, such as the USA, and countries with free access to healthcare, such as the UK, with its National Health Service). Fourth, all of the studies employed a cross-sectional design, and so are subject to potential methodological problems (such as differential recall or reporting of symptoms or of healthcare use); none prospectively followed a group of people with a given symptom to investigate how they dealt with their symptom over time.

This variability between studies limits the extent to which firm conclusions can be drawn about whether women and men differ in their healthcare utilization for the symptoms of headache and back pain and illustrates the need for well-designed studies which can accurately establish whether there are gender differences in consultation for specific symptoms and conditions. Despite these limitations, and given the strength of the assumptions that women consult more readily for common symptoms, what was striking was that the evidence for greater consultation amongst women was surprisingly weak and inconsistent, especially with respect to back pain.

Gender and consultation for chronic illness

In an analysis of general population data, Hunt and colleagues (1999) explicitly set out to examine gender differences in consultation when comparing 'like with like', as far as possible, by attempting to 'standardize' for presence and perceived severity of illness. This analysis used data from detailed face-to-face interviews with two cohorts (people born in the early 1930s and in the early 1950s, aged in their late thirties and late fifties when the data were collected for this analysis) of the West of Scotland Twenty-07 Study which included a much extended version of the British General Household Survey question on longstanding illness (LSI). Instead of asking simply whether a person had a longstanding illness and whether this caused limitation to their activities, further questions asked for the name of the conditions (so that LSI could be grouped to five condition groups [musculoskeletal, respiratory, digestive, cardiovascular and mental health] using the British Royal College of General Practitioners coding scheme [RCGP, 1986]), the frequency and severity of pain, and whether it had caused restriction to activities in the previous four weeks. As expected, overall women had consulted their GP more times on average than men in the previous twelve months – 3.48 vs 2.34 ($p < 0.01$) in the 1950s cohort; 4.38 vs 4.21 (NS) in the 1930s cohort; this included all consultations for any symptom, condition or advice.

However, a series of logistic regression analyses showed that amongst those who reported that they had a particular type of condition, women were no more likely to have consulted a GP for that condition in the past year for any condition group and *men* were *more* likely than women to consult if they reported a digestive condition (odds ratio 1.65, 95 per cent confidence limits (cls) 1.29–2.68). This pattern persisted when taking account of the severity of the condition. These results reinforced findings from an earlier analysis of participants in the Twenty-07 Study which examined consultation for 33 common symptoms (Wyke et al., 1998) and found that, when account was taken of who had experienced symptoms in the last month, there were no gender differences in GP consultation for any of the 33 symptoms in the 1930s cohort and gender differences for just three symptoms in the 1950s cohort (a female excess in consulting for headaches and skin problems, and a male excess for stomach problems or cramps). Hunt and colleagues concluded that:

... these data argue against the most widely accepted explanations for gender differences in consulting, namely that, once illness is recognised, women are more likely to consult than men ... It is important that the stereotype of women being more likely to respond to symptoms and chronic conditions by consulting general practitioners does not persist unchallenged. The limited evidence from ... studies which have controlled for underlying pathology or symptomatology ... lends little support to the view that women are more likely to over-rate and over-react to symptoms once recognised.

(1999: 98–9)

Gender and consultation prior to the diagnosis of colorectal cancer

One limitation of the study by Hunt and colleagues (1999) was that, although it was able to take account of self-perceived severity and restriction of daily activities (which are known to be important predictors of help-seeking), it was only able to control for type of morbidity within broad groupings of conditions, such as respiratory, cardiovascular and so on. An exemplar study comparing consultation in men and women with colorectal cancer, and specifically the time from their first recognition of symptoms to their diagnosis, was conducted over 20 years ago (Marshall and Funch, 1987). Few similar studies have been conducted since. This study (conducted in and around Seattle, USA) used population-based survey methods to identify people who had been diagnosed with colorectal cancer. Adult men and women with a definitive diagnosis (confirmed by a tissue biopsy) of non-recurrent colorectal cancer participated in an interview which investigated when they had first noticed their symptoms, any actions they took before they sought medical treatment, their reasons for seeking or waiting to seek treatment, and any problems they had in obtaining treatment. In all 154 men and 153 women were interviewed.

Marshall and Funch reported that the most common symptoms for both men and women were rectal bleeding, general weakness and abdominal pain. Neither the number of symptoms nor the prevalence of any prediagnostic symptom differed by gender. Similarly, the reported severity of symptoms was comparable between men and women. They concluded that 'overall, these findings suggest that, for colorectal cancer patients, males and females report the same symptoms, and describe them in a similar manner' (Marshall and Funch, 1987: 74). Men's and women's actions before consulting were also similar: they reported similar levels of use of over-the-counter drugs, and of talking to other people (including their spouse and friends) about their symptoms.

They then examined 'patient delay' (the number of days between first noticing symptoms and contacting a doctor about the symptoms) and 'diagnostic delay' (the time between the patient's first visit or call to the doctor and a definitive diagnosis) overall, and in people with cancer of the colon and cancer of the rectum separately. When both cancers were considered together, there was no difference between patient delay (mean number of days: 180.0 for men, 198.7 for women, t-value 0.72, NS). For colon cancer there was a suggestion that men delayed slightly longer (mean number of days: 198.4 for men, 179.5 for women), although this difference was not significant (t-value – 0.29). However, for cancer of the rectum *female* patients delayed on average more than 100 days longer than men (mean number of days: 149.3 for men, 254.9 for women, t-value 2.37, p = 0.02).

There was also a substantial difference in diagnostic delay for colorectal cancer (mean number of days: for men 67.0, for women 106.1, t-value = 2.35, p = 0.02), which was due entirely to the greater diagnostic delay experienced by women with colon cancer (mean number of days: for men 71.7, for women 125.7, t-value = 2.49, p = 0.01). Further investigation showed that women who had longer diagnostic delays had visited their doctor more times before their diagnosis was made. Marshall and Funch concluded that their study

> [lends] little support to the common claim that women are more likely than men to respond to symptoms of illness by seeking medical care. Female colorectal cancer patients did not . . . report with disease at earlier stages than those at which male colorectal cancer patients reported. Female colorectal cancer patients did not delay less than male patients in seeking medical care [. . .] They also experienced more delay than men securing definitive diagnosis subsequent to having consulted a clinician.
>
> (1987: 80)

Although this study was conducted more than two decades ago, it is clear that the conclusions have done little to dent the popular medical view that women are less likely to delay before presenting their symptoms to the medical profession. Furthermore, a recent systematic review of the influences on pre-hospital delay in the diagnosis of colorectal cancer concluded that there was no relationship between patient gender and the time between a patient first noticing a cancer symptom and presenting to primary care or between first presentation and referral to secondary care (Mitchell et al., 2008).

Conclusion

In this chapter we have attempted to demonstrate that the link between gender and help-seeking is much more complex than commonly portrayed. Whilst we recognize that many well-conducted studies of men recount numerous examples of men's reluctance to seek medical help when they experience symptoms or are worried that something may be wrong, we are concerned that there is a danger that an over-simplistic view of gender and healthcare use may lead to policies or interventions which may not best serve the health of either men or women. Failing to recognize contexts in which men engage in *timely* help-seeking consistent with their masculine identities may lead us to overlook ways that health practitioners and policy-makers could encourage more men to take more active care of their health.

However, we believe that there are more fundamental gaps in the evidence. Because most recent insights from research on men, masculinities and health have arisen from empirical studies of all-male samples, there is no opportunity to ask whether there are similar expressions of reluctance to seek healthcare amongst women. This is a surprising omission as some qualitative research (for recent examples, see Townsend et al., 2006; 2008) has shown that it is commonplace for both men and women (even those with high levels of morbidity) to represent their use of healthcare as a 'last resort' and to go to great lengths to present their management of their illness and their use of healthcare within a moral framework. Because of an often unconscious tendency to valorize distinctions rather than similarities between men and women, it is often presumed that *because* men are reluctant to consult, women are not, and because women are willing to use healthcare for some aspects of their lives (such as contraception and the monitoring of pregnancy and childbirth), they will be more willing to consult more quickly for all aspects of their health.

In the few examples that we have cited which have used gender-comparative methods to examine patterns of healthcare use in men and women with similar underlying morbidity, there is, at best, insufficient evidence that men consult less frequently or delay longer before consulting. The study by Marshall and Funch (1987), though over 20 years old, is not alone (Mitchell et al., 2008) in finding that men do *not* delay longer before consulting with symptoms of colorectal cancer, but is often overlooked. Their findings suggest that doctors may pay different attention to symptoms depending on the gender of the patient. Whilst this may often make good clinical sense (abdominal pain or bloating in a man could not be a symptom of cancer of the ovary in men, and frequent night-time urination could not be a symptom of prostate cancer in women, to take extreme examples), Arber and colleagues (2006) have found that a patient's gender may affect the initial assessment of the severity of symptoms and the need for further investigation. In an elegant experimental study, doctors assessing exactly the same presentation of potential symptoms of coronary heart disease by males and females asked fewer questions and recommended fewer examinations and further diagnostic tests when assessing female patients. They were less likely to think that their symptoms were due to CHD, and they had a lower threshold of certainty about their diagnosis. Arber and her colleagues (Arber et al., 2006; Adams et al., 2008) recognized that their findings may reflect stereotypical conceptualizations of CHD as a male disease. However, their results and those of Marshall and Funch (1987) could indicate that there is a danger that, because of the deep-rootedness of the assumption that women will consult more quickly and at lower levels of morbidity (despite a lack of robust scientific evidence), women's symptoms may be regarded as more trivial and less indicative of serious underlying disease than men's.

Appropriate use of healthcare is vital in maximizing individual health and longevity and in making the best use of resources that are increasingly overstretched with increasing burdens of chronic ill-health. The goal is to increase rapid consultation with early symptoms of serious underlying disease that could respond to early medical intervention, whilst discouraging consultations for more commonplace symptoms which are not amenable to medical treatment. More empirical research is needed that includes and compares both men and women, and which examines the diversity of experience and attitudes *amongst* men and *amongst* women if we are to avoid misleading essentialist assumptions that because 'men' behave in one way, 'women' will behave in another.

Summary

- Although, on average, women consult in primary care more than men, particularly during the peak reproductive years, there is little robust evidence comparing rates of consultation in men and women experiencing the same illnesses.
- Although gender-comparative studies are rare, according to current evidence men do not delay longer in seeking help for colorectal cancer, a major contributor to premature mortality.
- Studies with all-male samples have noted a reluctance to consult amongst men which has been widely attributed to a desire to conform to dominant representation of masculinity. However, qualitative research also shows that women also commonly present healthcare use as a 'last resort'.
- More critical gender-comparative research is needed to understand the ways in which men and women's help-seeking is similar or different to avoid medical bias in consultations (based on false premises about readiness to consult) and to develop gender-sensitive policy and practice on the most appropriate use of healthcare resources.

Key reading

Adams, A., C. D. Buckingham, A. Lindenmeyer, J. B. McKinlay, C. Link, L. Marceau and S. Arber (2008) 'The Influence of Patient and Doctor Gender on Diagnosing Coronary Heart Disease', *Sociology of Health and Illness*, 30 (1), 1–18.

Annandale, E., J. Harvey, D. Cavers and M. Dixon-Woods (2007) 'Gender and Access to Healthcare in the UK: A Critical Interpretive Synthesis of the Literature', *Evidence and Policy*, 3 (4), 463–86.

Galdas, P. (2009) 'Men, Masculinity and Help-seeking', in A. Broom and P. Tovey (eds), *Men's Health: Body, Identity and Social Context* (London: Wiley), 63–82.

O'Brien, R., K. Hunt and G. Hart (2005) 'Men's Accounts of Masculinity and Help-seeking: "It's Caveman Stuff, But That Is to a Certain Extent How Guys Still Operate"', *Social Science & Medicine*, 61 (3), 503–16.

References

Adams, A., C. D. Buckingham, A. Lindenmeyer, J. B. McKinlay, C. Link, L. Marceau and S. Arber (2008) 'The Influence of Patient and Doctor Gender on Diagnosing Coronary Heart Disease', *Sociology of Health and Illness*, 30 (1), 1–18.

Addis, M. E. and J. R. Mahalik (2003) 'Men, Masculinity, and the Contexts of Help Seeking', *American Psychologist*, 58 (1), 5–14.

Annandale, E., J. Harvey, D. Cavers and M. Dixon-Woods (2007) 'Gender and Access to Healthcare in the UK: A Critical Interpretive Synthesis of the Literature', *Evidence and Policy*, 3 (4), 463–86.

Arber, S., J. McKinlay, A. Adams, L. Marceau, C. Link and A. O'Donnell (2006) 'Patient Characteristics and Inequalities in Doctors' Diagnostic and Management Strategies Relating to CHD: A Video-Simulation Experiment', *Social Science & Medicine*, 62 (1), 103–15.

Cleary, P. D., D. Mechanic and J. R. Greenley (1982) 'Sex Differences in Medical Care Utilization: An Empirical Investigation', *Journal of Health and Social Behavior*, 23 (2), 106–19.

Connell, R. and J. W. Messerschmidt (2005) 'Hegemonic Masculinity. Rethinking the Concept', *Gender and Society*, 19 (6), 829–59.

Courtenay, W. (2000) 'Constructions of Masculinity and their Influence on Men's Well-Being: A Theory of Gender and Health', *Social Science & Medicine*, 50 (10), 1385–1401.

Emslie, C., K. Hunt and G. Watt (2001) 'Invisible Women? The Importance of Gender in Lay Beliefs about Heart Problems', *Sociology of Health and Illness*, 23 (2), 203–33.

Galdas, P. (2009) 'Men, Masculinity and Help-seeking', in A. Broom and P. Tovey (eds), *Men's Health: Body, Identity and Social Context* (London: Wiley), 63–82.

Galdas, P., F. Cheater and P. Marshall (2007) 'What Is the Role of Masculinity in White and South Asian Men's Decisions to Seek Medical Help for Cardiac Chest Pain?', *Journal of Health Service Research and Policy*, 12 (4), 223–9.

George, A. and P. Fleming (2004) 'Factors Affecting Men's Help-seeking in the Early Detection of Prostate Cancer: Implications for Health Promotion', *Journal of Men's Health and Gender*, 1 (4), 345–52.

Hunt, K., J. Adamson, C. Hewitt and N. Nazareth (2010) 'Do Women Consult More than Men? A Systematic Review of Gender and Consultation for Back Pain and Headache', unpublished manuscript.

Hunt K., G. Ford, L. Harkins and S. Wyke (1999) 'Are Women More Ready to Consult than Men? Gender Differences in General Practitioner Consultation for Common Chronic Conditions', *Journal of Health Services Research & Policy*, 4 (2), 96–100.

ISD – Information Services Division, NHS Scotland (2000) Consultation rates per 1,000 population. Scottish Health Statistics, Section L1 (Edinburgh: ISD).

McCormick, A., D. Fleming and J. Charlton (1995) *Morbidity Statistics from General Practice. Fourth National Study 1991–1992*, OPCS Series MB5 no. 3 (London: HMSO).

Marshall, J. R. and D. P. Funch (1987) 'Gender and Illness Behavior among Colorectal Cancer Patients', *Women & Health*, 11, 67–82.

Mechanic, D. (1976) 'Sex, Illness Behavior, and the Use of Health Services', *Journal of Human Stress*, 2, 29–40.

Mitchell, E., S. Macdonald, N. Campbell, D. Weller and U. Macleod (2008) 'Influences on Pre-hospital Delay in the Diagnosis of Colorectal Cancer: A Systematic Review', *British Journal of Cancer*, 98 (1), 60–70.

Nathanson, C. A. (1977) 'Sex, Illness and Medical Care: A Review of Data, Theory and Method', *Social Science & Medicine*, 11 (1), 13–25.

O'Brien, R., K. Hunt and G. Hart (2005) 'Men's Accounts of Masculinity and Help-seeking: "It's Caveman Stuff, But That Is to a Certain Extent How Guys Still Operate"', *Social Science & Medicine*, 61 (3), 503–16.

Robertson, S. (2003) 'Men Managing Health', *Men's Health Journal*, 2 (4), 111–13.

RCGP – Royal College of General Practitioners (1986) *The Classification and Analysis of General Practice Data* (London: Royal College of General Practitioners).

Saltonstall, R. (1993) 'Healthy Bodies, Social Bodies: Men's and Women's Concepts and Practices of Health in Everyday Life', *Social Science & Medicine*, 36 (1), 7–14.

Townsend, A., S. Wyke and K. Hunt (2006) 'Self-managing and Managing Self: Practical and Moral Dilemmas in Accounts of Living with Chronic Illness', *Chronic Illness*, 2 (3), 185–94.

Townsend, A., S. Wyke and K. Hunt (2008) 'Frequent Consulting and Multiple Morbidity: A Qualitative Comparison of "High" and "Low" Consulters of GPS', *Family Practice*, 25 (3), 168–75.

Tudiver, F. and Y. Talbot (1999) 'Why Don't Men Seek Help? Family Physicians' Perspectives on Help-seeking Behaviour in Men', *Journal of Family Practice*, 48 (1), 47–52.

West, C. and D. Zimmerman, D. (1987) 'Doing Gender', *Gender and Society*, 1 (2), 125–51.

White, A. and M. Johnson (2000) 'Men Making Sense of Their Chest Pain – Niggles, Doubts and Denials', *Journal of Clinical Nursing*, 9 (4), 534–41.

White, A. and K. Witty (2009) 'Men's Under Use of Health Services – Finding Alternative Approaches', *Journal of Men's Health*, 6 (2), 95–7.

Wilkins, D., S. Payne, G. Granville and P. Branney (2009) *The Gender and Access to Health Services Study* (London: Department of Health).

Wyke, S., K. Hunt and G. Ford (1998) 'Gender Differences in Consulting a General Practitioner for Common Symptoms of Minor Illness', *Social Science & Medicine*, 46 (7), 901–6.

58
GENDER AND ACCESS TO HIV TESTING AND ANTIRETROVIRAL TREATMENTS IN THAILAND
Why do women have more and earlier access?

*Sophie Le Cœur, Intira J. Collins,
Julie Pannetier and Eva Lelièvre*

Source: *Social Science & Medicine*, 69 (2009), 846–53.

Abstract

In the recent scale-up of antiretroviral treatment, gender differences in access to treatment have been reported. In Thailand, as the HIV epidemic became more generalised, there has been a shift from men being disproportionately affected to increased vulnerability of women. In 2007, the Living with Antiretrovirals (LIWA-ANRS 12141) study investigated the gender distribution of all adult patients receiving antiretroviral therapy ($N = 513$ patients) in four community hospitals in northern Thailand and factors influencing the disparities observed. From this retrospective life-event history survey, we found that proportionately more women (53%) were receiving antiretroviral therapy than men, an unexpected result for a country with a higher proportion of infections among men. They were more likely to initiate treatment within one year of diagnosis and were at a more advanced stage of the disease compared to women. This gender distribution is partly explained by the evolving dynamics of the HIV epidemic, initial prioritization of mothers for treatment and earlier access to HIV testing for women. These issues are also entangled with gender differences in the reasons and timing to HIV testing at the individual level. This study found that the majority of men underwent HIV testing for health reasons while the majority of women were tested following family events such as a spouse/child death or during pregnancy. Further qualitative research on gender specific barriers to HIV testing and care, such as perceived low risk of infection, poor access to medical care, lack of social support, actual or anticipated HIV/AIDS-related stigma would provide greater insight. In the meantime, urgent efforts are needed to increase access to voluntary counselling and testing inside and outside the family setting with targeted interventions for men.

© 2009 Elsevier Ltd. All rights reserved.

Introduction

Thailand was the first Asian country affected by the AIDS epidemic in the late 1980s. It is estimated that over 1 million of the 64 million population has been infected with HIV of which over 460,000 have died (UNDP, 2004). At the end of 2007, there were an estimated 610,000 persons living with HIV (UNAIDS & WHO, 2008).

Gender distribution among HIV infected persons in Thailand

In 1989, the initial wave of the epidemic developed very rapidly through mostly men intravenous drug users. The second wave was predominately spread among commercial sex workers while the third wave diffused into the general heterosexual population, initially from commercial sex workers to their clients, and then from the clients to their regular spouses (Weniger et al., 1991). The second and third waves of the epidemic were closely related to gender specific sexual norms (Brown, Sittitrai, Vanichseni, & Thisyakorn, 1994; Brown & Xenos, 1994; Ford & Koetsawang, 1991). For men, visits to commercial sex workers before marriage were widely accepted as a form of sexual initiation, while after marriage, visits to commercial sex workers often occurred in the company of peers and were generally tolerated by the spouse (Maticka-Tyndale et al., 1997; Saengtienchai, Knodel, Van-Landingham, & Pramualratana, 1999; Vanlandingham, Knodel, Saengtienchai, & Pramualratana, 1998). However, women were traditionally expected to be abstinent before marriage, and extramarital sexual relationships were considered socially unacceptable (Knodel, Saengtienchai, Vanlandingham, & Lucas, 1999).

While HIV prevalence rates in Thailand are remarkably well documented among specific populations such as pregnant women, military conscripts, men who have sex with men, direct and indirect sex workers and blood-donors, there is currently a lack of reliable data on the overall sex-ratio in HIV infected adults (UNAIDS & WHO, 2008). There is growing concern for the increased vulnerability of women following the dramatic decrease in the male to female sex-ratio of reported AIDS cases, from 6.8:1 in 1992 to 4.4:1 in 1996 (Rerks-Ngarm, 1997). This trend appears to be continuing with the sex-ratio of reported AIDS cases decreasing further to 2.4:1 in 1999 (World Bank, 2000) and to 1.6:1 in 2007 (Ministry of Public Health, 2008). This is close to the UNAIDS, 2007 estimate that 250,000 of the 600,000 adults living with HIV/AIDS in Thailand were women, which represents a male to female sex-ratio of about 1.4:1 (UNAIDS & WHO, 2008).

National AIDS program

The Thai government made considerable efforts to curtail the HIV epidemic with a multi-sectoral AIDS program implemented beginning in 1989. Among the preventive strategies, the 100% condom campaign was uniquely successful in limiting the number of new infections in the general population by increasing the use of condoms among commercial sex workers and reducing the frequency of commercial sex visits (Ainsworth, Beyrer, & Soucat, 2003; Hanenberg, Rojanapithayakorn, Kunasol, & Sokal, 1994; Nelson et al., 1996; Phoolcharoen, Ungchusak, Sittitrai, & Brown, 1998; Rojanapithayakorn & Hanenberg, 1996; UNAIDS, 2000). However, the prevalence remains high among the predominantly male high risk behavior populations such as injecting drug users, and men who have sex with men (Nelson et al., 2002; UNAIDS, 2007; van Griensven et al., 2005).

In terms of provision of antiretroviral treatment, the Department of Health piloted the Access to Care (ATC) treatment program in 2002, which prioritized HIV infected mothers. HIV infected pregnant women were identified at the antenatal clinic (ANC) through HIV screening and enrolled in the national Prevention of Mother to Child Transmission (PMTCT) of HIV program. This program, which had a very high antenatal HIV testing acceptance rate of 97%, led to a dramatic decrease in the number of pediatric AIDS cases (Amornwichet et al., 2002). The strong association between maternal and child health was the rationale for prioritizing HIV infected new mothers who, if treated, would be able to raise their children, therefore reducing the burden of orphans. The ATC program then expanded under the family centered approach of "PMTCT-Plus", which incorporated voluntary HIV counselling and testing and antiretroviral treatment for infected husbands/partners and children.

It is important to note that a major health care reform was implemented in 2001, with the introduction of a universal coverage system, providing health care at very low patient fees of "30-baht" (US$0.75) per hospital visit to all Thai citizens (Tangcharoensathien, Wibulpholprasert, & Nitayaramphong, 2004). The universal coverage system is predominately targeted towards low income families and runs in parallel with other existing health coverage schemes – the Social Security Scheme (SSS), the Workmen's Compensation Fund (WCF) for workers in the private sector, the Civil Servant Medical Benefit Scheme (CSMBS) for government employees and some private insurance programs. For HIV infected patients, the government launched the National Access to Antiretroviral Treatment Program (NAPHA) in 2003, providing free access to antiretroviral therapy (Chasombat, Lertpiriyasuwat, Thanprasertsuk, Suebsaeng, & Lo, 2006). This program was subsequently integrated with the universal coverage system. By the end of 2007, the scale-up of antiretroviral treatments was estimated to have reached 153,000 persons (UNAIDS & WHO, 2008).

Gender, HIV and antiretroviral treatment programs

There have been increasing reports of over-representation of women enrolled in antiretroviral treatments programs compared to men in lower or middle income countries, in proportion to the number of HIV infected persons by gender (Braitstein et al., 2008; Muula et al., 2007). In addition, it appears that men in these settings are more likely to present late for testing, at more advanced stages of the disease and with greater risk of mortality compared to women (Keiser et al., 2008; Lawn & Wood, 2006).

In Thailand, a full evaluation of the gender distribution among adults in the national antiretroviral program has not been conducted. It has been suggested that Thai women were either equally or over-represented in antiretroviral treatment programs (Braitstein et al., 2008; Leusaree, Srithanaviboonchai, Chanmangkang, Ying-Ru, & Natpratan, 2002). While there have been studies in Southern Africa (Muula et al., 2007) on the reasons for gender based differences in access to HIV care, there are limited data in the Asian setting (Braitstein et al., 2008; Keiser et al., 2008) and, to our knowledge, no comprehensive study in Thailand.

In this paper, we conducted a life-event history survey of all adults receiving antiretroviral therapy in four hospitals in a semi-urban population in Northern Thailand, from which we conducted a gender based descriptive analysis. This approach enabled us to relate the gender distribution in access to antiretroviral treatments with the reasons and timing of HIV testing in the context of the individual life-course and the evolving AIDS epidemic in Thailand.

Methods

Data were collected from the "Living with Antiretrovirals" study (LIWA), a socio-demographic and economic evaluation of the impact of access to antiretroviral treatments in northern Thailand, a region heavily affected by HIV. The study targeted all HIV infected adults receiving antiretroviral treatment in four community hospitals (Mae On, San Sai, Doi Saket and Sankaempeng Hospitals) in Chiang Mai province.

Life-event history survey

In order to assess the access to antiretroviral treatments and their socio-demographic impact on the lives of patients, several approaches could be envisioned. The epidemiological approach would follow prospectively a population of HIV infected individuals from the time of their diagnosis, and assess the changes in their situation by interviewing them at different time points, in particular after treatment initiation. However, such an approach has huge logistical requirements due to the long follow-up duration and would need to address issues of attrition related to loss to follow-up. An alternative approach, chosen here, is a retrospective life-event history survey where participants are interviewed about their personal history. This approach is derived from demographic studies (Courgeau & Lelievre, 1991). Individual life histories are considered as a continuum of events of various nature involving family, housing, occupation, health, etc. This technique allows the study of the occurrence of different types of events or situations and their interactions, and enables a comparison of different periods in a person's life-course: for example, a patient's situation or life events before and after HIV diagnosis and antiretroviral initiation. However, as AIDS is a fatal disease, there is a selection bias of respondents towards survivors.

Interview process

After explaining the purpose of the study and topics covered, *all* HIV infected adults registered in the hospitals, aged > 18 years, non perinatally infected,[1] and receiving antiretroviral treatments were offered the opportunity to be interviewed for the study. Interviews were conducted on a one-to-one basis in a private room dedicated for the study. In the interview process, participants were informed that all answers to the interview were strictly confidential and completely anonymous. It was stressed that participants were free to decline answering any questions and that there were no good or bad answers. After this introduction, willing participants were asked to provide written informed consent. Respondents were reimbursed for their transport costs and time. However, reimbursement was not used as an incentive, and the small sum (200 Baht or approximately US$5) was presented at the end of the interview. The interview was based on a standard questionnaire, and all dated events or periods of life were recorded on a calendar sheet (Lelièvre & Vivier, 2001). The median duration of the interviews was 50 min (ranging from 25 to 132 min).

Study setting and study population

The four community hospitals were selected based on their long-term provision of antiretroviral treatments, mostly since 2002. Consequently, they treat a large number of adults and are representative of community hospitals in semi-rural/sub-urban areas of the Northern region.

From August to November 2007, all adult patients on antiretroviral treatment at participating hospitals were contacted for an interview. Data on the socio-demographic (age, gender), clinical characteristics (disease stage as indicated by the immunologic status, as assessed by the most recent CD4 count, in cells/mm^3, as of the interview date and based on hospital records, and treatment regimen) and HIV disclosure status of both respondents and non-respondents were collected and compared.

Issues explored

We analyzed data from the life-event history survey exploring the following issues:

(1) Family history: all successive unions, births, separation and death of spouses, children; (2) Education; (3) Health: disease history—mode of infection, date of diagnosis; disease stage as assessed by the immunologic status before and after antiretroviral treatment (again assessed by CD4 cell count before treatment initiation, based on hospital records); treatment history, date of antiretroviral initiation, type of treatment; overall appreciation of health status before and after antiretrovirals.

Statistical analysis

Descriptive statistics were performed using Stata™ version 9. The percentages were compared using a Pearson's chi-square test or a Fisher's exact test according to the sample distribution. Means and medians were compared using the student t test, and Kruskal-Wallis test, respectively (medians and Kruskal-Wallis tests were only applied to variables with sufficient value range).

Ethical considerations

The study was reviewed and approved by the Ethics Committee of Chiang Mai University, Faculty of Associated Medical Sciences. Interviewers were psychiatric nurses, who received specific training on the life-event history survey process and HIV/AIDS counselling.

Results

A total of 578 patients on antiretroviral treatments were contacted for an interview; 513 agreed to participate, a response rate of 89%.

Population characteristics

Socio-demographic and clinical characteristics of respondents and non-respondents are reported in Table 1. There were slightly more men non-respondents than women (54% versus 46%, respectively), but the difference was not statistically significant ($p = 0.296$). Non-respondents were younger than respondents (median age of 37 versus 40 years respectively, $p = 0.015$). Immune status of the patients, before and after antiretroviral treatment, and treatment regimen were similar among the two groups. This indicates that there was no self-selection of the respondents according to their disease stage. Among the reasons provided for not participating in the study, unavailability due to work was reported by 61% of non-respondents while

Table 1 Comparison of the demographic and HIV characteristics of non-respondents and respondents.

	Non-respondents N = 65	Respondents N = 513	p Value
Sex	%	%	
Men	53.9	47.0	0.296
Women	46.1	53.0	
Current age[a] (in years)			
20–34	30.7	25.0	0.120
35–39	35.5	25.1	
40–44	16.1	23.6	
≥45	17.7	26.3	
Antiretroviral treatment			
Thai generic ARV combination	76.9	79.7	0.599
Others	23.1	20.3	
Patient's immune status			
CD4 < 50 cells/mm^3 before ARV initiation[b]	52.8	45.6	0.504
CD4 ≥ 200 cells/mm^3 after ARV treatment[c]	87.7	82.6	0.399
Reasons given for not responding[d]			
Working	60.9		
Concern about disclosure risk	21.7		
Others[e]	17.4		
HIV status disclosure	63.1	84.4	<0.001

	Median	Range	Median	Range	p Value
Age (in years)	36.7	19–58	40.0	23–70	0.015
CD4 before ARV initiation (cells/mm^3)	37.0	0–385	60.0	0–508	0.194
CD4 after ARV treatment (cells/mm^3)	381.0	0–904	352.0	6–1343	0.465

[a] N = 62 non-respondents, N = 513 respondents.
[b] CD4 cell count before ARV, as recorded in the hospital file. N = 61 non-respondents, N = 480 respondents.
[c] Most recent CD4 cell count, as recorded in the hospital file. N = 60 non-respondents, N = 480 respondents.
[d] N = 46 non-respondents (9 non-respondents did not give any reason).
[e] Including 2 patients who did not want to be interviewed; 3 could not come to the hospital because of illness, 3 who forgot to come to their appointment.

confidentiality concerns was reported by 22%. This is consistent with data on serostatus disclosure, showing non-respondents to be more reluctant to disclose their HIV status compared to respondents (37% versus 16% respectively, $p < 0.001$).

Data on the socio-demographic characteristics of the respondents by gender are provided in Table 2. The sex distribution was relatively balanced, with slightly more women than men, 53% versus 47%, respectively. The mean age of participants at the time of interview was 40 years for both sexes. Overall women had a lower education level than men ($p = 0.003$): 27% of women attended secondary school or more compared to 39% of men. This reflects the gender difference in education in the adult population of this age group in northern Thailand (National Statistical Office, 2007). The median individual income were 4000 baht for men (US$100) compared to 3000 baht for women (US$75) ($p < 0.001$). This is within the low income range for Thailand (National Statistical Office, 2007). The vast majority of the patients (91%) were receiving treatment under the universal coverage system with no difference by gender (Table 2).

Table 2 Comparison by gender, of the age and education level of the respondents.

	All respondents		Men		Women		
	N = 513		N = 241		N = 272		p Value
Current age (in years)	%		%		%		
20–34	25.0		24.5		25.4		0.759
35–39	25.1		24.5		25.7		
40–44	23.6		25.7		21.7		
≥45	26.3		25.3		27.2		
Education level							
None	3.7		1.7		5.5		0.003
Primary	63.6		59.8		67.3		
Secondary	22.6		24.5		20.6		
Vocational college	7.8		11.6		4.4		
University	2.3		2.4		2.2		
Health coverage							
Universal Coverage	91.2		91.3		91.2		0.965
Others[a]	8.8		8.7		8.8		
	Median	Range	Median	Range	Median	Range	p Value
Current age (in years)	40.0	23–70	40.2	23–70	39.8	23–63	0.953
Current Income (in bath)	3000	0–50,000	4000	0–50,000	3000	0–30,000	<0.001

[a] Including 1 patient who declared not having any health coverage, 27 patients who receive benefits from the Social Security Scheme, 11 patients who receive benefits from the Civil Servant Medical Benefits Scheme and 4 patients who have health coverage.

Characteristics relating to marital life and children are outlined in Table 3. "Spouses" were defined as people living in a cohabiting union for more than 6 months, mostly in marriage settings. The mean number of spouses reported was lower for men than women (1.5 versus 1.8, $p < 0.001$), although there was a wider range in men compared to women (0 to 12 spouses versus 0 to 4 spouses, respectively). A much higher proportion of men reported never

Table 3 Comparison by gender, of the marital and children history of the respondents.

	All respondents	Men	Women	
	N = 513	N = 241	N = 272	p Value
Number of spouse(s)	%	%	%	
0	6.4	13.3	0.4	<0.001
1	41.5	49.0	34.9	
2	35.9	24.0	46.3	
≥3	16.2	13.7	18.4	
Experienced a spouse's death(s)[a]				
0	54.4	77.9	36.2	<0.001
≥1	45.6	22.1	63.8	
Experienced a spouse's separation(s)[a]				
0	18.3	8.1	26.2	<0.001
1	44.8	56.0	36.2	
≥2	36.9	35.9	37.6	
Number of children				
0	34.9	51.9	19.9	<0.001
1	38.0	30.3	44.9	
≥2	27.1	17.8	35.2	
Experienced a child death(s)[b]				
0	91.9	89.7	93.1	0.316
≥1	8.1	10.3	6.9	

	Mean	Range	Mean	Range	Mean	Range	p Value
Number of spouse(s)	1.7	0–12	1.5	0–12	1.8	0–4	<0.001
Number of spouse's deaths	0.5	0–3	0.2	0–3	0.7	0–2	<0.001
Number of separations	1.3	0–12	1.4	0–12	1.2	0–4	0.002
Number of children	1.0	0–5	0.7	0–5	1.2	0–4	<0.001

[a] Number of respondents who ever had a spouse: N = 480 all respondents; N = 209 men; N = 271 women.
[b] Number of respondents who ever had a child: N = 334 all respondents; N = 116 men; N = 218 women.

having a spouse (13.3%) compared to only one woman (0.4%). Importantly, among the respondents who ever had a spouse, women were more likely to have experienced a spouse death (64% versus 22%, $p < 0.001$), while men were more likely to have been divorced or separated (92% versus 74%, $p < 0.001$). Sixty-five percent of women had had more than one spouse compared to 38% of men. Whether the second union occurred before or after widowhood – mostly AIDS-related – needs to be investigated further. In a previous study in Thailand performed at a time when antiretroviral treatments were not available, we observed that HIV infected persons often to remarry within the people living with HIV networks (Le Cœur, Im-Em, Koetsawang, & Lelièvre, 2005).

The average number of children was significantly different for women and men (1.2 versus 0.7 respectively; $p < 0.001$). Less than a quarter of women had no children compared to more than half of the men (20% versus 52% respectively, $p < 0.001$). We investigated if these contrasting family situations could explain differences in HIV test-seeking behaviors.

Reasons for undergoing HIV test, route of infection

To better assess the difference in HIV test-seeking behavior by gender, we analyzed the age of respondents at the time of HIV test, the year of test and the reasons for having a test. In cases where participants had more than one HIV test, this refers to the test which first confirmed their HIV-positive status.

Women were about one year younger than men at the time of HIV diagnosis (mean age 33.8 years versus 35.0 years, respectively, $p = 0.110$) (Table 4). Interestingly, more women than men tested for HIV before or during 2003, the turning point for the national scale-up of free access to antiretroviral treatment, while more men were tested after this date (Table 4). This suggests that the scale-up of antiretroviral treatment boosted health-seeking behavior for HIV testing among men. As shown on Fig. 1, the reasons reported for HIV testing differed significantly according to gender ($p < 0.001$): health problems in 65% of men versus 38% of women; spouse or child death in 11% of men versus 34% of women; voluntary HIV counselling and testing – with no specific reason reported – was similar among men and women (7% and 8%, respectively); 9% of men and 2% of women had the test for social reasons such as to take a loan, a job application, blood donation or during military service. Interestingly, antenatal testing accounted for 17% of HIV tests in women compared to 7% in men. Premarital testing was the reason for very few tests, only 1.5% of the tests in women and 2.0% in men.

These gender differences highlight that over two-thirds of men (65%) underwent HIV testing due to health problems, i.e., when symptomatic, while the majority of women (52%) sought an HIV test in relation to either their spouse's

Table 4 Comparison by gender, of the age at HIV diagnosis, the mode of infection of the respondents.

	All respondents N = 513	Men N = 241	Women N = 272	p Value
Age at HIV diagnosis (in years)	%	%	%	
15–29	30.6	27.0	33.8	0.109
30–34	24.0	22.0	25.7	
35–39	20.1	23.2	17.3	
≥40	25.3	27.8	23.2	
Year of the HIV diagnosis				
<1999	28.8	24.4	32.7	<0.001
1999–2001	15.4	10.0	20.2	
2002–2003	20.7	22.0	19.5	
2004–2005	22.2	27.0	18.0	
2006–2007	12.9	16.6	9.6	
Reported mode of infection[a]				
Sexual	88.5	81.7	94.4	<0.001
Injected Drug Use	4.1	8.3	0.4	
Medical procedure	3.9	5.0	3.0	
Not sure/don't know	3.5	5.0	2.2	

	Mean	Range	Mean	Range	Mean	Range	p Value
Age at HIV diagnosis (in years)	34.4	17–66	35.0	18–66	33.8	17–62	0.110

[a] N = 510 Total respondents; N = 240 men; N = 270 women.

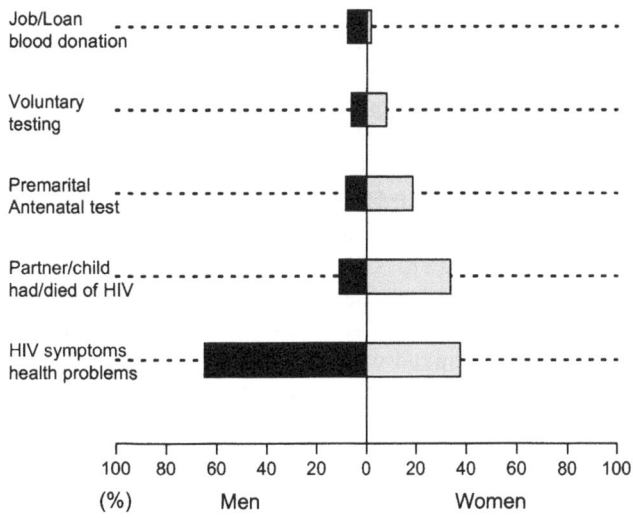

Figure 1 Reasons for HIV testing among men and women.

illness/death, or through premarital/antenatal testing, at a time when they were generally asymptomatic.

Table 4 shows the reported mode of infection: In both sexes, the large majority were sexual transmission, injection drug use was much higher in men (8.3%) than women (0.4%), which is consistent with other studies from Thailand (Razak et al., 2003).

Antiretroviral treatment initiation

The mean age at antiretroviral initiation was 37.4 years for men and 37.0 for women ($p = 0.67$) (Table 5). The delay between the HIV-positive test and treatment initiation was about one year shorter in men compared to women ($p = 0.004$). Interestingly, before 2004, significantly more women had started antiretroviral treatment than men (42% versus 31.0%), while more men initiated treatment after, when free access to treatment was widely available. Fifty-four percent of men initiated treatment within one year of diagnosis, compared to 33% of women. This is most likely due to the fact that more men were symptomatic at time of diagnosis, while most women were tested earlier in the course of infection. This was reflected in the clinical condition at time of initiation of treatment: a higher proportion of men had CD4 cell count less than 50 cells/mm^3 (55% in men versus 38% in women, $p < 0.001$) and their median CD4 count was 45 cells/mm^3 compared to 84 cells/mm^3 in women ($p < 0.001$) (Table 5). In contrast, the most recent median CD4 count did not significantly differ by gender, suggesting comparable efficacy of treatment. Finally, the more advanced disease stage in men was also reflected in the patients' health status perception at time of treatment initiation, which was significantly poorer in men compared to women ($p = 0.038$) (Table 6).

Discussion

Our results show a higher proportion of women receiving antiretroviral treatments compared to men. While over-representation of women has been reported in sub-Saharan Africa, where there are generally higher proportions of women in need of treatment than men (UNAIDS, 2006), it is surprising for Thailand where there is a higher proportion of HIV infected men (UNAIDS & WHO, 2008). Our findings are consistent with two reports on adults on antiretroviral treatment in Thailand, (Braitstein et al., 2008; Leusaree et al., 2002), however a selection bias towards women is possible in these studies partially linked with PMTCT-Plus programs.

A key strength of our study was that adults were treated in a community hospital setting providing standard of care and that we were exhaustive in reaching all patients. The percentage of non-respondents was low (about 10%) and when recalculating the sex-ratio taking into account the gender of non-respondents, the gender balance remains unchanged (52% women). One

Table 5 Comparison by gender, of the age at ARV initiation, delay between HIV diagnosis and ARV initiation, and patient's immune status before and after ARV initiation.

	All respondents N = 513		Men N = 241		Women N = 272		p Value
Age at ARV initiation (in years)	%		%		%		
15–29	17.1		15.4		18.8		0.686
30–34	23.6		22.8		24.3		
35–39	22.8		23.6		22.1		
≥40	36.5		38.2		34.9		
Year at ARV treatment initiation							
< 2002	9.8		9.4		9.9		0.028
2002–2003	27.0		21.6		32.0		
2004–2005	40.2		46.2		34.9		
2006–2007	23.0		22.8		23.2		
Delay between HIV diagnosis and ARV initiation[a]							
< 1 year	42.9		53.9		33.1		<0.001
1 year	12.1		11.6		12.4		
2 to 4 years	16.6		11.2		21.3		
5 to 7 years	14.4		9.5		18.8		
≥ 8 years	14.0		13.7		14.3		
Duration of the ARV treatment							
Less than 2 years	23.0		22.8		23.2		0.018
2 to 4 years	40.2		46.1		34.9		
≥ 5 years	36.8		31.1		41.9		
Patient's immune status							
CD4 <50 cells/mm^3 before ARV initiation[b]	45.6		55.3		37.6		0.001
CD4 ≥ 200 cells/mm^3 after ARV treatment[c]	82.6		75.7		88.3		<0.001
	Mean	Range	Mean	Range	Mean	Range	p Value
Age at ARV initiation (years)	37.2	18–66	37.4	20–66	37.0	18–62	0.666
Delay between HIV diagnosis and ARV initiation (years)	2.6	0–14	2.3	0–14	2.9	0–13	0.017
Duration of the ARV treatment (years)	3.1	0–13	2.9	0–13	3.2	0–13	0.051
CD4 before ARV initiation (cells/mm^3)	60.0	0–508	45.0	0–508	84.0	0–417	<0.001
CD4 after ARV treatment (cells/mm^3)	352.0	6–1343	304.0	6–1338	399.5	6–1343	0.314

[a] Total respondents $N = 509$; $N = 238$ men; $N = 272$ women.
[b] Total respondents $N = 480$; $N = 219$ men; $N = 261$ women.
[c] Total respondents $N = 482$; $N = 226$ men; $N = 256$ women.

Table 6 Comparison by gender, of the health status perception before and after ARV treatment.

	All respondents	Men	Women	
	N = 513	N = 241	N = 272	p Value
	%	%	%	
Health status perception before ARV initiation				
Very poor	27.7	33.2	22.8	0.038
Poor	28.4	29.1	27.9	
Fair	23.0	20.3	25.4	
Good	12.3	9.1	15.1	
Very good	8.6	8.3	8.8	
Health status perception after ARV treatment (current)				
Very poor	0.5	0.4	0.7	0.784
Poor	5.4	6.6	4.4	
Fair	27.7	26.6	28.7	
Good	45.4	44.8	46.0	
Very good	20.8	21.6	20.2	

limitation may be that, for confidentiality reasons, some patients chose to be treated in hospitals outside of their residence area or in private hospitals and therefore were not included in this study. Under both circumstances, patients would no longer receive free care and would have to pay for the cost of the treatments by themselves, options not readily available for a population whose income is generally low, although men's incomes are slightly higher than women's. This is because the cost of the cheapest antiretroviral treatment is 1200 baht (US$30) per month, not including the cost of outpatient visits and monitoring. However, our study population is likely to be representative of adults receiving antiretroviral therapy in public hospitals in semi-rural Northern Thailand. There are regional variations in the HIV epidemic trends (UNAIDS & WHO, 2008), therefore one should be cautious in extrapolating the results on gender balance to the rest of the country. A study on a random sample of hospitals throughout the country would be ideal, but problems of cost and logistics would have to be resolved.

Many factors at the population and individual level may explain the gender distribution observed in our study. At the population level, one should consider the evolving dynamics of the HIV epidemic, the initial prioritization of mothers for treatment and earlier access to HIV testing for women. These issues are entangled with gender differences at the individual level in the reasons and timing to HIV testing.

Firstly, as explained in the introduction, women were late comers in the epidemic: the HIV epidemic wave among women in the general population started a few years after the epidemic wave among men and was of a lower magnitude. Therefore the mortality peak occurred earlier and reached a higher level among men (Surasiengsunk et al., 1998). This was confirmed in our study by the higher proportion of women (64%) who experienced a spouse death, mostly assumed to be AIDS-related, compared with men (22%). Due to this time lag, it is possible that, in the course of the epidemic, we stand precisely at a time when there is a diminishing gap between the number of surviving men and women in need of treatment, particularly in northern Thailand, which was the first region affected by the HIV epidemic and the most hard hit (Surasiengsunk et al., 1998). In the absence of reliable data on the HIV prevalence by age and gender in the general population for the Chiang Mai region, it is difficult to assess the extent to which men are underrepresented in our population on antiretroviral treatment. However, as there are still more men than women living with HIV in Thailand, this epidemiologic factor does not fully explain the gender balance of patients on antiretroviral treatment.

Secondly, the initial prioritization of HIV infected mothers for antiretroviral treatment may partly explain the lower proportion of men in the care system. Indeed, at a time when antiretroviral treatments were limited, the Access to Care program, first prioritized mothers, then women mostly seen as victims of the epidemic, and lastly men who were perceived as those who brought HIV into the family/community. This is confirmed by our data showing that before 2003, when access to antiretrovirals was severely limited, patients who received therapy were mostly women.

A third factor may be the earlier HIV diagnosis and treatment initiation in the course of the disease observed in women compared to men. Indeed, symptomatic patients represent only the tip of the iceberg, i.e., 10–20% of the HIV infected population. Asymptomatic patients are more numerous and generally unaware of their HIV status. Therefore, earlier diagnosis and treatment initiation contributes towards a higher proportion of women on antiretrovirals.

One key strength in our study methodology, retracing the life histories of the patients, is the ability to assess gender differences in access to treatment but also to disentangle their relationships to access to HIV testing at the individual level.

Men and women underwent HIV testing in very different circumstances. The large majority of women in this study had been married and had children while men were more likely to never had a spouse and children. This key difference in family situation may partly explain the gender differences in HIV test-seeking behavior. As part of their family responsibilities, as in most countries, women have more contact with the health care system, where HIV testing is more likely to be suggested to them (Mane & Aggleton, 2001). For example, over one-third of women were tested for HIV while caring or grieving for a spouse or child, and interestingly, more women (47.4%) whose spouse had passed away reported that they were tested because of their spouse's death compared to men (36.1%) in the same circumstances. Women are often under significant social and family pressure to be tested following a suspected AIDS-related spousal death, particularly in semi-rural villages, hit hard by the epidemic, as they are assumed to be HIV infected unless proven otherwise.

During their life-course, women also have access to HIV testing during pregnancy and uptake for testing at this point is very high in Thailand (Amornwichet et al., 2002). This was the reason for HIV testing in 17% of women in this study, enabling them to be identified and followed up prior to onset of AIDS-related disease. The strong incentive to accept the routine HIV testing during pregnancy to preserve the child's health—at a time when PMTCT is widely available—may help overcome women's own fear of being tested. The PMTCT-Plus strategy attempts to extend this incentive from "motherhood" onto "parenthood", aiming at protecting the welfare of the family as a whole and targeting future fathers for HIV testing. However, our data show that although a non-negligible proportion of men (7%) underwent HIV testing during their spouse's pregnancy, the majority of men had no children and a significant proportion had never had a spouse, and therefore would be excluded from such targeted interventions.

In contrast, two-thirds of men underwent HIV testing due to their own health problems, often when symptomatic. A small proportion of men (4%) were tested under institutional circumstances – job or loan application, to become a member of an association, or at military service. These policies, discriminatory in essence, and where confidentiality is not systematically protected, generate fear of testing in the population and do not improve people's access to treatment as there is no referral to health care services for follow-up.

To ensure equal access to HIV care, interventions to improve access to and uptake of voluntary HIV testing should be promoted. Indeed, contrary to women who are offered testing while already *inside* the medical setting, somehow captive of it, for men, testing requires a more personal motivation. Interestingly, our data indicate the percentage of patients diagnosed through voluntary testing to be similar among men and women, when ideally a larger proportion of men should be tested in this setting due to lack of alternative systematic channels.

Finally, other barriers to HIV testing and care such as low risk perception of disease prognosis, poor access to medical care, lack of social support, and actual or anticipated HIV/AIDS-related stigma have been mentioned (Krawczyk et al., 2006; Mane & Aggleton, 2001; Muula et al., 2007). For example, Muula and colleagues (Muula et al., 2007) argue that in sub-Saharan countries, women are less stigmatized when seeking HIV testing as it is widely perceived that women acquired HIV from a spouse, while men are perceived to have acquired the infection outside of marriage. In addition, HIV test-seeking behavior was perceived as an expression of weakness in some settings where male strength was expected (Greig & Lang, 2000). Further barriers may include denial of the risk of HIV infection or fear of confidentiality breach. While such obstacles probably apply in Thailand, qualitative research is needed to further assess their level of influence on access to HIV testing and care and how they may be overcome.

In our study, women appear to have a double advantage in both diagnosis and treatment. However, if men had been diagnosed and treated earlier, HIV transmission to their spouse may have been avoided and their spouse may not have been widowed. In terms of policy implications, there is an urgent need for a concerted effort to promote voluntary HIV counselling and testing both inside and outside of the family setting, with interventions specifically targeted for men. Both women and men stand to benefit from lessening of gender stereotypes and their attached stigma, as it would ensure better equity in the access to antiretroviral treatments.

Acknowledgements

Financial support for the Living with Antiretroviral Study (LIWA) was provided by the Agence Nationale de recherche sur le Sida et les Hépatites Virales (ANRS) and Oxfam GB. Intira Collins received an International Fellowship from the American Association of University Women Educational Foundation 2007–2008. We would like to thank Dr Marc Lallemant and the two anonymous reviewers for their helpful comments.

Note

1 Per protocol, individuals with perinatal infections had to be excluded so as to ensure a homogeneous study population. However, among patients aged > 18 years, there were no cases of perinatal infection.

References

Ainsworth, M., Beyrer, C., & Soucat, A. (2003). AIDS and public policy: the lessons and challenges of "success" in Thailand. *Health Policy*, *64*(1), 13–37.

Amornwichet, P., Teeraratkul, A., Simonds, R. J., Naiwatanakul, T., Chantharojwong, N., Culnane, M., et al. (2002). Preventing mother-to-child HIV transmission: the first year of Thailand's national program. *JAMA*, *288*(2), 245–248.

Braitstein, P., Boulle, A., Nash, D., Brinkhof, M. W., Dabis, F., Laurent, C., et al. (2008). Gender and the use of antiretroviral treatment in resource-constrained settings: findings from a multicenter collaboration. *Journal of Women's Health (Larchmt)*, *17*(1), 47–55.

Brown, T., Sittitrai, W., Vanichseni, S., & Thisyakorn, U. (1994). The recent epidemiology of HIV and AIDS in Thailand. *AIDS*, *8*(Suppl. 2), S131–S141.

Brown, T., Xenos, P. (1994). AIDS in Asia: the gathering storm. Asia Pacific Issues Analysis from the East–West Center, 16(August), 1–15.

Chasombat, S., Lertpiriyasuwat, C., Thanprasertsuk, S., Suebsaeng, L., & Lo, Y. R. (2006). The national access to antiretroviral program for PHA (NAPHA) in Thailand. *The Southeast Asian Journal of Tropical Medicine and Public Health*, *37*(4), 704–715.

Courgeau, D., & Lelievre, E. (1991). The event history approach in demography. *Population*, *3*, 63–79.

Ford, N., & Koetsawang, S. (1991). The socio-cultural context of the transmission of HIV in Thailand. *Social Science & Medicine*, *33*(4), 405–414.

Greig, A., & Lang, J. (2000). *Men, masculinity and development: Broadening our work towards gender equality*. In: *Gender and development monograph series, vol. 10*. Geneva: United Nations Development Programme.

Hanenberg, R. S., Rojanapithayakorn, W., Kunasol, P., & Sokal, D. C. (1994). Impact of Thailand's HIV-control programme as indicated by the decline of sexually transmitted diseases. *Lancet*, *344*(8917), 243–245.

Keiser, O., Anastos, K., Schechter, M., Balestre, E., Myer, L., Boulle, A., et al. (2008). Antiretroviral therapy in resource-limited settings 1996 to 2006: patient characteristics, treatment regimens and monitoring in sub-Saharan Africa, Asia and Latin America. *Tropical Medicine & International Health*, *13*(7), 870–879.

Knodel, J., Saengtienchai, C., Vanlandingham, M., & Lucas, R. (1999). Sexuality, sexual experience and the good spouse: views of married Thai men and women. In S. Press (Ed.), *Genders and sexuality in modern Thailand Chiang Mai*. Silkworm Press.

Krawczyk, C. S., Funkhouser, E., Kilby, J. M., Kaslow, R. A., Bey, A. K., & Vermund, S. H. (2006). Factors associated with delayed initiation of HIV medical care among infected persons attending a southern HIV/AIDS clinic. *South Medicinal Journal*, *99*(5), 472–481.

Lawn, S. D., & Wood, R. (2006). How can earlier entry of patients into antiretroviral programs in low-income countries be promoted? *Clinical Infectious Diseases*, *42*(3), 431–432, author reply 432–433.

Le Cœur, S., Im-Em, W., Koetsawang, S., & Lelièvre, E. (2005). Living with HIV in Thailand: assessing vulnerability through a life-event history approach. *Population*, *60*(4), 551–568.

Lelièvre, E., & Vivier, G. (2001). Evaluation d'une collecte à la croisée du quantitatif et du qualitatif: l'enquête Biographies et entourage. *Population*, *56*(6), 1043–1073.

Leusaree, T., Srithanaviboonchai, K., Chanmangkang, S., Ying-Ru, L., & Natpratan, C. (2002). The feasibility of HAART in a Northern Thai cohort: 2000–2001. In: *14th International AIDS Conference, Barcelona, Spain, July 7–12*.

Mane, P., & Aggleton, P. (2001). Gender and HIV/AIDS: what do men have to do with it? *Current Sociology*, *49*(23).

Maticka-Tyndale, E., Elkins, D., Haswell-Elkins, M., Rujkarakorn, D., Kuyyakanond, T., & Stam, K. (1997). Contexts and patterns of men's commercial sexual partnerships in northeastern Thailand: implications for AIDS prevention. *Social Science & Medicine*, *44*(2), 199–213.

Ministry of Public Health. (2008). *Section Bureau of Epidemiology*. Department of Disease Control.

Muula, A. S., Ngulube, T. J., Siziya, S., Makupe, C. M., Umar, E., Prozesky, H. W., et al. (2007). Gender distribution of adult patients on highly active antiretroviral therapy (HAART) in Southern Africa: a systematic review. *BMC Public Health*, *7*, 63.

National Statistical Office. (July–September 2007). *The labour force survey.* Quarter 3.
Nelson, K. E., Celentano, D. D., Eiumtrakol, S., Hoover, D. R., Beyrer, C., Suprasert, S., et al. (1996). Changes in sexual behavior and a decline in HIV infection among young men in Thailand. *The New England Journal of Medicine, 335*(5), 297–303.
Nelson, K. E., Eiumtrakul, S., Celentano, D. D., Beyrer, C., Galai, N., Kawichai, S., et al. (2002). HIV infection in young men in northern Thailand, 1991–1998: increasing role of injection drug use. *Journal of Acquired Immune Deficiency Syndromes, 29*(1), 62–68.
Phoolcharoen, W., Ungchusak, K., Sittitrai, W., & Brown, T. (1998). Thailand: lessons from a strong national response to HIV/AIDS. *AIDS, 12*(Suppl. B), S123–S135.
Razak, M. H., Jittiwutikarn, J., Suriyanon, V., Vongchak, T., Srirak, N., Beyrer, C. et al. (2003). HIV prevalence and risks among injection and noninjection drug users in northern Thailand: need for comprehensive HIV prevention programs. *Journal of Acquired Immune Deficiency Syndromes, 33*(2), 259–266.
Rerks-Ngarm, S. (1997). Sex-ratio patterns of AIDS patients. *Journal of Medical Association of Thailand, 80*(1), 34–46.
Rojanapithayakorn, W., & Hanenberg, R. (1996). The 100% condom program in Thailand. *AIDS, 10*(1), 1–7.
Saengtienchai, C., Knodel, J., VanLandingham, M., & Pramualratana, A. (1999). Prostitutes are better than lovers: wives's views on the extramarital sexual behavior of Thai men. In N. C J. Peter (Ed.), *Genders and sexuality in modern Thailand Chiang Mai.* Silkworm Press.
Surasiengsunk, S., Kiranandana, S., Wongboonsin, K., Garnett, G. P., Anderson, R. M., & van Griensven, G. J. (1998). Demographic impact of the HIV epidemic in Thailand. *AIDS, 12*(7), 775–784.
Tangcharoensathien, V., Wibulpholprasert, S., & Nitayaramphong, S. (2004). Knowledge-based changes to health systems: the Thai experience in policy development. *Bulletin of the World Health Organization, 82*(10), 750–756.
UNAIDS. (2000). *Case study, evaluation of the 100% condom programme in Thailand.*
UNAIDS. (2006). *Report on the global AIDS epidemic.* Geneva: Joint United Nations Programme on AIDS 2006.
UNAIDS. (2007). *Aids Epidemic Update.* Asia.
UNAIDS, & WHO. (2008). *Epidemiological fact sheet on HIV and AIDS, 2008 update.*
UNDP. (2004). *Thailand's response to HIV/AIDS: progress and challenges.* Thematic MDG report, June 2004, Bangkok.
van Griensven, F., Thanprasertsuk, S., Jommaroeng, R., Mansergh, G., Naorat, S., Jenkins, R. A., et al. (2005). Evidence of a previously undocumented epidemic of HIV infection among men who have sex with men in Bangkok, Thailand. *AIDS, 19*(5), 521–526.
Vanlandingham, M., Knodel, J., Saengtienchai, C., & Pramualratana, A. (1998). In the company of friends: peer influence on Thai male extramarital sex. *Social Science & Medicine, 47*(12), 1993–2011.
Weniger, B. G., Limpakarnjanarat, K., Ungchusak, K., Thanprasertsuk, S., Choopanya, K., Vanichseni, S., et al. (1991). The epidemiology of HIV infection and AIDS in Thailand. *AIDS, 5*(Suppl. 2), S71–S85.
World Bank. (2000). *Thailand's response to AIDS: Building on success, confronting the Future.* Washington: Oxford University Press.

59
GENDER, SEXUALITY AND EMBODIMENT
Access to and experience of healthcare by same-sex attracted women in Australia

Jane Edwards and Helen van Roekel

Source: *Current Sociology*, 57:2 (2009), 193–210.

Abstract

This article identifies the way same-sex attracted women negotiate healthcare in a rural Australian setting. In-depth interviews were conducted with 10 women. Respondents choose general practitioners (GPs) carefully, 'interviewing' them to see if they hold acceptable attitudes to same-sex attraction. However, sexuality is not the only evaluative criteria women use. Some women invoke gender-based discourse, evaluating GPs by how well they treat women's bodies. In other instances, women utilize a framework based on sexuality; good healthcare is associated with how the practitioner dealt with same-sex attraction. Sometimes women evaluated care by reference to a model of the body that did not implicate gender or sexuality and GPs are evaluated on the basis of clinical knowledge. This shows that women do not define themselves in a unitary way in relation to gender or sexuality. They selectively and strategically employ discourses of gender, sexuality and embodiment to structure and evaluate healthcare.

Introduction

Despite the well-documented evidence that same-sex attracted (SSA) women have poorer health status than their heterosexual counterparts and are less likely than them to use health services, little is known about SSA women's experience of healthcare. Specifically, there are few accounts of how SSA women seek out a general practitioner (GP) with whom they can establish a therapeutic relationship. Having identified an acceptable GP, how do women handle information related to their sexuality in interaction with practitioners? In what ways does sexuality structure SSA women's use of, and satisfaction with, health services? This article reports the results of a qualitative study that explored these issues among SSA women living in a rural area in Australia.

Population-based data on the mental health status of SSA women indicate relatively high levels of affective disorder, substance abuse and suicidal ideation or behaviour (Pitts et al., 2006; Welch et al., 2000). Available data on the physical health of SSA women are also relatively scarce, but suggest they are less likely than heterosexual women to utilize routine screening services (Diamant et al., 2000; Mathieson et al., 2002: 187; Pitts et al., 2006), and are more likely to use tobacco, to be obese and to engage in high-risk levels of alcohol consumption (Diamant et al., 2000). Same-sex attracted women are less likely than the general population of women to report good health status (Pitts et al., 2006: 29–33). It must be recognized, however, that the evidence related to SSA women's health status and health service needs derives almost exclusively from western settings.

Same-sex attracted women, at least within the setting of western healthcare systems, are frequently 'invisible' (McNair, 2000). Concern about having to disclose sexual orientation often prevents women accessing services until the problem can no longer be avoided (Mathieson et al., 2002; Pitts et al., 2006). Those who do use health services may not divulge their sexuality, which may mean information relevant to treatment is not provided (McNair, 2000). Alternatively, where healthcare providers know their patient's sexual orientation, stereotyped views may lead to suboptimal treatment (Meyer, 2001). Misperceptions about the health needs of SSA women are entrenched; for instance, that they are not at risk of sexually transmissible diseases (Mathieson et al., 2002) or that they do not require screening for cervical cancer (McNair, 2000). Further, in many western settings, same-sex attracted women report encountering overt discrimination by healthcare professionals: in Britain (McColl, 1994), New Zealand (Welch et al., 2000), Canada (Mathieson et al., 2002), the US (Meyer, 2001) and Australia (McNair and Medland, 2002). The fear or experience of insensitive treatment, or of blatant discrimination, therefore, is a major barrier to accessing appropriate and acceptable healthcare (Pitts et al., 2006).

For their part, health professionals may be unaware that some of their patients are SSA (McNair, 2000; Meyer, 2001). Even if they know of their clients' sexuality, doctors may feel unsure about the healthcare needs of SSA women, since most have received little training in this area. Same-sex attracted women are likely to have special needs associated with relationship problems, sexual problems, grief following relationship breakdown or the death of a partner, familial relationships, domestic violence and issues related to parenting and the inclusion of partners in healthcare settings (McNair and Harrison, 2002; Pitts et al., 2006). Many health professionals may lack adequate information about SSA women and their 'culture' and 'lifestyle' and may be uncertain about their capacity to provide care (Rabin et al., 1986). These factors are likely to be exacerbated in rural settings, which, in Australia, are more conservative than urban areas in relation to gender and sexuality. Furthermore, the markedly reduced number of specialist medical services and a smaller pool of general medical practitioners than exists in metropolitan areas are likely to reduce women's capacity to find an 'SSA-friendly' GP. In rural settings, the lack of an SSA community, or its relative invisibility should it exist, hampers the informal dissemination of information about general practitioners that are known to be accepting of SSA women (Tiemann et al., 1998).

Despite the documentation of SSA women's relatively poor health status and their difficulty in using health services, little is known about how sexuality shapes the seeking and utilization of health services and how SSA women define their satisfaction with them. In their research in rural North America, Tiemann at al. (1998) discerned four strategies among SSA women to manage information about their sexuality when utilizing health services. The first – screening – refers to women seeking information that allows them to choose a practitioner from whom they believe they can access acceptable healthcare. This can entail asking other SSA women about healthcare providers or by asking healthcare workers themselves for referrals to 'SSA-friendly' providers. A second 'technique' is that women disclose their sexuality during consultation to a healthcare provider in an unplanned way. Conversely, women may have a policy of always revealing their sexuality because they feel it is relevant and necessary information for healthcare providers or because non-disclosure feels uncomfortable. Planned disclosure is much more likely to occur if women have screened a practitioner and are confident that they will not be met with a negative response. Finally, some women make a deliberate decision not to disclose their sexuality to healthcare providers (Tiemann et al., 1998: 71–3).

Available research suggests that when women do disclose their sexuality in the clinical encounter they may be met with a range of responses ranked from positive to negative (Saulnier, 2002). At the negative end of the continuum are responses conceptualized as homophobic or heteronormative. Homophobia is a disapproving reaction by a health practitioner to a woman's disclosure that she is SSA, while heteronormativity encapsulates health professionals' assumptions that women are heterosexual, thus making same-sex attraction invisible. Tolerance occupies the midpoint and is best described as non-discriminatory behaviour. At the positive end of the spectrum is healthcare provider behaviour that is 'SSA-sensitive' in that it acknowledges women's sexuality in an accepting manner. Finally same-sex attraction affirmative healthcare providers offer specific services or create environments that make SSA women feel welcomed (Saulnier, 2002: 360–2).

The dissatisfaction of the general population of women with the care they receive from healthcare professionals, notably medical practitioners, has been extensively documented (see BWHBC, 1985; Broom, 1991; Lorber and Moore, 2002). While the history of women's oppressive medical treatment is a long one, medicine's conceptualization and treatment of women came under sustained challenge in the late 1960s and early 1970s as part of second wave feminism. This social movement helped generate the women's health movement (WHM), articulating a theoretical critique of women's treatment at the hands of mainstream services and spawning a political movement aimed at transforming healthcare.

The WHM continues to provide some useful benchmarks against which to evaluate the care women receive from GPs. Notwithstanding local differences, some common complaints were made about women's health and its treatment at the hands of medicine in North America, the UK and Australia. The WHM defined women's health as linked with difference; a framework that has dominated scholarship on gender and health until recently (see Annandale and Riska, this issue, pp. 00–00). It made clear that women had distinctive health needs based on their embodiment and their social location (Broom, 1991: 33–4). The WHM unequivocally demonstrated how profound gender was in shaping the aetiology of ill health and the experience of healthcare (Annandale and Hunt, 2000: 3–21; Broom, 1991: 47–53). Gender is not just a social status existing in isolation from other social structures and processes. Lorber and Moore point to the existence of a gendered social order that not only shapes an individual's sense of identity, but which specifies the social status they are accorded and the way in which they are treated in many domains of life (Lorber and Moore, 2002: 3–5).

The WHM facilitated a thorough exposé of how gendered the experience of health and healthcare was, and remains (Broom, 1991; Lorber and Moore, 2002: 37–51). It arraigned mainstream medicine for its unwillingness or inability to respond adequately to women's needs. The doctor–patient relationship, critics charged, was permeated with the patriarchal power imbalance that characterized wider society (Broom, 1991: 40–1). Access to effective contraception and safe abortion were frequently denied to women by a male-dominated profession reluctant to create conditions in which women could exercise sexual agency (Broom, 1991: 34–5). Another of women's most vociferously voiced charges was that doctors failed to listen to them adequately. They resented the medical encounter, alleging that they were treated condescendingly, given insufficient information and that their questions went without adequate answers. Furthermore, women began to challenge the power of medicine to label them as ill, or as dangerous and to preside over some of their legal rights, such as access to children (Broom, 1991: 40–3; BWHBC, 1985: 141–6; Lorber and Moore, 2002: 74–81).

The seeming inability of individual practitioners to listen comprehensively to their female 'patients' was matched by a kind of epistemological deafness in 'hearing' the causes of women's ill health. Women's differential access to the labour market and education, their role in the family and their informal work in the private sphere generated distinct patterns of ill health (Annandale and Hunt, 2000: 22–7). In addition, the experience of poverty and racism also contributed to women's ill health (BWHBC, 1985: 559–60). These factors gave rise to women bringing different kinds of complaints than those of men to their practitioners; problems that should have generated complex and multifaceted responses, but which frequently generated only a prescription for medication (Lorber and Moore, 2002: 71).

Medicine's capacity to define women's physiology, in tandem with its incapacity to listen respectfully to women's accounts of their embodied experience, left many women feeling alienated from their own bodies This complaint was allied with a critique about the medicalization of routine life events undergone by many women; menstruation, childbirth, menopause and ageing. The dissection of medicalization also dovetailed with a wider movement challenging the efficacy of medicine. Much medical intervention in menstruation or childbirth, for example, harmed rather than helped women, it was claimed. Insensitive or rough treatment during pelvic examinations, for example, was held out as further evidence of medicine's inability to cater for the unique aspects of women's bodies (Broom, 1991: 37; BWHBC, 1985: 555–60). While women's bodies were ill-treated in some contexts, in others they were overlooked. Many of women's symptoms were underinvestigated and psychological causation was frequently presumed. It has been documented that when men and women present with similar complaints, men's symptoms are more thoroughly investigated. Moreover, male patients are given more thorough explanations of their symptoms and treatment options than female patients (Broom, 1991: 39–44). All of this was (justly) taken as evidence that medicine could not respond to women's difference.

Intuitively it might be expected that SSA women would experience even greater alienation from, and less satisfaction with, the medical encounter than their heterosexual counterparts since they manifest double 'deviance'. Almost uniformly, SSA women fear disclosing their sexuality, believing it will lead to them receiving poorer care (Lorber and Moore, 2002: 43; Thompson, 1998: 112; BWHBC, 1985: 152–3). There is evidence to suggest that some health professionals view same-sex attraction as pathological and interpret SSA women's symptoms through this distorting lens (Thompson, 1998: 113). North American data indicate that SSA women find the care they receive from male medical practitioners less satisfactory than that provided by female doctors. Their dissatisfaction with male medics centres on their dignity not being respected, their concerns being overlooked, their intellectual capacities being denigrated and their bodily safety being compromised. Gender congruity between consumer and practitioner is a powerful predictor of SSA women's satisfaction with care (Lorber and Moore, 2002: 42).

Material and methods

This article reports the results of a qualitative investigation of SSA women's utilization of, and satisfaction with, healthcare in a rural Australian setting. Ten SSA women were interviewed. The interviews, lasting between 30 and 60 minutes, were semi-structured and audio-taped. The tapes were transcribed verbatim. The analysis developed in three steps. First, three transcripts were independently analysed by each of the authors for emergent themes. This analysis was undertaken manually rather than with a software package. Second, we then refined the list of emergent themes and used them as the basis for independently coding another two transcripts. These transcripts were then exchanged between the two authors so that we could be confident that the codes validly described the data and that they were being applied reliably. Third, having completed this process, one of the authors (JE) coded the remaining transcripts. This process conforms to criteria that promote rigorous analysis of qualitative data (Liamputtong and Ezzy, 2005: 270–3). This phase of the analysis identified themes that we wished to explore in greater depth and all the women were contacted and a second interview was sought; all the women consented and most interviews took place within two months. The second set of interview transcripts were analysed in the same way as the first round.

The women interviewed range in age from 18 to 61 years, though most were in their fifties. All but one of the participants, an Indigenous Australian, are from English-speaking backgrounds. Most are employed in professional or semi-professional fields of employment; two women are semi-retired. Most women live in a small town (under 1000 inhabitants) about 40 minutes' drive from the nearest large population centre, Greenways (to protect the anonymity of respondents, all place and person names are pseudonyms). Three of the women live in Greenways itself, which is a town of approximately 14,000 inhabitants, about 700 km from the state capital. Its economic foundations are agriculture and aquaculture. Australian rural communities, particularly agricultural ones, are, generally speaking, conservative cultures enforcing more traditional views of gender than metropolitan settings. In addition, they are frequently homophobic and SSA women usually try to keep their sexuality relatively invisible to protect themselves from rejection, harassment or violence (Edwards, 2005).

There is a small network of SSA women centred in and around Greenways. Information about the study was circulated through this network and women interested in participating made contact with one of the authors (HvR) and a time and place for interview was arranged. The network consists of about 20 women who meet from time to time for social and recreational purposes. They are also undertaking some lobbying and advocacy designed to improve the lives of SSA women and gay men in Greenways. The network is an important source of information and support for SSA women, who feel the constraints of their community and their relative invisibility, along with their isolation from the more well-developed and active SSA community in the state capital.

Greenways has a relatively good supply of GPs, but few resident specialist services. The nearest clinical services devoted to women's health, for example, are 700 km distant. Likewise specialist services related to family planning and sexual and reproductive health are a full day's drive away. For the most part, then, women seeking routine medical care in Greenway will consult a local GP. These practitioners possess an undergraduate degree and, while they may undertake further training, they are not specialist physicians. Despite the fact that most GPs operate on a fee-for-service basis, they are the mainstay of primary healthcare in Australia. They are the health professional most likely to be consulted in the first instance and they are the most frequently consulted type of health professional within the Australian system (Gray, 2006: 192). They act as gatekeepers to specialist practitioners. Unless people present directly at publicly funded hospitals, it is necessary to have a referral from a GP to consult a specialist. The fee-for-service system is a powerful economic incentive for GPs to have a high number of consultations. It is routine for consultations to last 10 minutes, thwarting attempts by either practitioner or patient to establish a therapeutic relationship that can respond to complex problems (Shorne et al., 2001–2).

In Australia as a whole, male practitioners constitute approximately two-thirds of the GP workforce; the percentage of women GPs practising in rural and remote areas is lower than the rate of female practice in urban settings (Gray, 2006: 196–8). The number of male practitioners in the study setting far outnumbers female practitioners and the capacity to consult a female GP is harder in Greenways than it is in metropolitan locations. Cost is not a significant issue in accessing GP services. Australia's government-sponsored health insurance scheme (Medicare) means services are provided at no direct cost to consumers, or, at most, require payment of a 15 percent fee that bridges the gap between the scheduled consulting charge and the Medicare rebate (Gray, 2006: 191). While gender played a part in choice of GP, the cost of accessing medical care was irrelevant for the women in our sample.

Results

'Screening': identifying and 'interviewing' a doctor

Women attach importance to the relationship they have with their GP. Several of the women testified to the gravity they attached to finding an acceptable general practitioner. For example, whereas Colleen reported that she would pick a plumber or electrician from the telephone book, like all the women interviewed, she was far more rigorous in seeking out a GP. This suggests that GP consultations are not routine transactions in the way consulting, say, an accountant might be. Our respondents reveal the degree to which encounters with GPs place them in a position of great vulnerability. Poor past experiences of healthcare had given some a perpetual wariness about disclosing their sexuality. Both Judy and Mary had experiences with health professionals in the past who had been discriminatory. Mary had a male GP who was verbally offensive and physically rough while conducting a vaginal examination. Judy recalls a GP who wanted to 'treat' her same-sex attraction after she presented at his practice with a minor infection. However, even women who had not experienced such egregious behaviour expressed a need to protect themselves from insensitive practitioners. Kathy sums up this sensibility, 'Doctors can be scary sometimes, you know.' Colleen confides similar feelings, 'yeah, it isn't an easy thing to do I find, finding a doctor and finding somebody you like, you sort of put yourself on the line a bit'.

Colleen goes on to suggest that her wariness about GPs is partly because she feels that encounters with them have the potential to treat her insensitively as a woman. However, her sexuality is a factor that could also inspire frank malice:

> I find it scary to step out and find a doctor you're happy with or feel comfortable with for a few reasons. One, probably being in the profession [Colleen is a nurse], I am actually pretty hard on them because I see a lot of not very helpful or not really that interested, and the other side is, yeah, doing the women's checks. You do have to expose who and what you are and it is never easy. You know regardless of the fact that at the end of the day we are all a lot more enlightened and we can tell people to go to hell, you really don't ever want to expose yourself to people's nastiness I guess.

Colleen comments on the possible fate of women who do not, or can not, select a GP carefully, 'I suspect there's a couple of people [local doctors] you'd want to stay away from too ... if you are somebody who doesn't look into it and stumble on someone it could be a pretty nasty experience I should think.'

Given the risk of encountering a discriminatory doctor, it is not surprising that women exercise considerable agency in choosing a GP. With one exception, all the women exercise screening (Tiemann et al., 1998). That is, they utilize their social networks to gain information about potential practitioners before contacting them. Anne, for example, is likely to choose a practitioner on the basis of information provided through the local SSA women's community, 'I'm most likely to choose a female doctor that I've heard good reports of from others in the community'. This process has worked well for her in the past and has shielded her from unpleasant encounters with unaccepting practitioners. Anne, 'found out about the ones who were family friendly or gay friendly. So [I have had] no bad experiences that I can recall.'

However, using networks to identify potential GPs is only the beginning of the process for some women; they then subject GPs to considerable scrutiny before making a decision about establishing an ongoing relationship with them. Judy is overt about how active she is in selecting a GP, 'Well, I actually interview them.' Kathy explains the somewhat convoluted process she employs in selecting a suitable practitioner:

> I tend to pick my GP pretty well before I, I don't just pick anyone and go to them. I will ask around and a get a good feel for the doctor... you have to ask around. My mum had gone to this GP as well and a couple of other people we know and they said he was really good and I went in to meet him first and just to have a chat and see how it was going... what he was like and I was comfortable with him the first time.

For Jackie, developing a sense of confidence in, and comfort with her GP is a layered process. If she is happy with the way they respond to the outer layers she presents, she will then reveal deeper levels:

> Um, I tend to start off with the physical things and if I feel comfortable that they have addressed that and they're actually genuinely concerned then, you know, little by little you sort of open up a bit more. I am like that, I have a lot of walls and you have to get through a fair few... they have to perform for me... and if I am not happy with everything then I move on.

In choosing a GP, the term 'comfortable' was ubiquitous. Every woman interviewed spontaneously used the term to describe how they wanted to feel about the relationship. Being comfortable entails a GP's willingness to listen and to engage in a relationship extending beyond purely clinical foci. Maggie comments on these factors:

> ...my doctor is a woman and I have a lot of confidence in her because I find her to be, she talks to me, you know, sits down with me and sits there and listens to me most of the time.

Other women comment that an asymmetry in doctor–patient interaction is incompatible with a comfortable relationship. An egalitarian bond with her practitioner is essential in Stacey's view, 'Doctors are to be on first name terms with.' For Judy, an equal relationship entails the GP's willingness to respect her experience:

> ...she will allow me to go along with how my body is feeling and what I believe I need. And I might not always be right in some of

the things that I say but mostly I think we all have to know what we are doing with our bodies. So she is really good that way.

'Good' practitioners

Many women said that they felt more comfortable with women GPs because they considered them more capable of empathizing. Colleen sums up this sentiment, 'I am not saying that all women are gentle and thoughtful but I think you can usually find a little more empathy... [with them]'. Jackie suggests that women practitioners are more likely to respect emotions:

> I feel more comfortable with a woman. Um, only because I, you know, you tend to connect more with a woman because they know how we think and how we feel and that you know they won't dismiss anything that's emotional. Men tend to dismiss that side of you... I am not embarrassed to go and see a man, it is more the connection side of it that I prefer to see a woman.

Most women commented spontaneously on the personal and relational attributes that they deem desirable in a practitioner. However, it is clear that the knowledge and skill level of their GP is also very important. Anne, for instance, wants, 'a GP that is expert in women's health issues. I want to feel that... I wouldn't necessarily ask what their qualifications are but [I want someone] particularly skilled in Pap smears and gynae [gynaecological] examinations.' Colleen elaborates on the technical knowledge and skills that a 'good' GP should possess:

> ... for women's health, that they have done the extra bits of quals [qualifications]. It is quite a skill to know how to touch me, breast checks, and women's health in a sense of what they require for menopause and birth control and all those other bits that go along with it. I suppose someone that has done those women's health certificates and the gynae [gynaecological] training.

However, knowledge and skill are insufficient criteria for being a 'good' GP; attitudes and interpersonal characteristics are an inextricable part of the evaluation. For Judy, an Indigenous woman, GPs must have a commitment to social justice, 'if they don't have those values, well I am not interested. Even if they're reputed to be the best doctor in the world that would not suit me.' Colleen also points out that she needs to feel a personal connection to her practitioner because they do not only deal with only the 'technical' aspects of her life, 'if I didn't have a sense that they were a nice person, it wouldn't matter how good you were and I suppose that it is because that somebody is going to be dealing with my personal stuff.'

Feeling comfortable with, or about, a GP is a reciprocal process, however. Some women insisted that doctors had to feel comfortable with them as SSA women to establish an optimal therapeutic relationship. As Chantelle says, 'For me to go to the doctor, like especially a male, ahm, we need to feel very comfortable with who we choose and we need for them to feel comfortable about us as well.' Anne also conveys how she wants a GP that will not recoil from her disclosing her sexual orientation, 'if I go in and they ask me am I on the contraceptive pill and I say no, I need to know that they are not going to keel over in horror'.

Mind and body

As the previous discussion demonstrates, most women rate a good GP as someone who cares for them in a holistic sense by listening to them, treating their emotions respectfully and being interested in them as a 'whole' person. However, a good GP is also someone who is knowledgeable and skilful; they can successfully undertake the 'technical' aspects of practice. Yet while most women applaud GPs who treat them as 'whole people', not all of the women define themselves, and the relationship between their mind and body, in a unitary way. Accordingly, not all women want 'holistic' care that pays attention to mind and body, and to the relationship between them. For Jo, the healthcare that she wants from her GP is centred on physical issues. Hence, in some situations, Jo conceptualizes herself as embodying a Cartesian separation of psyche and soma. Moreover, for her, the demarcation of mind and body is aligned with a medical division of labour; GPs treat her body and specialists attend to her psyche, 'That is what doctors are for [physical issues]; you go and see your psychiatrist if there is anything else. I have done that. I have seen a psychiatrist and psychologist for the other stuff.'

Mary, likewise, would not talk to a GP about non-physical issues, 'I'd go to a psychologist I think'. By contrast, Jackie clearly regards physical and emotional issues as inextricably linked and is dismayed by practitioners who will not link the two. Doctors, she suggests, focus on corporeal issues, neglecting the life lived in and through her body. Clearly, Jackie wants a GP who regards mind, body and emotions as unified:

> ... and being the size I am they put everything down to weight – 'it's just your weight, go and fix it up' – they are not interested in looking into why things are happening ... that's what I look for, someone that is genuinely interested in what's happening because there is so much more, you know stress and emotional stuff that contributes.

While most women laud holistic care, they are also capable of conceptualizing themselves in fragmented ways in relation to healthcare they utilize. Within the clinical encounter, women can accentuate their sexuality or their gender in some contexts, while, on other occasions, they can define themselves without overt reference to gender and sexuality. Women act as bricoleurs, drawing on different discursive frameworks, to define their healthcare needs and shape their interaction with doctors accordingly. In some instances, their same-sex attraction is a factor that is relevant to their healthcare, while in other cases they deem it irrelevant.

Sexuality and embodiment

Jo, for instance, does not consider that her sexuality has a role in her interaction with her doctor. She has not told her GP that she is SSA because her experience of routine healthcare does not, she feels, implicate her sexuality, 'it is not relevant for anything that I have been in for'. Anne, likewise, distinguishes situations in which her sexuality is relevant and those in which it is not. Some ailments entail an understanding of her body to which sexuality has little, if any, relationship:

> Only if it was relevant I suppose. If I've got a sore throat it might not be relevant to say, 'oh, by the way, I am a lesbian'. Just with a sore throat. Like I saw the dentist yesterday, it wasn't actually relevant to tell him about my private life.

Women define encounters with their GPs in phenomenological ways. Anne is clearly making a judgement that a sore throat is a 'neutral' phenomenon and does not require information about more private, intimate domains of her life. Yet, in other instances, Anne suggests that it is important that her doctor should know about her and her life, 'if they are a good doctor they should want a more comprehensive history – family histories and things and all that sort of stuff. They should see more of the whole person.' A sore throat is construed as a physical condition that has, at best, a tenuous relationship with Anne's life-world. However, in the case of other conditions, information about her sexuality and her relationship with her partner would be relevant, she considers.

In some cases, women define their interaction with GPs as centred on a physical state that can be meaningfully extricated from the wider context of their lives. Anne, for instance, defines a sore throat as a somewhat atomized occurrence that need not invoke other information. In this instance, mind/life-world and body are conceptualized as distinct and information about her identity is not relevant to the bodily problem of a sore throat. In other instances, however, the domain of relevant information is extended to include 'comprehensive history' and the 'whole person'. Women define how particular ailments or aspects of embodiment have meanings that may or may not, in their opinion, implicate their sexuality; this then shapes what is considered relevant information.

Stacey also relates how information about her sexuality is related to which part of her body is involved in some clinical encounters, but not in others. Some complaints, which in the opinion of the affected women do not implicate gender or sexuality, rule out the relevance of information about sexuality. However, in Stacey's opinion, screening for cervical cancer warrants routinely disclosing her sexuality:

> Oh I normally do it [disclose her sexuality] during screening for a Pap smear and that sort of thing and they ask about my sexual history. If I feel it is information they need, I give it to them. I wouldn't tell her that if I had got a sore throat or something ... but in general conversation I might have.

Stacey defines a Pap smear or her sexual history as something that implicates her sexuality. A sore throat is construed as a gender- and sexuality-neutral affliction, implicating an apparently gender-neutral and asexual body that can be considered in relative isolation from her life-world. It does not, in Stacey's judgement, require information about her sexuality. It is interesting that Stacey considers that she may have mentioned her sexuality in 'general conversation'. A general conversation is, by definition, general and will establish links between bodily issues and an individual's wider life; sexuality clearly has a place in this ambit.

Sexuality and a gendered division of labour

Several of the women interviewed defined some parts of their body, and some ailments, as inextricably linked to gender and sexuality, while other bodily parts and illnesses were given a more apparently neutral definition. This differentiation between issues related to gender and sexuality and issues that are more 'neutral' means that some practitioners are utilized for some domains and not others. Mary, for example, construes some things as gender and sexuality specific and will consult a female practitioner about them, while she is content to have other illnesses treated by male doctors. In her words, 'I mean I have had lots of male doctors, like oncologists and that kind of thing, yes. But for Pap smears and things, I've had females.' Pap smears clearly implicate gender and sexuality; as such, they are something for which it is inappropriate to consult a male doctor. Mary suggests that cancer (evidenced by reference to the oncologist) is somehow more gender-neutral than a Pap smear and she feels relatively at ease with it being treated by a male oncologist. Mary's cancer was in her breast and yet she is able to define that as less associated with her gender and sexuality than a Pap smear and, therefore, as something to which a male doctor can legitimately attend.

Like about half the women we interviewed, Maggie divides her body between highly gender-specific arenas, requiring a female practitioner, and 'other' dimensions that can be cared for by a male GP, 'I had a male doctor as well but he was for all the other things. I got a woman for all the things "down there".' Colleen's definition of whether a 'complaint' implicates her gender and sexuality has a direct influence on the gender of the practitioner she consults:

> ... if I had a virus or flu or sinusitis or something I used to go to Julian, the female stuff I did at family planning. . . . I didn't think about it, but I did split things. He [Julian, the doctor] was alright for everyday stuff, you know routine.

Conclusion

Annandale and Riska observe that feminist approaches to health and healthcare have inadvertently enforced binary concepts of gender, thus perpetuating heterosexism. A move away from a concern with 'gender as difference' to a focus on gender and health, they suggest, might expand the conceptual repertoire of 'male' and 'female' to encompass multiple femininities and masculinities (Annandale and Riska, this issue, pp. 00–00). The evidence from this study suggests such a move would be a welcome conceptual advance in explaining the healthcare experiences of SSA women. Lorber suggests that there is a general recognition of at least four gender identities; heterosexual women, lesbians, heterosexual men and gay men (Lorber, 1994: 58–9). While this helps to erode the male–female binary, it still implies a unitary identity; the 'lesbian' or 'heterosexual man', for instance. Our data, however, indicate that some SSA women do not define themselves by a unitary concept of either gender or sexuality. Rather, notions of gender and sexuality are utilized in complex and shifting ways in an attempt to receive satisfactory healthcare. Indeed, what constitutes satisfactory healthcare is partly an outcome of the way in which this group of women selectively deploy concepts of gender and sexuality in interaction with GPs.

The women in this study do not define themselves either as women or as SSA in an essentialist way; neither gender nor sexuality occupies master-narrative status in the way they configure their sense of self in interaction with GPs. In fact, this group of women has what might be termed kaleidoscopic identities. Their capacity to receive healthcare they find satisfactory is largely dependent on their adroitness in strategically highlighting and veiling themes related to their gender and to their sexuality. At times, they identify themselves primarily in relation to gender and their concerns echo many of those first articulated by the women's health movement. They want practitioners who have special knowledge about women and their bodies and who exercise technical skill when undertaking procedures such as breast checks and Pap smears. A respectful and competent engagement with the distinctive features of women's embodiment is thus an important criterion of good practice. These are concerns that could be articulated by most women, not only SSA ones. However, the women in this study also want empathetic GPs who regard them as whole people; that is, as unified bodies and psyches, and as individuals with a life-history and a life-world that deserve respectful treatment when recounted to GPs. Again, this demand is common to many women and formed a key platform of the WHM's agenda.

While the women in our study, for the most part, want their life-histories and life-worlds – that is, their identities – treated with civility, part of that identity is being a same-sex attracted woman. For SSA women, gender and sexuality are not synonymous or interchangeable concepts in the context of healthcare utilization. These women want the kind of open, reciprocal relationship with GPs that feminists have long-called for, yet their sexuality may work against developing the kind consumer–practitioner relationship they desire. As women, they want openness, but as SSA women they may choose to conceal information about their identities and their lives to ensure their psychological safety. For these women, gender and sexuality stand as tensions requiring active management, not as stable components of a unified identity. Likewise, the women in our sample do not define their embodiment in an essentialist or unitary way. While most rate the capacity of practitioners to respond to the unity of body and mind an important criterion in evaluating care, it is clear that women make strategic decisions about the circumstances in which this will occur.

Women do not have a unitary definition of their bodies as either women, or as SSA women, that they bring to the medical encounter. Women define aspects of their embodiment, or their presenting 'complaint', in highly phenomenological ways; neither has a fixed meaning that is uniformly invoked in consulting GPs. It is therefore unhelpful to tie gender identity to embodiment in a fixed, linear fashion because the women we interviewed reveal how complex and fluid the relationship between the two concepts may be. A fixed understanding of gendered identity and embodiment will not put an analytical spotlight on how selectively women emphasize various aspects of their identity and embodiment in dealing with doctors. Binary or unitary understandings of gendered identity will exhibit some conceptual myopia in their capacity to understand the experience of SSA women in negotiating satisfactory healthcare.

The literature on gender and healthcare has not thus far formulated the relationship between gender, sexuality and embodiment in theoretically or empirically adequate ways. Sexuality is often treated as an 'add-on' to gender and the relationship between them is frequently conceptualized as a kind of arithmetical formula: gender + minority sexuality = compounded disadvantage. This approach has been useful in broadening the category of 'women' to give explicit attention to the experience of those who are not heterosexual. It has thus been fruitful in allowing examination of the poor and discriminatory healthcare inflicted on SSA women. However, it has done little to advance an understanding of how women deploy definitions of sexuality and gender to negotiate healthcare with which they are satisfied. Even attempts to recognize 'lesbian' as a 'stand-alone' gender identity (Lorber, 1994) convey a sense that this identity is unitary and fixed; our evidence suggests this may not always be so. Moreover, an analysis of the variable deployment by SSA women of notions of gender and sexuality within the medical encounter allows an examination of the processes SSA engage when negotiating satisfactory healthcare. The women in our study do not report negative experience of healthcare because they do not define their gender, sexuality or embodiment as fixed, immutable entities, rather they deftly manage them in kaleidoscopic fashion.

While these groups of women are largely satisfied with the care they receive, it does not mean that it produces good health outcomes. It may be that the ways in which women accentuate or veil different facets of their identities and lives in medical encounters leads to less than optimum health outcomes for them. It is possible that the information women do not disclose to their GPs, or the unwillingness of some to provide comprehensive histories, may inadvertently compromise their health; further research is needed on this topic. Moreover, while the women in this study were adept at the strategic management of information relating to gender, sexuality and embodiment within the clinical encounter, the pervasive influence of homophobia and heterosexism in shaping this process should not be overlooked. Women engage in the process of information management because they wish to protect themselves from discriminatory practice. Hence, while the move to a more inclusive approach to gender and health, stressing diversity rather than difference and encompassing the notion of kaleidoscopic identities, has the promise to promote a more finely textured understanding of gender and health, the insights of the WHM not be discarded. Gender inclusive approaches can easily be hijacked by gender 'mainstreaming'. Kuhlmann (this issue, pp. 00–00) shows how 'mainstreaming' can overlook important elements of the feminist agenda, such as egalitarian 'patient'–practitioner relationships and empowerment through open information exchange. The ideals of the WHM have the potential to improve the healthcare that is delivered to men, to women and to those with other gendered identities. An intellectual and political commitment to these goals, together with an analytical framework that can move beyond the male–female binary – accentuated by a focus on 'difference' – to one that can recognize diverse and fluid identities, promises a way forward.

Acknowledgements

We gratefully acknowledge the funding for this research provided by the Division of Health Sciences, University of South Australia. Our thanks to the reviewers for the comments and suggestions they offered about this article. Finally, our gratitude goes to the women we interviewed for their willingness to share their time, their experiences and their insights.

References

Annandale, Ellen and Hunt, Kate (2000) 'Gender Inequalities in Health: Research at the Crossroads', in Ellen Annandale and Kate Hunt (eds) *Gender Inequalities in Health*, pp. 1–35. Buckingham: Open University Press.

Broom, Dorothy (1991) *Damned if We Do: Contradictions in Women's Health Care*. North Sydney: Allen and Unwin.

BWHBC (Boston Women's Health Book Collective) (1985) *The New Our Bodies, Ourselves*. Ringwood, Melbourne: Penguin.

Diamant, Allison, Wold, Cheryl, Spritzer, Karen and Gelberg, Lillian (2000) 'Health Behaviours, Health Status, and Access to and Use of Health – A Population Based Study of Lesbian, Bisexual and Heterosexual Women', *Archives of Family Medicine* 9(10): 1043–51.

Edwards, Jane (2005) 'Invisibility, Safety and Psycho-Social Distress among Same-Sex Attracted Women in Rural South Australia', *Rural and Remote Health: The International Electronic Journal of Rural and Remote Health, Research, Education, Practice and Policy* 5: 343; at: rrh.deakin.edu.au (accessed March 2007).

Gray, David (2006) *Health Sociology: An Australian Perspective*. Frenchs Forest: Pearson Education Australia.

Liamputtong, Pranee and Ezzy, Doug (2005) *Qualitative Research Methods*, 2nd edn. South Melbourne: Oxford University Press.

Lorber, Judith (1994) *Paradoxes of Gender*. Binghampton, CT: Yale University Press.

Lorber, Judith and Moore, Lisa (2002) *Gender and the Social Construction of Illness*, 2nd edn. Walnut Creek, CA: Altamira Press.

McColl, Peter (1994) 'Homosexuality and Mental Health Services', *British Medical Journal* 308: 550–1.

McNair, Ruth (2000) 'Lesbian Sexuality: Do GPs Contribute to Lesbian Invisibility and Ill Health?', *Australian Family Physician* 29(6): 514–16.

McNair, Ruth and Harrison, Jo (2002) 'Life Stage Issues within GLBTI Communities', in Department of Human Services, Victoria (ed.) *What's the Difference: Health Issues of Major Concern to Gay, Lesbian, Bisexual, Transgender and Intersex (GLBTI) Victorians*, pp. 37–43. Melbourne: Ministerial Advisory Council on Gay and Lesbian Health.

McNair, Ruth and Medland, Nick (2002) 'Physical Health Issues for GLBTI Victorians', in Department of Human Services, Victoria (ed.) *What's the Difference: Health Issues of Major Concern to Gay, Lesbian, Bisexual, Transgender and Intersex (GLBTI) Victorians*, pp. 13–20. Melbourne: Ministerial Advisory Council on Gay and Lesbian Health.

Mathieson, Cynthia, Bailey, Natasha and Gurevich, Maria (2002) 'Health Care Services for Lesbian and Bisexual Women', *Health Care for Women International* 23: 185–96.

Meyer, Ilan (2001) 'Why Lesbian, Gay, Bisexual, and Transgender Public Health?', *American Journal of Public Health* 91(6): 855–6.

Pitts, Marion, Smith, Anne, Mitchell, Anne and Patel, Sunni (2006) *Private Lives: A Report on the Health and Well-Being of GLBTI Australians*. Melbourne: Australian Research Centre in Sex, Health and Society, La Trobe University.

Rabin, Jack, Keefe, Kathleen and Burton, Michael (1986) 'Enhancing Services for Sexual Minority Clients: A Community Mental Health Approach', *Social Work* 31(4): 294–9.

Saulnier, Christine (2002) 'Deciding Who to See: Lesbians Discuss Their Preferences in Health and Mental Health Care Providers', *Social Work* 47(4): 355–65.

Shorne, Lesley, McCaul, Moira and Gunn, Jenny (2001–2) '"Beam me up Scotty": Trekking from Women's Health to General Practice', *New Doctor* 76: 22–5.

Thompson, Jan (1998) 'The Health of Lesbian Women', in Cath Rogers-Clark and Angie Smith (eds) *Women's Health: A Primary Health Care Approach*, pp. 100–19. Sydney: Maclennan and Petty.

Tiemann, Kathleen, Kennedy, Sally and Haga, Myrna (1998) 'Rural Lesbian's Strategies for Coming out to Health Care Professionals', *Journal of Lesbian Studies* 2(1): 61–75.

Welch, Sarah, Collings, Sunny and Howden-Chapman, Phillippa (2000) 'Lesbians in New Zealand: Their Mental Health and Satisfaction with Mental Health Services', *Australian and New Zealand Journal of Psychiatry* 34(2): 256–63.

60

CHOOSING CESAREAN

Feminism and the politics of childbirth in the United States

Katherine Beckett

Source: *Feminist Theory*, 6:3 (2006), 251–75.

Abstract

This article uses the US debate over elective Cesarean section to re-consider some of the more contentious issues raised in feminist debates about childbirth. Three waves of feminist commentary and critique in the United States are analysed in light of the ongoing debate over whether women should be able to choose Cesarean for non-medical reasons. I argue that the alternative birth movement's essentialist and occasionally moralistic rhetoric is problematic, and the idea that some women's preference for high-tech obstetrics is the result of a passive 'socialization' into 'dominant values' is theoretically inadequate. On the other hand, the invocation of women's choice and appreciation of high-tech childbirth serves as a weak foundation for a feminist perspective on childbirth. By limiting their analysis to the rhetorical and discursive nature and functions of 'the medical' and 'the natural', post-structuralist critics of the alternative birth movement obscure the connection of these discourses to practices that have very different consequences for maternal and infant health and, most importantly, for the consumption of health care resources.

Introduction

Although popularly conceived as a biological and personal experience, childbirth is also a cultural and political phenomenon, one that is both embedded in and consequential for gender relations (Jordan, 1983; Davis-Floyd, 1992; Davis-Floyd and Sargent, 1997; Rothman, 1982, 1989; Kitzinger, 1981; Leavitt, 1983, 1984; Oakley, 1980, 1993). As a result, feminist scholars and activists have taken an active interest in childbirth over the years. In the early 20th century, feminists in the United States and elsewhere struggled to overcome medical opposition to the use of pain relief during labour (Canton, 1999; Leavitt, 1984). In the 1960s and 1970s, the 'alternative birth movement' catapulted childbirth to the front pages of women's, parenting, and even some news magazines once again. Drawing their inspiration from the women's health and counter-cultural movements, second wave birth activists offered a powerful critique of conventional birthing practices and advocated alternative approaches to childbirth, especially home birth and midwifery services.

In the United States, this alternative/natural birth movement has come under attack from quite disparate parties. On the one hand, the alternative birth movement has been vigorously opposed by organized medicine, most recently by a segment of the medical community arguing that women should have the right to choose Cesarean section for personal (rather than medical) reasons. At the same time, some feminists are also challenging aspects of the alternative birth movement's rhetoric and goals. These critics have been especially concerned about the alternative birth movement's tendency to valorize 'natural' birth and its associated failure to deconstruct the dualisms (such as nature/culture and nature/technology) that underpin patriarchal ideology.

In what follows, I use the US debate over elective Cesarean section to explore these and other theoretical issues. I argue that the alternative birth movement's essentialist and occasionally moralistic rhetoric is problematic, and the idea that some women's preference for high-tech obstetrics is the result of a passive 'socialization' into 'dominant values' is theoretically inadequate. On the other hand, the invocation of women's choice and appreciation of high-tech childbirth ignores the social and political processes through which those choices are made and serves as a weak foundation for a feminist perspective of childbirth. By limiting their analysis to the rhetorical and discursive nature and functions of 'the medical' and 'the natural', post-structuralist critics of the alternative birth movement obscure the connection of these discourses to different sets of practices that have different consequences for maternal and infant health and, most importantly, for the consumption of health care resources.

This article unfolds in five parts. The first section briefly synthesizes secondary accounts of the 20th century transformation of childbirth in the United States and describes the first and second waves of feminist activism around it. The second section provides an account of recent feminist criticism of the alternative birth movement's rhetoric, vision, and goals. The third section describes medical advocacy of elective Cesarean and the debate it has engendered. The fourth section reflects on the theoretical dilemmas raised by the debate over elective Cesarean for feminist analysts of childbirth, and evaluates recent feminist criticism of the alternative birth activism in this context. A conclusion summarizes the main arguments and highlights their theoretical and political implications.

Childbirth in the United States: transformation and critique

Throughout the 19th century, most women living in the United States delivered their babies at home, typically with a midwife in attendance (Donegan, 1984; Scholten, 1984). After the turn of the 20th century, the location of birth changed rapidly, and by 1939, over half of all birthing women delivered their child in the hospital. Since the 1970s, hospital birth has become normative across racial and demographic groups, with roughly 90 per cent of all US births taking place in hospitals under the supervision of physicians (Rooks, 1997). Many feminist accounts of the relocation of childbirth from the home to the hospital emphasize the political machinations of the emerging medical profession and the impact of the profession's propaganda on women's beliefs and preferences. According to these analysts, doctors used their growing political and cultural authority to redefine childbirth as a dangerous, pathological event, to denigrate and eliminate midwives, and to fuel the perception that middle and upper class women were less able to withstand the challenges of childbirth (e.g. Daly, 1978; Ehrenreich and English, 1973; Oakley, 1980; Sullivan and Weitz, 1988).

While medical propaganda may indeed have shaped popular perceptions of childbirth and helped to associate doctors and hospitals with safety, historical scholarship indicates that women had long expressed a great deal of fear and trepidation about the potential pain (and danger) of childbirth. Indeed, many first wave feminist activists saw the right to pain relief as an important political issue (Leavitt and Walton, 1984; Leavitt, 1984, 1986; Reissman, 1983; Wertz and Wertz, 1977) and argued strenuously for women's right to relieve their suffering – and hence gain control of the birthing process – through the use of drugs, and specifically, scopolamine. These activists were outraged by obstetricians' reluctance to provide pharmacological pain relief, and saw this reluctance as indicative of physicians' tendency to place their own interests ahead of those of their female patients (Leavitt, 1984: 177). In this sense, first wave feminists' efforts to transform childbirth were less a campaign for drugs than for responsive and respectful medicine, expanded choices in childbirth, and control over one's body and reproductive life.

Scopolamine was eventually shown to be quite harmful to infant health, and its use subsequently declined. However, the use of other forms of anaesthesia became widespread after the 1940s. The legacy of first wave activism around childbirth is thus a mixed one: on the one hand, women won the right to pain relief and compelled obstetricians to at least consider women's preference for it; on the other hand, women arguably lost control over the process of childbirth, as well as the comforts of home and support of female relatives, friends, and midwives (Leavitt 1984, 179).[1]

Second wave birth activism: origins

As hospital birth and pain-relieving medication became ubiquitous, modern childbirth came under critical scrutiny once again. Beginning in the 1960s, increasing numbers of women began to wonder aloud if childbirth had to be 'a time of alienation from the body, from family and friends, from the community, and even from life itself' (Wertz and Wertz, 1977: 173). Advocates of 'natural birth' – in which a woman was 'awake and aware' throughout the birth process – emerged in this context. As early as 1940, these critics decried the impersonality, isolation, and passivity that now characterized childbirth. In 1944, the English obstetrician Grantly Dick-Read published *Birth Without Fear* in the United States, which argued that much of the pain associated with childbirth was a product of fear. These ideas spawned what became known as the 'natural childbirth' movement (Rothman, 1982). And in 1956, seven Chicago-area women founded La Leche League to advocate for more natural forms of childrearing, including 'natural' birth and breastfeeding (Rooks, 1997). Although hardly couched in feminist rhetoric, these early criticisms – replete with the idiom of 'the natural' – had a significant impact on second wave activism around childbirth (Umansky, 1996).

The alternative birth movement emerged as an increasingly coherent and united movement in the United States and other industrialized countries in the late 1960s and early 1970s. Although many activists drew their inspiration from the women's health and counter-cultural movements, a few in the US were also influenced by more conservative childbirth and childrearing philosophies (Umansky, 1996). The alternative birth movement has nevertheless offered a fairly coherent critique of the conventional approach to childbirth, one that emphasized the importance of treating childbirth as an important life experience and family event rather than a medical emergency; the right of women and families to choose their birth setting and attendants; the inhumane and impersonal nature of many routine hospital procedures; and the counter-productive nature of the 'high-tech, low-touch' approach to childbirth. In what follows, I explicate these themes and consider recent criticism of the alternative birth movement's discourse and goals.

Birth as a natural phenomenon

As was discussed previously, second wave feminist birth activists and scholars place a great deal of emphasis on the role of the (male) medical profession in the relocation and transformation of childbirth (see Daly, 1978; Ehrenreich and English, 1973; DeVries, 1996; Leavitt, 1983, 1984; Oakley, 1993; Sullivan and Weitz, 1988). According to these accounts, obstetricians argued 'again and again that normal pregnancy and parturition are exceptions and that to consider them to be normal physiologic conditions was a fallacy' (Kobrin, 1984); this re-definition of childbirth as pathological served to justify and legitimate the expansion of medicine's jurisdiction to include childbirth. As a result, resistance to medical control of childbirth has been framed in the language of 'normality' or the idiom of 'natural' (Kobrin, 1984; Michie and Cahn, 1996). Still today, birth activists' emphasis on the 'normality' and 'naturalness' of birth is best understood as part of an effort to contest medical control of birth and to challenge the increasingly narrow definitions of normality that prevail in hospital settings.

Similarly, the rhetoric of the 'normal' and 'natural' reflects concern about diagnostic technologies that overstate the risks of childbirth. The widespread use of the Electronic Foetal Monitor (EFM), for example, leads to a dramatic overestimation of foetal distress (estimates of the rate of false positives run as high as 98 per cent) and has therefore contributed significantly to rising levels of Cesarean section (Lent, 1999). In short, the development and deployment of the idioms of 'the natural' and 'the normal' can be understood in historical and political terms as a response to the medical profession's pathologization of birth, as well as to the use of technology and application of norms that render birth a 'high risk' event.

Many second wave scholars and activists argue that the conceptualization of childbirth as a pathological process and treatment of it as a (high risk) medical event eroded not only midwives' claim to expertise, but birthing women's as well (see especially Arms, 1994; Davis-Floyd, 1992; Rothman, 1982; Leavitt, 1984). For example, when women give birth in hospital settings, their capacity to act upon their preferences (such as eating or drinking, moving about, and so forth) is limited. In addition, procedures that made labour and delivery more comfortable for physicians – and more difficult for women – were adopted.

Some birth activists argue that the widespread use of such procedures reflects not only the prioritization of doctors' comfort over that of birthing women, but also the 'ideology of technology' which connotes order, rationality, predictability, and control, and treats women's bodies as a (malfunctioning) machine that must be oriented toward these goals (see especially Davis-Floyd, 1992; Martin, 1992; Rothman, 1989). (Here, the implicit contrast is not between nature/pathology, but between nature/technology.) These procedures are also thought to stem from a patriarchal devaluing of women's bodies, and the tendency to conceive of the foetus/newborn as a 'second patient', separate from – and in need of protection from – their mother (Rothman, 1989; Hubbard, 1990).

Birth activists also cite evidence of the safety of home birth to justify their emphasis on the normality and 'naturalness' of birth. Indeed, many epidemiological studies indicate that planned home births attended by trained midwives are as safe or safer than physician-attended hospital births for 'low risk' women (for summaries of these literatures, see Goer, 1995; Rooks, 1997; Wagner, 2000). Birth activists conclude that since midwives, operating from a conception of birth as 'natural', are able to match or exceed doctors' safety record at lower cost, the pathologization of birth is not just unnecessary, but epistemologically and empirically incorrect.

The iatrogenic and dehumanizing nature of medical intervention

Second wave birth scholars and activists emphasize that the vast majority of births involve high – and increasing – levels of technological intervention. Indeed, nearly all US hospital births are now monitored electronically; approximately one in five births is artificially induced; more than one in four is surgical in nature; and four of the eight most common US surgical procedures are obstetric in nature (Keefe, 2002; Moon, 2002). These rates far exceed World Health Organization standards for maternity care, and are, therefore, the subject of much controversy (Wagner, 1997, 2000). As was discussed previously, high levels of intervention are considered problematic because obstetric intervention often results from misleading indicators of risk or narrowed definitions of normality, and because they may diminish women's capacity to make meaningful choices regarding their birth deliveries. Critics also point out that these interventions do not appear to have improved the safety of childbirth: despite its highly interventionist approach, the US boasts higher maternal and infant mortality rates than all other developed, and some developing, nations (Keefe, 2002).[2]

Second wave birth activists make sense of this apparent contradiction by arguing that although sometimes necessary and life-saving, medical intervention is frequently unnecessary, and often causes harm to women and babies. These critics also stress that each intervention makes another more likely.[3] Further, there is evidence that few women are aware of these possible effects when they choose or consent to the procedures that increase the likelihood of subsequent interventions (Goer, 1995).

Some birth activists also register concern about the loss of intimacy that resulted from the modernization and bureaucratization of birth: hospital births, replete with 'the cool penetration of needles, the distant interpretation of lines on a graph' deprive women of 'the warm exchange of breath and sweat, of touch and gaze, of body oils and emotions that characterize births in which there is an intimate connection between the mother and her caretaker' (Davis-Floyd and Davis, 1997: 315). As this quote suggests, the loss of familiar, female supporters during birth and the intimacy of home is a pervasive theme in the literature of the alternative birth movement (see also Leavitt, 1984).

A few more radical critics see the high-tech nature of childbirth and poor women's lack of access to prenatal care as two sides of the for-profit health care coin. As political activist and scholar Angela Davis put it at a hearing on the issue in California in 1981:

> As growing numbers of medically indigent women are forced to go without prenatal care and proper nutrition, thus producing very low birth weight babies, every effort is made to keep those infants alive ... through the use of expensive, profit-making technology ... The medical establishment's solution to an embarrassingly high rate of infant mortality in this country's poor and Third World communities is increased reliance on the technological miracles that keep low birth weight babies alive, many of whom are born prematurely because their mothers could not obtain early, meaningful and respectful prenatal care.
>
> (quoted in Edwards and Waldorf, 1984: 175)

Davis thus situated high-tech obstetrics (and paediatrics) in the context of a health care system that uses its resources in a highly inequitable and injudicious fashion. Such a system ignores the under- and uninsured, and creates incentives to over-treat those with private insurance. This argument has found support in empirical studies: women of higher socio-economic status, who give birth in private hospitals and have private insurance, are more likely to give birth surgically, despite having 'lower risk' pregnancies and deliveries (Gould et al., 1989; Sakala, 1993: notes 91–8; Wagner, 2000).

Midwifery and women's right to choose

Women's right to choose the place and circumstances of their birth deliveries is also stressed by birth activists. Given that physician-attended birth has become the norm, this has largely meant the right to choose a midwife-attended, out-of-hospital birth. As Ina May Gaskin, author of *Spiritual Midwifery* and current President of the Midwives Alliance of North America (MANA) put it, 'We feel that returning the major responsibility for normal childbirth to well-trained midwives rather than have it rest with a predominantly male and profit-oriented medical establishment is a major advance in self-determination for women' (1975: 11).[4] To deny this choice is to allow the state to limit reproductive freedom and treat women as mere vessels of the foetus (Rothman, 1989).

Though simple, the rhetoric of choice is one of the most powerful weapons deployed by birth activists in their campaign to increase access to alternative childbirth choices (see Beckett and Hoffman, 2005) and, ironically, links first wave advocates of pain medication to second wave critics of the widespread use of that medication and other medical interventions. However, as critics of the alternative birth movement note, this emphasis on choice does sit somewhat uneasily with the movement's pervasive and quite damning critique of the medical management of childbirth. (What if women actively choose medical intervention?)

In addition, many birth activists argue that midwives offer quality – even superior – care throughout pregnancy and childbirth. Some, invoking the essentialist logic that is so irksome to their critics, stress the overwhelmingly female nature of the profession and the (apparently related) fact that midwifery is rooted in a 'holistic' rather than 'mechanistic' philosophy. According to this line of reasoning, midwives develop more empathic relations with their clients, rely usefully and wisely on their intuition, and trust women's 'embodied' knowledge as well as objective diagnostic data (see Davis-Floyd, 1992; Davis-Floyd and Davis, 1997). This argument implicitly – and sometimes explicitly – relies on an essentialist conception of femaleness by assuming women's greater capacity for intuition and empathy.

Others avoid this essentialism by emphasizing the institutional organization of midwifery practice rather than its gender composition. In particular, midwives' intensive and comprehensive approach to prenatal care is contrasted with obstetricians' perfunctory care (Beckett and Hoffman, 2005). These advocates also point out that midwives use far less technology during labour and delivery, and therefore offer a cost-effective form of obstetrical care (National Organization of Women, 1999).

Natural birth, empowerment, and pain

More controversially, some birth activists argue that the high-tech approach to birth – and especially the use of pharmacological pain relief – denies women the experience of childbirth and the sense of empowerment that results from knowing that one is capable of bringing forth life. Because this argument is typically accompanied by the claim that medical intervention is medically harmful to women and newborns, it is not clear how pervasive the notion that the experience of the pain (and pleasure) of birth endows some spiritual or psychic benefit actually is among birth activists. It appears, though, that withstanding/experiencing the pain of childbirth is seen by at least some in the alternative birth community as a positive occurrence, one that allows women to fully appreciate the power of the birthing body, the drama that is childbirth, the inherent connection between joy and suffering, and the satisfaction that may result from surrendering oneself to a force more powerful than one's conscious will. Thus, women who choose home birth 'supervalue nature and their natural bodies over science and technology ... regard the technocratic destruction of birth as harmful and dangerous ... and desire to experience the whole of birth – its rhythms, its juiciness, its intense sexuality, fluidity, ecstasy, and pain' (Davis-Floyd and Davis, 1997: 316; see also Biesele, 1997: 488). The assumption that women can (or should) find this kind of surrender empowering reveals the influence of a 'strong version' of radical/cultural feminism that celebrates women's life-bearing capacities and the commitment to motherhood they embody (see Annandale and Clark, 1996).

Feminist critics of the alternative birth movement

In recent years, medical opponents of the alternative birth movement have been joined by a small number of feminist critics who have expressed concern about aspects of the alternative birth movement's rhetoric and goals. Some such critics ground their arguments in their own (less than positive) experience of the alternative birth culture. Others, drawing on post-structuralist theory, are especially critical of the alternative birth movement's tendency to celebrate women's reproductive capacities and invert the categories through which women have historically been denigrated. For lack of a better term, I will refer to this body of criticism as the 'third wave' critique, much of which centres on the idiom of 'the natural'.

Deconstructing 'the natural'

Many contemporary feminist critics worry about the influence of cultural feminism on the birth movement and the related tendency to invoke the ideal of 'the natural' (see especially Annandale and Clark, 1996; Michie and Cahn, 1996; Treichler, 1990). The legacy of Derrida is apparent here. For Derrida, 'women have always been defined as a subjugated difference within a binary opposition: man/woman, culture/nature, positive/negative, intuitive/analytical. To assert an essential gender difference as cultural feminists do is to re-invoke this oppositional structure' (cited in Alcoff, 1994: 104). From this perspective, the alternative birth movement's veneration of 'the natural' mistakenly seeks to overturn male domination by super-valuing the denigrated categories with which women have long been associated rather than by deconstructing and destabilizing these hierarchical constructions (Annandale and Clark, 1996; Treichler, 1990). Furthermore, the valorization of 'the natural' leads to the perception of births that do not conform to the 'natural' ideal as 'unnatural', and therefore denies women who experience such births both agency and humanity (Michie and Cahn, 1996).

These critics also point out that the juxtaposition of 'the natural' and 'the medical' obscures the fact that 'the natural' also does cultural work: 'natural childbirth discourse itself serves as cultural initiation' (Michie and Cahn, 1996: 46). Indeed, these analysts argue, childbirth has no meaning or essence outside of its construction through this and other discourses. In short, third wave critics argue that the idealization of 'natural childbirth' rests on the assumption that both women and childbirth have a true essence or nature that is respected by the natural childbirth movement but violated by the medical establishment: birth activists then 'assert a nature to which birthing women must conform' (Michie and Cahn, 1996: 49). By contrast, third wave critics argue that we cannot know what childbirth 'really is', as 'discourse itself is the site in which birth becomes knowable' (Treichler, 1990, quoted in Annandale and Clark, 1996: 31).

Technology

According to these critics, the second wave critique of high-tech obstetrics also reflects a troubling construction of technology as inherently patriarchal (Annandale and Clark, 1996: 35). In addition, these critics point out that women can and do find the use of obstetric technology to be an empowering experience (1996: 35). To ignore this, they argue, is not only to reproduce restrictive dualisms, but to treat some women's use appreciation of technology as indicative of a kind of false consciousness, a violation of their true (essential) nature. Thus, while second wave feminists tend to see women's seeking/enjoyment of technological intervention as indicative of the ubiquity and power of patriarchal, technocratic, and medical discourses (e.g. Davis-Floyd, 1992; Campbell and Porter, 1997), third wave feminists argue that women's choice/positive experience of high-tech births confirms that technology is not inherently male, and can serve women's needs and purposes.

Domesticity

Some third wave critics are also troubled by what they see as the idealization of domesticity in the rhetoric of the alternative birth movement. As one analyst writes: 'In much of the literature of the home-birth movement, as well as in feminist and proto-feminist accounts of home birth in more general contexts, home functions . . . as a synecdoche for female autonomy; it becomes the place not only of comfort, but of freedom and power' (Michie, 1998: 261). Michie notes that this idealization of the home is an implicit contrast to the alleged sterility, inhumanity, and isolation of the hospital, and that it reverses the medical narrative that equates hospitals with technology and safety and homes with danger and disease. But this veneration of the home, she argues, not only reiterates a long-standing association of women with the private sphere, but also obscures the ways in which power operates in domestic spaces, and particularly the ways in which 'home' may limit young, poor, and abused women's autonomy: 'home might be an especially fraught term for a teenage unwed mother trying to hide her pregnancy from her family by delivering in the bathroom' (p. 264).

The politics of midwifery

Birth activists' tendency to treat midwifery as synonymous with feminism and to overlook possible conflicts between midwives and birthing women is also a source of concern. Some critics argue, for example, that birth activists' emphasis on midwives' provision of continuous care during labour and delivery obscures the fact that the provision of such care may be very difficult for – even exploitative of – midwives (Annandale and Clark, 1996). Others point out that where they exist, (North American) licensure requirements do not recognize midwives who acquire their training elsewhere or indigenous midwives, and therefore exclude immigrant midwives and reproduce racial and ethnic hierarchy in the profession (Nestle, 2000). Finally, these critics argue that licensure requirements in these developed countries lead aspiring midwives to exploit Third World women. In Ontario, for example, licensure requirements have given rise to 'midwifery tourism' in which aspiring First World midwives travel to impoverished countries to gain the experience they need to satisfy those requirements (Nestle, 2000).

Pain and the experience of natural childbirth

Pain is a recurring issue for feminist analysts of childbirth (as well as for countless numbers of women anticipating the experience). First wave feminists saw the right to pain relief during childbirth as an important political issue. Second wave feminists also sought to render women's voices more powerful, this time by asserting their right to choose a non-medicated and otherwise 'natural' birth for both medical and psychological/spiritual reasons. But some third wave scholars, drawing on their experiences with alternative 'birth culture', have criticized the alternative birthing community's knee-jerk rejection of (pharmacological) pain relief and understand this rejection as indicative of a kind of machisma, a belief that birth is 'an extreme sport' (Shapiro, 1998; Talbot, 1999). 'Isn't it interesting', one such writer comments, 'that the movement that's supposedly feminist is the one that insists on women feeling pain?' (Shapiro, 1998). Another suggests: 'Today's natural childbirth purists don't see moral punishment in pain but they do see moral superiority in refusing pain relief' (Talbot, 1999: 19).

According to these critics, the tendency of 'birth junkies' to valorize the experience of natural (i.e. painful) childbirth is not only moralistic, but unrealistic. One writer, citing a childbirth educator warning that women with quick deliveries might be disappointed that they were not able to savour the experience, counters that 'If I could get away with delivering a baby in five minutes, I'd jump at the chance' (Shapiro, 1998). The idea that women do (or should) savour, enjoy, or feel empowered by the experience of labour and delivery, they argue, romanticizes women's roles as life-bearers and mothers, and assumes an emotional and physical reality (or posits an emotional and physical norm) that does not exist for many. Echoing their poststructuralist counterparts, these critics argue that the emphasis on birth as a defining moment in women's lives is deeply problematic: 'all this emphasis on keen awareness means exalting the moment of childbirth as the moment at which a woman is most authentically, "naturally", a woman, most in tune with her evolutionary destiny' (Talbot, 1999: 20).

In short, some feminists perceive the alternative birth movement as rigid and moralistic, insistent that giving birth 'naturally' is superior and, indeed, is a measure of a 'good mother'. The perceived moralism of this stance is quite troubling to some; according to one feminist critic, the 'natural' philosophy espoused in an alternative birth centre is as tyrannical and prescriptive as the medical model, but pretends not to be by emphasizing women's right to individualized and alternative births (cited in Treichler, 1990: 129–30).

These and other sources of disagreement among feminist analysts of childbirth are not easily resolved, and I do not attempt any final resolution here. Rather, in what follows, I use the debate over whether or not women should be able to choose to deliver their babies surgically for non-medical reasons as a means of exploring the strengths and limitations of both second wave and third wave critiques. I begin with a brief account of the debate over elective Cesarean.

Cesarean section: from problem to choice

The alternative birth movement was perceived at the outset as a serious threat by organized medicine (DeVries, 1996: 53; Edwards and Waldorf, 1984). Organized medicine has also responded aggressively to widespread criticism of the increase in surgical delivery (i.e. Cesarean section (C-section)). Much to the chagrin of consumer, public health, feminist, and governmental organizations, the US C-section rate rose from about 5 per cent in 1970 to nearly 25 per cent by the late 1980s (Grisanti, 1989). This Cesarean 'epidemic' was widely discussed in women's magazines and other media outlets.

Despite disagreement about why C-section rates were increasing, there was, until recently, widespread consensus that this development was problematic. Medical research indicates that unnecessary Cesarean sections are extremely costly and pose significant risk of harm to both foetuses and women (see Goer, 1995; Rooks, 1997; Wagner, 2000). As a result, government and public health agencies such as the Department of Health and Human Services and the World Health Organization included lowering the rate of Cesarean section in their goals, and medical organizations such as the AMA (American Medical Association) and ACOG (American College of Obstetricians and Gynecologists) largely accepted the need to do so. But efforts to reduce the Cesarean section rate were only temporarily successful. After declining to just under 20 per cent in the late 1980s and early 1990s, the incidence of surgical birth began to increase again in the mid 1990s, this time quickly and dramatically. By 2002, an estimated 26 per cent of all US babies were delivered surgically (Moon, 2002).

It was in this context that some obstetricians, including former ACOG President Benjamin Harer, began to argue that high rates of surgical birth are not problematic, but rather are medically and philosophically defensible, even optimal. These outspoken and controversial physicians claimed that such intervention is often chosen by birthing women, and that obstetricians should respect their patients' preferences for surgical birth. The debate over elective Cesarean has received significant media attention, especially after a popular Spice Girl announced her plan to have an elective Cesarean and was dubbed 'Too Posh to Push' by the English press.

Two kinds of argument are marshalled to support the argument that women should be allowed to choose Cesarean. The first is the empirical claim that C-sections have become safer, and that the risks of vaginal birth have been underestimated. Indeed, proponents of elective Cesarean argue that surgical birth is now almost always safer than vaginal birth for the foetus/newborn, and that the short term risks of surgery (including risk of infection, adverse drug reaction, uterine rupture, and death) for women are offset by the long term risks of vaginal delivery, which include the increased likelihood of incontinence and diminished vaginal 'tone' (Walters, 1998; see also Elliott, 2001; Young, 2001). (I will return to this controversial point shortly.) These and related claims have been vigorously disputed by other analysts, and many medical researchers and public health organizations continue to stress the risks of elective Cesareans and point out that many of the alleged 'risks' of vaginal birth (such as incontinence) are easily and inexpensively remedied through behavioural techniques (i.e., Kegels) (see Goer, 2001; Grobman, 2002; Sakala, 1993; Wagner, 2000).

Second, although organized medicine has actively opposed women's right to choose to give birth in birth centres or at home and has supported physicians' authority to compel women to deliver surgically against their will, medical proponents of elective Cesarean make the philosophical argument that women have the right to choose Cesarean section for non-medical reasons.[5] This argument is couched in terms of patients' right to choose the form of medical care they receive; thus, women's right to choose to give birth surgically is said to be analogous to their right to choose between mastectomy and lumpectomy for treatment of breast cancer (Walters, 1998). Opponents of elective Cesarean argue that this analogy assumes that childbirth is, like breast cancer, a disease, and is, therefore, misleading. By contrast, they aver, to permit women to choose Cesarean birth for non-medical reasons is analogous to allowing a healthy person to 'choose' a kidney transplant or to give antibiotics to a person with a viral infection. In both cases, they argue, the 'treatment' is unnecessary, potentially harmful and costly to the wider community (Wagner, 2000).

Feminism and childbirth reconsidered

The debate over elective Cesarean brings to the fore many of the issues and concerns raised in the feminist literatures on childbirth regarding choice, technology, and medicalization. In what follows, I discuss these three issues and offer some concluding thoughts regarding the (re)construction of a feminist politics and theory of childbirth.

Complicating 'choice' and 'experience'

As was discussed previously, third wave feminist critics stress that the use and experience of technology during pregnancy and birth may be empowering for women, and conclude that medicalization is not necessarily incompatible with feminism and/or women's interests. Furthermore, because technology is not inherently 'male', women's preference for/enjoyment of it ought not to be seen as a kind of false consciousness or, in Bourdian terms, misrecognition. This argument reflects the post-structuralist emphasis on the need to destabilize rather than invert oppressive dualisms, as well as an appreciation for the diversity of women's experiences and desires.

The fact that many birthing women choose and experience positively pharmacological pain relief provides compelling evidence for this argument. This option was made available as a result of feminist agitation, and many women continue to choose it when possible. Given that many women have feared and sought to minimize the pain of childbirth, that midwives have historically worked to alleviate it, and that many women now choose and appreciate pharmaceutical pain relief, it seems quite reasonable to conclude that medical technology can serve women's interests and feminist purposes.

On the other hand, there is evidence that women make choices regarding medical technology – including pharmaceutical pain relief – on the basis of very partial and biased information about their risks and benefits. For example, US physicians are increasingly inducing labour, sometimes at the behest of pregnant women, but very few of the doctors who use Cytotec® to do so inform their patients that its use for this purpose has been contraindicated by both the manufacturer and the Food and Drug Administration. More generally, studies indicating that considerations of both convenience and profitability shape patterns of medical intervention suggest that doctors often shape and withhold relevant medical information when communicating with their patients (Wagner, 2000). It is also evident that diagnostic technologies frequently overstate the risks posed to the foetus (Lent, 1999). Even when these factors are relevant, patients choose or consent to this intervention in the vast majority of cases. The question thus arises: what if a woman is pleased with her 'choice' to induce labour or deliver surgically but did so because the risks of continuing to labour to herself, or, more likely, her foetus/baby were significantly overstated?

Further complicating matters, the normative and emotional grounds upon which some women choose obstetrical interventions such as labour induction and Cesarean delivery may be reflective of, and perpetuate, patriarchal values. For example, one of the main arguments for elective Cesarean section is that vaginal delivery poses long term risks to the mother, including (and, it appears, especially) the loss of 'vaginal tone' and therefore of sexual pleasure. For obvious reasons, it is widely assumed that what is really at stake here is (some) men's preferences for more 'toned' vaginas. What if women feel pleased with or empowered by their choice to deliver surgically because they believe that this choice will ensure their partner's sexual pleasure? Should this experience be treated as evidence of the empowering potential of medical technology? In short, ignoring the grounds upon which women make their choices may not be compatible with feminists' commitment to minimizing the influence of patriarchy and other systems of inequality on women's lives.

It is somewhat ironic that those feminists who adopt the most radically constructionist position ignore the social construction of women's desires, preferences and choices. As Hirschmann argues, social constructionism is not simply concerned with rhetoric, but 'requires us to think about the context in which choices are made' (2003: 39). This kind of 'deep constructionism' also goes well beyond the idea that women are simply socialized to accept and internalize 'dominant values'. Such theories of 'oppressive socialization' assume that patriarchy (and technocracy) pervert a prior and natural reality, and are frequently, and appropriately, criticized as treating women's choice to utilize technology as a kind of false consciousness. By contrast, deep social constructionism allows us to think about the complex ways in which women's assessments of risk, their hopes, and their aspirations are socially produced (Hirschmann, 2003: 80). There is ample reason to suspect that both the devaluation of women and medical interests are relevant to those processes.

The question then becomes how to assess women's choices, for if choice can never express an authentic or pre-social self, on what grounds can we assess women's choices to elect (or not) obstetric technology? Third wave critics are correct, I think, to argue that we cannot assess the validity of the idioms of 'the natural' or 'the medical' by ascertaining which of these idioms more closely approximates the 'reality' of women's bodies or childbirth; these are conceptual and cultural categories rather than empirically testable propositions. On the other hand, the historical context, political purposes, bodily effects, and material consequences of these discourses cannot be ignored. Consideration of these consequences allows us to begin to assess the validity of the 'high-tech' approach to childbirth.

Contextualizing medicine and medicalization

One of the most powerful aspects of the third wave critique is the recognition that 'the natural' is as much a cultural category as 'the medical', and that attempts to revive traditional birthing practices or legitimate new ones *on the grounds that those practices more closely approximate 'nature'* are misguided. Thus, we cannot choose between the notion that childbirth *is* natural or that it *is* disease-like on philosophical or abstract grounds. Rather, birth *is* natural for those who define and experience it as such; it *is* medical for those who define and experience it in that manner (Treichler, 1990).

On the other hand, the practices associated with treating childbirth *as if* it were medical or natural in nature can and should be evaluated. Many women want to know, for example, what the medical research shows about the risks and benefits of elective Cesarean section (the existence of which rests on the notion that C-section and vaginal delivery are alternative medical treatments), as well as pharmacological pain relief, induction, and other common obstetric procedures. Although inevitably partial and imperfect, the information that accrues from evaluations of these procedures is crucial to women hoping to make informed choices regarding the place and manner of their birth deliveries, as well as to the development of sound public health policy.

Yet there is ample evidence that this information cannot be communicated (or obtained) in anything approaching Habermas's free speech conditions. Most women depend on their doctors for information about the risks and benefits associated with different birthing practices, but physicians and hospitals have their own set of interests (inconvenience, profitability, liability reduction) that shape the way this information is packaged and presented to birthing women (Armstrong, 2000). In addition, medical research is reinterpreted in highly selective ways to support current obstetrical dogma (Goer, 1995, 2001). The fact that much existing medical research suggests that high levels of obstetric intervention do cause a great deal of harm, and evidence that women are not informed of these risks, is not addressed by third wave critics of the alternative birth movement. In sum, although the rhetoric of 'the natural' and the notion that medical technology is inherently male are problematic, limiting the feminist critique to these discursive issues does not address women's quite practical need for information regarding various birthing options or the difficulty of providing women with access to that information in a disinterested fashion.

Similarly, the third wave critique fails to address the ways in which the idioms of 'the medical' and 'the natural' support and sustain quite different professional/political projects. Although third wave critics are prescient to point out that midwifery is not synonymous with feminism or birthing women's interests, it would be a mistake to therefore assume that there is no association between the two, for two reasons. First, in the United States and most other Western countries, physician-attended hospital birth is the norm, and the option of midwife-attended home birth is highly restricted by law as well as by health and malpractice insurance practices. Because definitions of 'normal' birth are comparatively narrow and the use of technology common in hospitals, medical knowledge derives from bodies that birth in more circumscribed ways (Rothman, 1982). The preservation of midwifery and home birth is therefore crucially important for the generation of an alternative body of knowledge that allows us to subject obstetrical knowledge to analysis and critique.

For example, doctors now routinely diagnose a woman who has been in labour for 10 to 12 hours as having 'dystocia' (i.e. prolonged labour), and this diagnosis has become one of the leading indications for Cesarean section. Midwives working in out-of-hospital settings can effectively challenge this diagnosis by pointing out that many women, and a majority of first-time mothers, labour 'successfully' for longer than 10 hours. Without this kind of comparative information, the ability to critically assess obstetrical knowledge and the way that it reflects both obstetrical practices and interests is severely compromised.

Of course, the preservation of midwifery and out-of-hospital birth is also important because women should have the right to choose the place and manner of their birth deliveries; this is an important dimension of reproductive autonomy. The need to protect this choice is all the more important for the epistemological reasons just outlined. In short, the preservation of midwifery and out-of-hospital birth is necessary to ensure reproductive choice and because these practices give rise to an alternative body of knowledge that enables us to critically assess the viability of medical knowledge about women's bodies. In what follows, I discuss the importance of doing so.

Contextualizing medical technology

As has been discussed, third wave critics argue that medical technology is not inherently patriarchal or male, and can therefore be used by women for emancipatory purposes. Yet one need not make the argument that medical technology is *inherently* patriarchal or male to make the case that this emancipatory potential is, in the current social context, limited.

As many analysts have pointed out, the meanings, purposes, and effects of technology largely, though not exclusively, reflect the context in which that technology is developed and used. As one author put it, technologies 'do not fall from heaven ... and they are not neutral. In other words, a "technology" is not objective: it carries embedded in it a vision of the world and of what is considered important and valuable for the particular society where it is developed' (Arditti et al., 1984: xii). Although users may alter technologies, their usage, their meanings, and their effects (Akrich, 1992; Winner, 1986), this indeterminacy is not infinite. In this case, the importance of reproductive technology in the re-emergence of 'foetal polities', to the establishment and perpetuation of medical authority and profitability, and to the inequitable allocation of health care resources necessarily complicate its emancipatory potential. Each of these constraints is considered below.

Noting that the image of the foetus as a person separate from the mother-to-be is a central component of patriarchal ideology, many feminist analysts have argued that recent advances in reproductive technologies have played a crucial role in reviving and strengthening this conception of women's role in the reproductive process (as well as the related notion that the primary threat to foetal health comes from its 'maternal environment') (Rothman, 1987). In the images generated by many of these technologies, the foetus is separated from rather than connected to the pregnant woman, and the split between the foetus and mother – so prominent in patriarchal ideology – is reified (Hubbard, 1990; Spallone, 1989). The conception of the foetus as a 'second patient' has, in turn, given rise to a conception of pregnancy as a conflict of rights between a woman and her foetus and the sense that the primary threat to foetal health comes from pregnant women (Arney, 1982; Blank, 1984; Hubbard, 1990; Rothman, 1987; Spallone, 1989).

The debate over elective Cesarean invokes much of this imagery. There is evidence that some women choose Cesarean section – either in anticipation of their labour or in response to unanticipated developments during it – because they are told that this choice ensures the safety of their foetus/newborn. Not only does this advice often overstate the risks of vaginal delivery and understate those associated with surgical delivery, it plays on, and contributes to, the sense that 'good mothers' are willing to assume the risks of a surgical delivery. As one obstetrician and mother wrote in a high profile women's magazine, 'Maternal deaths due to C-sections are two to four times greater than those due to vaginal deliveries', but . . . 'when the rare problem occurs during a vaginal birth, it's the baby who's most likely to be harmed'. The choice of elective Cesarean section, she explains, 'gave her kids the best possible chance for a safe birth' (Freiman, 2000). The (quite controversial) study upon which Dr Freiman based her claims went on to calculate the number of infants who could be saved from 'birthing disasters' if more women elected to give birth surgically for the sake of their children. (Apparently, maternal death does not constitute a birthing disaster.)

Although controversial, this argument rests on a pervasive cultural logic; indeed, a recent editorial in a high-ranking medical journal argued that all women should deliver surgically in order to enhance the well-being of newborns. This proposal is not likely to be taken seriously, at least in the near term, but the message it reflects and conveys is both popular and powerful: good mothers make sacrifices for their children, and surgical birth may be one of those sacrifices. As Barbara Katz Rothman (1982) suggests in her discussion of prenatal testing, the increasing ubiquity of reproductive technology makes it more difficult to refuse it, for doing so is likely to be constructed and perceived as a 'selfish' choice that puts the foetus/newborn at risk.

The role of medical technology in the establishment and perpetuation of medical authority also complicates women's efforts to deploy obstetric technologies for their own purposes. Medical authority and control is partially sustained by doctors' expertise in the administration and interpretation of medical technology. As Jordan has argued, the medical 'ownership' of obstetric technology and technical procedures 'simultaneously defines and displays who should be seen as possessing authoritative knowledge, and consequently as holding legitimate decision-making power' (1997: 61; see also Rothman, 1989; Weir, 1996). To note the historical and political context in which obstetric technology is deployed does not imply that women cannot meaningfully choose and/or benefit from the utilization of obstetric technology. On the other hand, the recognition that technology is not inherently patriarchal does not mean that it is neutral. Medical technology may not be essentially male, but its development and use under existing historical conditions means that its use for feminist purposes is necessarily fraught with difficulty.

Perhaps the most important reason why an untempered emphasis on the emancipatory potential of obstetric technology is problematic is this: widespread use of this technology contributes significantly to the unequal distribution of health care resources, the existence of which is often overlooked in debates over the elective use of obstetrical technologies. For example, some supporters of elective Cesarean assert that the grounds upon which women choose to deliver surgically are irrelevant, and that their right to choose the mode of their delivery is absolute: 'In Brazil, C-sections are routinely done for aesthetic and sexual reasons... Many American women would dismiss this thinking as superficial, and maybe it is. But every woman has the right to make her birthing decision based on what's most important to her' (Freiman, 2000). This position overlooks the fact that many Brazilian women choose Cesarean for fear of the consequence of highly interventionist care during vaginal delivery, the epistemological and political issues raised previously, and the fact that obstetric technologies, including elective Cesarean, are quite costly. As one prominent opponent of elective Cesarean explains:

> A CS [Cesarean section] which is done because a woman chooses it requires a surgeon, possibly a second doctor to assist, an anesthesiologist, surgical nurses, equipment, an operating theatre, blood ready for transfusion if necessary, a longer post-operative hospital stay, etc. This costs a good deal of money and, equally importantly, a great deal of training of health personnel, most of which is at government expense, even if the CS is done by a private physician in a private hospital. If a woman receives an elective CS simply because she prefers it, there will be less human and financial resources for the rest of health care.
>
> (Wagner, 2000: 1679)

Researchers investigating the costs of unnecessary C-section have concluded 'The high cesarean section rate in the United States is a major public health problem, one that is having and will continue to have a major impact on health care delivery. If the $800 million that could be saved by reducing the cesarean section rate by 5% were spent instead on prenatal care and preventative programs, dramatic effects on maternal and child health would be seen' (Sachs, 1989: 38). Not surprisingly, high rates of Cesarean section in Brazil are associated not only with escalating rates of maternal mortality, but also with increasing inequities in the delivery of health care (Wagner, 2000). The Brazilian case, though extreme, is quite relevant, as Western countries aggressively export the high-tech approach to health care and childbirth in particular, and many developing countries seek to emulate its example.

In short, even if, somehow, women's choice of/consent to obstetric intervention were based on full understanding of the attendant medical risks and on criteria consistent with the feminist commitment to women's integrity and autonomy, the cost of elective obstetric intervention would worsen the already unjust distribution of health care resources, a pattern that has very real and important consequences in both the United States and elsewhere. Recognition of women's capacity to experience technology as empowering ought not to preclude consideration of broader areas of justice and equity, and of the need for the judicious use of health resources.

Conclusion

Although offering quite disparate analyses, each of the three waves of feminist reflection on childbirth in the United States is aimed at empowering birthing women and destabilizing dominant understandings of childbirth. This preoccupation with challenging previously hegemonic assumptions and practices reflects the feminist commitment to enhancing women's capacity to make meaningful choices, and to increasing the likelihood that women will be supported in and empowered by those choices. Here, though, the feminist consensus regarding childbirth appears to end.

There is much to be said for recent feminist criticism of the alternative birth movement. That movement's invocation of 'the natural', while understandable in historical terms, is often essentialist, and critics are right to point out that its invocation reproduces the cultural categories and assumptions that have historically justified male domination. The related notion that the widespread use of pharmaceutical pain relief is a consequence of obstetric propaganda and women's attendant lack of confidence in their (natural) bodies clearly oversimplifies the matter: midwives have historically used many techniques to minimize the pain of childbirth, and women have long expressed a great deal of trepidation and anxiety about it (Leavitt, 1983, 1986; Leavitt and Walton, 1984; Wertz and Wertz, 1977). The insistence that women can/should/do find the pain of childbirth to be empowering neglects the diversity of women's bodies and experiences, and deflects rather than grapples with the possibility that medical technology may, in some instances, serve women's interests.

On the other hand, unreflective invocations of women's choice and positive experience of technology as a corrective to the idiom of 'the natural' are a fragile foundation upon which to build an alternative feminist politics of childbirth. As Alcoff (1994) argues, the emphasis on the importance of resisting and deconstructing the binary categories that have buttressed male domination is not sufficient, for, alone, it leaves us with only a 'negative' feminism, the capacity to deconstruct, but an inability to construct. Further, it is not just abstract discourses that cry out for deconstruction and analysis, but also the social and political contexts in which women make choices. Although the choice/positive experience of obstetric technology ought not to be construed as false consciousness or women's misrecognition of their true nature, it is clear that women often (though not always) make such choices based on inadequate and interested sources of information, as well as subtle and not-so-subtle invocations of women's obligation to make significant sacrifices on behalf of their sexual partners and children-to-be. The situations in which women make these choices therefore require analysis and critique; the failure to do so obscures the way in which the quest for profit, medical interests, and the legacy of patriarchy complicate women's efforts to use technology for their own purposes and continue to influence women's definition of what those purposes are and should be.

This argument does not imply that technology can never be used to advance feminist purposes. In fact, many women's appreciation of pharmaceutical pain relief, despite awareness of some of its less positive consequences, suggests that women are sometimes able to influence medical practice and technological development, and to deploy that technology for their own ends. But it is important to recognize that the actualization of this possibility is inevitably fraught with danger: the danger that women's positive assessment of their experience with medical technology is based in part on a lack of awareness of its risks, and that women's choices may be shaped by social relations and dynamics that subordinate women's needs and interests.[6]

Third wave critics of the alternative birth movement also overstate the equivalence of medical rhetoric and the idiom of the natural. These discourses *are* analogous in the sense that they serve to render birth comprehensible and meaningful, and insofar as they reflect and sustain various childbirth practices. But as Foucault reminds us, discourses serve primarily to legitimate *practices* that have very real bodily and material consequences. Indeed, the discourses of 'the natural' and 'the medical' reflect and sustain different childbirth practices that generate different knowledges about women's bodies and have very different consequences for women and their babies, as well as for the distribution of health care resources. These consequences must also be considered, and if the available evidence is even partially correct, medicalization per se might be problematic after all. Indeed, there is overwhelming evidence that the social organization and practices of independent midwifery are more consistent with women's interest in their own health and well-being, the health and well-being of their babies, and, more indirectly, all consumers of health care resources that are affected by the injudicious use of those resources. Its existence also generates a body of knowledge that can be used to assess and critique obstetrical knowledge of birthing women; without it, the capacity to do so would be undermined.

Moreover, the notion that the alternative birth movement/culture has successfully challenged medical hegemony is misleading. Although the discourse and values of the alternative birth movement may have more cultural representation and appeal than its proponents aver (and may, as a result, induce guilt in some), the overwhelming majority of births remain highly medicalized, and even women who aspire to 'natural birth' experience significant medical intervention in the end (Declercq et al., 2002). In short, medicalization at the epistemological/cultural level is not the same as medicalization at the level of practice; in the realm of the latter, medicalization is stronger than ever.

Although childbirth has become comparatively safe for most women living in developed countries, some contemporary obstetrical practices pose serious threats to women and newborns and, by consuming significant medical resources, contribute to inequities in health and health care. Furthermore, Western obstetrical practices are aggressively promoted around the globe, and, if adopted, contribute to the injudicious use of health care resources in even more profound ways. While the essentializing and moralistic rhetoric of the alternative birth movement should be abandoned, its critique of contemporary obstetrics, commitment to women's and children's health, and thoughtful use of health care resources are essential to the reconstruction of a feminist politics of and theoretical approach to childbirth.

Notes

1 While some feminists focused their attention on women's right to pain relief during labour, other women's and public health organizations were more concerned about unequal access to obstetric services, and advocated increased government funding for maternity care to remedy this situation.
2 International comparisons also support this argument. At a time when the British Cesarean section rate was half that in the US (12% versus 24 per cent), its prenatal mortality rate was lower than that of the US (8.0 versus 9.6 per 1,000). Even more dramatically, a 5 per cent Cesarean section rate in the Netherlands was associated with a perinatal mortality rate of 6.5 per 1,000 (Kubasek, 1997).
3 Medical research generally supports this contention: women who opt for an epidural have lower rates of spontaneous vaginal delivery, longer labours, and are more likely to have intra-partum fever; their infants are at increased risk of sepsis (Lieberman and O'Donoghue, 2002). Similarly, induction of labour increases the risk of uterine rupture and the likelihood of Cesarean section (Goer, 1995; Wagner, 2000; Walling, 2000).
4 Recently, a small number of renegade birth activists in the United States have identified unassisted birth as a more natural and empowering alternative to midwife-attended home birth (see http://www.freebirth.com and http://www.unassistedbirth.com).
5 Nearly half of all physicians surveyed believe that judicial force should be used to impose treatment of unconsenting pregnant women if persuasion is unsuccessful (Ouellette, 1994).
6 In making this argument, I implicitly accept hooks' (1989) contention that not every woman with a theory is feminist, and that 'the "anything goes" approach to the term [feminism] renders it practically meaningless'. See also Lublin (1998).

References

Akrich, Madeleine (1992) 'The De-inscription of Technical Objects', pp. 205–24 in Wiebe E. Bijker and John Law (eds) *Shaping Technology/Building Society*. Cambridge, MA: MIT Press.

Alcoff, Linda (1994) 'Cultural Feminism versus Post-Structuralism: The Identity Crisis in Feminist Theory', pp. 96–122 in Nicholas B. Dirks, Geoff Eley and Sherry Ortner (eds) *Culture/Power/History: A Reader in Contemporary Social Theory*. Princeton, NJ: Princeton University Press.

Annandale, Ellen and Judith Clark (1996) 'What is Gender? Feminist Theory and the Sociology of Human Reproduction', *Sociology on Health & Illness* 18(1): 17–44.

Arditti, Rita, Renate Duelli Klein and Shelly Monden, eds (1984) *Test Tube Women*. London: Pandora Press.

Arms, Suzanne (1994) *Immaculate Deception II: Myth, Magic, & Birth*. Berkeley, CA: Celestial Arts.

Armstrong, Elizabeth M. (2000) 'Lessons in Control: Prenatal Education in the Hospital', *Social Problems* 47(4): 583–605.

Arney, William Ray (1982) *Power and the Profession of Obstetrics*. Chicago: University of Chicago Press.

Beckett, Katherine and Bruce Hoffman (2005) 'Challenging Medicine: Law, Resistance, and the Cultural Politics of Childbirth', *Law and Society Review* 39(5): 125–69.

Biesele, Megan (1997) 'The Ideal of Unassisted Birth: Hunting, Healing, and Transformation Among the Kalahari Ju/hoansi', pp. 474–92 in Robbie E. Davis-Floyd and Carolyn F. Sargent (eds) *Childbirth and Authoritative Knowledge: Cross-Cultural Perspectives*. Berkeley, CA: University of California Press.

Blank, Robert (1984) *Redefining Human Life: Reproductive Technologies and Social Policy*. Boulder, CO: Westview Press.

Campbell, Rona and Sam Porter (1997) 'Feminist Theory and the Sociology of Childbirth: A Response to Ellen Annandale and Judith Clark', *Sociology on Health & Illness* 19(3): 348–58.

Canton, Donald (1999) *What a Blessing She Had Chloroform: The Medical and Social Response to the Pain of Childbirth from 1800 to the Present*. New Haven, CT: Yale University Press.

Daly, Mary (1978) *Gyn/Ecology: The Metaethics of Radical Feminism*. Boston, MA: Beacon Press.

Davis-Floyd, Robbie E. (1992) *Birth as an American Rite of Passage*. Berkeley, CA: University of California Press.

Davis-Floyd, Robbie E. and Elizabeth Davis (1997) 'Intuition in Midwifery and Home Birth', pp. 315–49 in Robbie E. Davis-Floyd and Carolyn F. Sargent (eds) *Childbirth and Authoritative Knowledge: Cross-Cultural Perspectives*. Berkeley, CA: University of California Press.

Davis-Floyd, Robbie E. and Carolyn F. Sargent, eds (1997) *Childbirth and Authoritative Knowledge: Cross-Cultural Perspectives*. Berkeley, CA: University of California Press.

Declercq, Eugene R., Carol Sakala, Maureen P. Corry, Sandra Applebaum and Peter Risher (2002) *Listening to Mothers: Report of the First National U.S. Survey of*

Women's Childbearing Experiences. Conducted by Harris Interactive for the Maternity Center Association.

DeVries, Raymond (1996) *Making Midwives Legal: Childbirth, Medicine, and the Law,* 2nd edn. Columbus, OH: Ohio State University Press.

Dick-Read, Grantley (1959) *Birth Without Fear,* 2nd edn. New York: Harper & Row.

Donegan, Jane B. (1984) '"Safe Delivered," but by Whom? Midwives and Men-midwives in Early America', pp. 302–17 in Judith Walzer Leavitt (ed.) *Women and Health in America: Historical Readings.* Madison, WI: University of Wisconsin Press.

Edwards, Margot and Mary Waldorf (1984) *Reclaiming Birth: History and Heroines of American Childbirth Reform.* New York: The Crossing Press.

Ehrenreich, Barbara and Deirdre English (1973) *Witches, Midwives, and Healers: A History of Women Healers.* Old Westbury, NY: The Feminist Press.

Elliott, Victoria Stagg (2001) 'Ob-gyns Address Pressure to Lower C-Section Rate', *American Medical News* 28 May, pp. 14–15.

Freiman, Jennie (2000) 'Why I Wanted a C-section', *Self (New York)* 22(6): 96.

Gaskin, Ina May (1975) *Spiritual Midwifery,* 3rd edn. Summertown, TN: The Book Publishing Company.

Goer, Henci (1995) *Obstetric Myths versus Research Realities: A Guide to the Medical Literature.* Westport, CT: Bergin & Garvey.

Goer, Henci (2001) 'The Case against Elective Cesarean Section', *Journal of Perinatal and Neonatal Nursing* 15(3): 23–38.

Gould, Jeffrey B., Becky Davey and Randall S. Stafford (1989) 'Socioeconomic Differences in Rates of Cesarean Section', *New England Journal of Medicine* 321(4): 233–9.

Grisanti, Mary Lee (1989) 'The Cesarean Epidemic', *New York* 22: 56–61.

Grobman, William (2002) 'Broad-based Conversion to Elective Cesarean Not Justified', *Female Patient* 27(5): 19 and 25.

Hirschmann, Nancy J. (2003) *The Subject of Liberty: Toward a Feminist Theory of Freedom.* Princeton, NJ: Princeton University Press.

hooks, bell (1989) *Talking Back: Thinking Feminist, Thinking Black.* Boston: South End Press.

Hubbard, Ruth (1990) *The Politics of Women's Biology.* New Brunswick, NJ: Rutgers University Press.

Jordan, Brigette (1983) *Birth in Four Cultures,* 2nd edn. Montreal: Eden Press.

Jordan, Brigette (1997) 'Authoritative Knowledge and its Construction', pp. 55–79 in Robbie E. Davis-Floyd, and Carolyn F. Sargent (eds) *Childbirth and Authoritative Knowledge: Cross-Cultural Perspectives.* Berkeley, CA: University of California Press.

Keefe, Carolyn (2002) 'Overview of Maternity Care in the U.S.' URL: http://www.cfmidwifery.org/pdf/OverviewofMatCare2000data1.pdf.

Kitzinger, Sheila (1981) *Sheila Kitzinger's Birth Book.* New York: Grosset and Dunlap.

Kobrin, Frances E. (1984) 'The American Midwife Controversy: A Crisis of Professionalization', pp. 318–26 in Judith Walzer Leavitt (ed.) *Women and Health in America: Historical Readings.* Madison, WI: University of Wisconsin Press.

Kubasek, Nancy K. (1997) 'Legislative Approaches to Reducing the Hegemony of the Priestly Model of Medicine', *Michigan Journal of Gender and Law* 4: 375–442.

Leavitt, Judith Walzer (1983) 'Science Enters the Birthing Room: Obstetrics in America since the Eighteenth Century', *The Journal of American History* 70(2): 281–304.

Leavitt, Judith Walzer (1984) 'Birthing and Anesthesia: The Debate Over Twilight Sleep', pp. 175–84 in Judith Walzer Leavitt (ed.) *Women and Health in America: Historical Readings*. Madison, WI: University of Wisconsin Press.

Leavitt, Judith Walzer (1986) 'Under the Shadow of Maternity: American Women's Responses to Death and Debility Fears in Nineteenth-Century Childbirth', *Feminist Studies* 12(Spring): 129–54.

Leavitt, Judith Walzer and Whitney Walton (1984) 'Down to Death's Door: Women's Perceptions of Childbirth in America', pp. 155–65 in Judith Walzer Leavitt (ed.) *Women and Health in America: Historical Readings*. Madison, WI: University of Wisconsin Press.

Lent, Margaret (1999) 'The Medical and Legal Risks of the Electronic Fetal Monitor', *Stanford Law Review* 51(April): 807.

Lieberman, E. and C. O'Donoghue (2002) 'Unintended Effects of Epidural Analgesia During Labor: A Systematic Review', *American Journal of Obstetrics and Gynecology* 186(May): 78–80.

Lublin, Nancy (1998) *Pandora's Box: Feminism Confronts Reproductive Technology*. Oxford: Rowman & Littlefield.

Martin, Emily (1992 [1987]) *The Woman in the Body: A Cultural Analysis of Reproduction*, 2nd edn. Boston: Beacon Press.

Michie, Helena (1998) 'Confinements: The Domestic in the Discourse of Upper-Middle Class Pregnancy', pp. 258–73 in Susan Hardy Aiken, Ann Brigham, Sallie A. Marston and Penny Waterston (eds) *Making Worlds*. Tucson, AZ: University of Arizona Press.

Michie, Helena and Naomi R. Cahn (1996) 'Unnatural Births: Cesarean Sections in the Discourse of the "Natural Childbirth" Movement', pp. 44–55 in Carolyn F. Sargent and Caroline B. Brettell (eds) *Gender and Health: An International Perspective*. Englewood Cliffs, NJ: Prentice Hall.

Moon, Susanna (2002) 'C-section Rebirth; Procedure Making Strong Comeback After a Decade', *Modern Healthcare* 32: 18.

National Organization of Women (1999) 'Resolution: "Expansion of Reproductive Freedom to Include Midwives Model of Care"'. URL: http://www.cfmidwifery.org/Resources/item.aspx?ID=25† (accessed 11 July 2005).

Nestle, Sheryl (2000) 'Delivering Subjects: Race, Space, and the Emergence of Legalized Midwifery in Ontario', *Canadian Journal of Law and Society* 15(2): 187–215.

Oakley, Ann (1980) *Women Confined: Towards a Sociology of Childbirth*. New York: Schocken Books.

Oakley, Ann (1993) *Essays on Women, Medicine and Health*. Edinburgh: Edinburgh University Press.

Ouellette, Alicia (1994) 'New Medical Technology: A Chance to Re-Examine Court-Ordered Medical Procedures during Pregnancy', *Albany Law Review* 57–119.

Reissman, Catherine Kohler (1983) 'Women and Medicalization: A New Perspective', *Social Policy* 14(1): 3–18.

Rooks, Judith Pence (1997) *Midwifery and Childbirth in America*. Philadelphia, PA: Temple University Press.

Rothman, Barbara Katz (1982) *In Labor: Women and Power in the Birthplace*. New York: W.W. Norton.

Rothman, Barbara Katz (1987) 'Reproduction', pp. 154–70 in Beth B. Hess and Myra Marx Ferree (eds) *Analyzing Gender: A Handbook of Social Science Research*. Beverly Hills, CA: SAGE Publications.

Rothman, Barbara Katz (1989) *Recreating Motherhood: Ideology and Technology in Patriarchal Society*. New York: W.W. Norton.

Sachs, Benjamin (1989) 'Is the Rising Rate of Cesarean Sections a Result of More Defensive Medicine?', pp. 27–40 in Victoria P. Rostow and Roger J. Bulger (eds) *Medical Professional Liability and the Delivery of Obstetrical Care*. Committee to Study Medical Professional Liability and the Delivery of Obstetrical Care, Division of Health Promotion and Disease Prevention, Institute of Medicine. Washington, DC: National Academy Press.

Sakala, Carol (1993) 'Medically Unnecessary Cesarean Section Births', *Social Science & Medicine* 37(10): 1177–98.

Scholten, Catherine M. (1984) 'On the Importance of the Obstetrick Art: Changing Customs of Childbirth in America, 1760–1825', pp. 426–45 in Judith Walzer Leavitt (ed.) *Women and Health in America: Historical Readings*. Madison, WI: University of Wisconsin Press.

Shapiro, Nina (1998) 'Birth Control', *Seattle Weekly* 26 September.

Spallone, Patricia (1989) *Beyond Conception: The New Politics of Reproduction*. Westport, CT: Bergin and Garvey.

Sullivan, Deborah A. and Rose Weitz (1988) *Labor Pains: Modern Midwives and Home Birth*. New Haven, CT: Yale University Press.

Talbot, Margaret (1999) 'Pay on Delivery', *New York Times Magazine* 31 October, pp. 19–20.

Treichler, Paula A. (1990) 'Feminism, Medicine, and the Meaning of Childbirth', pp. 129–38 in Mary Jacobus, Evelyn Fox Keller and Sally Shuttleworth (eds) *Body/Politics: Women and the Discourses of Science*. New York: Routledge.

Umansky, Lauri (1996) *Motherhood Reconceived: Feminism and the Legacy of the Sixties*. New York: New York University Press.

Wagner, Marsden (1997) 'Confessions of a Dissident', pp. 366–98 in Robbie E. Davis-Floyd and Carolyn F. Sargent (eds) *Childbirth and Authoritative Knowledge: Cross-Cultural Perspectives*. Berkeley, CA: University of California Press.

Wagner, Marsden (2000) 'Choosing Cesarean Section', *The Lancet* 356(9242): 1677–80.

Walling, Anne D. (2000) 'Elective Cesarean Doubles Cesarean Delivery Rate', *American Family Physician* 61(4): 1173–6.

Walters, D. Campbell (1998) *Just Take it Out: The Ethics and Economics of Cesarean Section and Hysterectomy*. Mt Vernon, IL: Topiary Publishing.

Weir, Lorna (1996) 'Recent Developments in the Government of Pregnancy', *Economy and Society* 25(3): 372–92.

Wertz, Richard W. and Dorothy C. Wertz (1977) *Lying In: A History of Childbirth in America*. New York: The Free Press.

Winner, Langdon (1986) *The Whale and the Reactor: A Search for Limits in the Age of High Technology*. Chicago: Chicago University Press.

Young, Diony (2001) 'Maternal Choice and Elective Cesarean', *Network News* July/August.

61
DOING HEALTH, DOING GENDER
Teenagers, diabetes and asthma

Clare Williams

Source: *Social Science & Medicine*, 50 (2000), 387–96.

Abstract

Although most research linking health disadvantage with gender has focused on women, recent work indicates that hegemonic masculinities can also place the health of men at risk. The importance of comparing the experiences of women and men has been emphasised and this paper focuses on the ways in which the social constructions of femininities and masculinities affect how teenagers live with asthma or diabetes. The majority of girls incorporated these conditions and the associated treatment regimens into their social and personal identities, showing a greater adaptability to living with asthma or diabetes. However, this could have detrimental effects in terms of control, as girls sometimes lowered expectations for themselves. In addition, two aspects of the treatment regimens, diet and exercise, were found to disadvantage girls and advantage boys, because of contemporary meanings of femininities and masculinities. The social construction of femininities meant that these conditions were not seen as the threat that they were by the majority of boys interviewed, who made every effort to keep both conditions outside their personal and social identities by passing. The majority of boys maintained a 'valued' identity by feeling in control of their body and their condition. However, for the small minority of boys who were no longer able to pass the impact of chronic illness led to a 'disparaged' identity. The interaction of gender and health is seen as a complex two-way process, with aspects of contemporary femininities and masculinities impacting on the management of these conditions, and aspects of these conditions impacting in gendered ways upon the constructions of gender.

© 1999 Elsevier Science Ltd. All rights reserved.

Introduction

This paper explores the interaction of gender with the management of chronic illness during adolescence, focusing on the ways in which the social constructions of femininities and masculinities affects how young people live with asthma or diabetes. The majority of research linking health disadvantage with gender has focused on women (Nathanson, 1975), but more recent research such as that by Cameron and Bernardes (1998) indicates that hegemonic masculinities can also place the health of men at risk, both in terms of being a risk factor in the aetiology of disease, and in the ways in which men manage illness. The importance of comparing the experiences of women and men has recently been highlighted (Verbrugge, 1997) and Charmaz (1995, p. 287) states:

> As the research in chronic illness grows, studying men and women comparatively in conjunction with marital, age and social class statuses, in addition to type of illness, can substantially refine sociological interpretations of the narratives of chronically ill people.

The paper aims to make a contribution to the literature by exploring how teenage girls and boys live with and manage two different conditions. Young people with asthma or diabetes were interviewed as they are both conditions requiring high levels of self-care, which can also have similar high levels of personal responsibility for 'juggling' treatment (Bytheway and Furth, 1996). In terms of the control of both asthma and diabetes, it appears that the mid-teens is a critical time when control worsens, particularly for young women (Gregg, 1983; Pond et al., 1996), which fits in with the overall pattern of a gradual emergence of excess morbidity in females during adolescence (Sweeting, 1995).

A central theme to be explored is the way in which the teenagers in this study incorporated asthma and diabetes into their personal and social identities. These terms were developed by Adams et al. (1997) based upon Mead's (1961) analysis of the self, particularly his dialectic between the 'I' which they termed "personal identity" and the 'me' or "social identity", conceptualised as "the sum of an individual's group memberships, interpersonal relationships, social positions and statuses" (Adams et al., 1997, p. 199). This is a key issue because the gendered ways in which specific illnesses impact on the personal and social identities of individuals can affect how they choose to live with the illness, including the management of medication regimens. As Saltonstall (1993, p. 12) states:

> ... the doing of health is a form of doing gender. This is not because there is an essential difference between male and female body healthiness, but because of social and cultural interpretations of masculine

and feminine selves — selves which are attached to biological male and female bodies. Health activities can be seen as a form of practice which constructs the subject (the 'person') in the same way that other social and cultural activities do.

It has been argued that chronic illnesses, with their unpredictable trajectories and uncertainties (Bury, 1991) may particularly threaten dominant masculinity, which is characterised by self-control, independence and self-sufficiency (Seidler, 1998). Arguably the threat may be greatest during adolescence, which Prendergast (1995) describes as the time when heterosexual values are most powerfully pursued and enforced. However Miller et al. (1993) found the social practice of masculinities to be beneficial in key aspects of cystic fibrosis management. For example, because of the importance of sport and exercise to the social construction of masculinities, many of the boys interviewed were engaged in considerable amounts of exercise, which benefited their condition. Although all of the young people were aware of their reduced life expectancy, the young men dealt with this by 'putting it to one side' and by generally being less willing than the girls to incorporate cystic fibrosis into their social identities. The young men were also found to maintain a more positive attitude in their everyday experiences of living with cystic fibrosis, expressing a greater sense of control over their health and lives than did the girls.

When exploring the effect of chronic illness on the gendered identity of adults, Charmaz (1995) found that the social construction of masculinities could have both beneficial and adverse effects. Many of the men she interviewed attempted to conceal their illness, particularly in public settings, and drawing on the work of Connell (1987) to help explain their behaviour, she states that chronic illness can "relegate a man to a position of 'marginalized' masculinity in the gender order" (Charmaz, 1995, p. 268). Charmaz (1995, p. 286) also argues that although traditional assumptions of male identities can encourage men to recover from illness, such assumptions can lead to a narrow range of 'credible' behaviours for men, in that "an uneasy tension exists between valued identities and disparaged, that is, denigrated or shameful ones".

In contrast, women are often perceived as more able to cope with ill health than men because of the stereotypical expectations of femininity as being adaptive and passive (Coppock et al., 1995). Charmaz (1995) found that women with a chronic illness generally showed a greater adaptability than men, and that women "rarely persisted in tying their futures to recapturing their past selves when they defined physical changes as permanent" (Charmaz, 1995, p. 280). However, Miller et al. (1993) found that the teenage girls in their study were less likely than the boys to experience a sense of positiveness in relation to their everyday experience of living with cystic fibrosis, which they felt was due to the social practice of femininity. This led to passivity, feelings of powerlessness and an emphasis on attractiveness which in turn led to a decline in health status, with the lack of physical activity and the need to be attractive rather than active having a powerful adverse effect on morbidity.

Stigma is closely linked with gender and illness management. In his research on children, Prout (1989) found the stigmatising effects of illness to be gendered. For boys, illness could be an isolating and threatening experience and Prout (1989, p. 350) noted the accusation of 'skiving' which greeted almost every boy on his return to school, stating that, "it underlined a basic feature of the boys' culture, that being physically fit and tough was highly valued and that sickness... was a stigmatising form of weakness and incompetence". In contrast, Prout (1989) found that sickness was seen as something quite different for girls, with the 'best friend' group being mobilised and visits being made to the girl's home. Goffman (1963) described a variety of coping strategies which related mainly to whether or not the stigma was obvious to others (discrediting), or could be hidden from others (discreditable). Someone with a potentially stigmatising condition such as diabetes or asthma has the option of trying to hide it, and one of the main coping strategies which Goffman (1963) described as being used in this situation is 'passing', which entails trying to pass as 'normal' with the constant risk of exposure.

The extent to which individuals choose to pass may also impact on adherence to treatment regimens. Much of the professional literature on 'non-compliance' is based on the premise that it is deviant behaviour, leading to the blaming of patients (Donovan and Blake, 1992), with the 'compliance' of young people identified as particularly problematic by health care professionals (Klingelhofer, 1987; Pond et al., 1996). In contrast, Conrad (1985) argues that from the patient's viewpoint, altering medication can be seen as an attempt by the individual to assert some control over their illness, and he sees the modification of medicine as 'active self-regulation' rather than non-compliance.

It appears that the social constructions of femininities and masculinities may interact in complex ways with overarching concepts impacting on chronic illness, such as stigma and compliance, as well as with more specific aspects relating to the management of particular chronic illnesses. By exploring the extent to which teenage girls and boys incorporate asthma and diabetes into their identities, and how this impacts on the ways in which they live with and manage these different conditions, the paper aims to help begin unravelling these issues.

The study

This paper reports on part of a larger project which explored how teenagers with asthma or diabetes negotiated responsibility for self-care with their main carer, usually their mother (Williams, 1998). In depth interviews were conducted with 20 young people aged between 15 and 18 years with asthma, and 20 with diabetes (10 females and 10 males in each group). Interviews were also carried out with the parent most involved in helping the young person manage the chronic illness, who in all cases except one was the mother. The young person and parent were interviewed separately, usually consecutively, and all (except one) of the interviews were conducted in their homes.

Nearly all cases of diabetes occurring in children and young people are of the insulin-dependent, or 'Type 1' category. All of the young people interviewed had insulin-dependent diabetes, where there is a severe lack of insulin, and daily insulin injections are necessary for survival. Asthma is a more variable condition than diabetes, so young people were recruited who had been diagnosed as having moderate or severe asthma, and who were prescribed regular anti-inflammatory inhalers (preventers) in addition to inhaled bronchodilators (relievers). Although asthma and diabetes both have specific treatment regimens, there is arguably more leeway in the management of asthma, in that it may be possible to be more flexible with treatment, in the short term at least. In contrast, ketoacidosis due to lack of insulin in diabetes can rapidly lead to coma and death if untreated.

Just over half of the sample of young people was located through five hospitals in South West London. In addition, 13 were identified through seven GPs in the same area and four through young people who had been interviewed. The respondents were mainly white (one quarter came from various ethnic minority groups) and all social classes were represented, although the majority were middle-class. In order to increase the diversity of the sample, a letter was placed in 'Balance', a magazine for people with diabetes published by the British Diabetic Association which resulted in contact being made with two mother/son pairs. In addition, interviews were carried out with the mothers of three young men who were concerned about their sons' poor control of diabetes, but the young men themselves declined to be interviewed.

The interviews were conducted as flexible, semi-structured 'guided conversations' (Lofland and Lofland, 1984) in an attempt to increase the likelihood that respondents' own accounts and meanings would take priority. The interview guide consisted of a series of prompts relating to topics such as treatment, stigma, and illness management, and this was updated as new areas for discussion emerged from the interviews. With permission, the interviews were taped and fully transcribed.

Transcripts were read several times and were coded using a system of open coding, described by Strauss and Corbin (1990, p. 61) as: "the process of breaking down, examining, comparing, conceptualizing and categorizing data". A grounded theory approach was taken, which allowed themes and concepts to emerge from the data and inform the theoretical framework (Charmaz, 1990). The coded data was compared for similarities and differences in the experiences of the people interviewed, and over time the codes were grouped into broader, conceptual themes, which eventually became part of the larger theoretical framework. In the following sections I have quoted from the transcripts of the recorded interviews, the quotes being illustrative of the particular perspective being discussed.

Chronic illnesses and identities

In this study, the vast majority of girls interviewed were found to incorporate asthma or diabetes into their social identities. This manifested itself in various ways, including girls telling people about their condition and being prepared to treat themselves in public settings:

> Jemma: "I was quite happy to tell people because I think if you can educate people then there won't be these problems, and people saying, 'Oh, why is she wanting to inject herself?' They'll understand it, and I think if you shy away from it then other people will as well and they'll tend to be embarrassed about it."
>
> Viri: "No, I always tell everyone, just in case (asthma)."

In contrast, most of the boys with diabetes or asthma made it as invisible or as small a part of their lives as possible, particularly in public settings. They managed this in many ways, including not talking about their condition in public, even with close friends, and not allowing the treatment regimens to 'spill over' into their public lives. As a consequence, the condition was not seen as an integral part of their social identities, but as something separate:

> Scott: "I just carry on as normal, one injection in the morning, one in the evening. It hasn't affected my life at all, hasn't changed anything, nobody really knows except my family."
>
> Jack: "It's not what boys talk about really — not being sexist, but that's the sort of thing that girls talk about, problems and things. At school a boy might ask quickly about it [asthma] and I'd say, 'oh, it's OK', but they'd never ask questions like what happens when I get it, anything like that... at school it was, 'right, I've got asthma, I'll keep it to myself and the people that know, they know, and the people that don't know it won't affect them sort of thing'."

It was difficult for boys to express why they behaved in this way, and the impression given was that it was just 'natural' behaviour. For example, Richard had a friend and classmate who also had diabetes, but when I asked him if they discussed diabetes, he laughed, saying:

Richard: "No, we don't discuss diabetes at all ... that's your business if you're diabetic sort of thing."

Sometimes the interviews with mothers could help throw some light on the issue. For example, when interviewed, Martin said he did not have any problems in terms of his diabetes treatment, but according to his mother:

"He won't do them [blood sugars] at school now, he absolutely refuses, he won't even do an injection at school. He's on three injections a day and the hospital would like him to go on to four but he won't do it in front of his friends, and he doesn't like the fact that he is diabetic in that respect, he wants to be normal."

There were also differences in how the impact of asthma and diabetes was perceived by teenage girls and boys. Girls appeared more likely to think about and worry about their condition, as Reena and Sharon illustrate:

Reena: "It just means you've got to control your sugar level, your diet and everything... You've got to put a lot of effort into it and — it's horrible, it's dreadful, I hate it."

Sharon: "You've just got to have it [asthma] there at the back of your mind, all the time."

In contrast, the boys generally tried to ignore their condition, and to think about it as little as possible:

Martin: "I don't really think about it [diabetes] because I'm used to it, it's kind of natural."

Donald: "I just try and forget about it [asthma], you know, put it aside, try and put it aside and get on with things. I don't think it affects my life that much ... I'm not too worried about things."

In many ways these findings support those of Miller et al. (1993), and it seems that the extent to which the teenage girls and boys interviewed incorporated their conditions into their identities reflects the differential gendered meanings of chronic illness. If, as Adams et al. (1997) suggest, social and personal identities are "irrevocably interconnected", the fact that the majority of girls accepted being 'asthmatic' or 'diabetic' as part of their social identities would also mean that these conditions were assimilated into their personal identities. In contrast, most of the boys did not accept the social (or personal) identities of having asthma or diabetes. Although boys found it hard to articulate why they managed in this way, it seemed that signs of illness were seen by them as potentially stigmatising. This led to boys working hard to pass in public settings wherever possible (Goffman, 1963), and one of the main ways this was achieved was in the use of specific strategies relating to diabetes and asthma regimens.

Treatment regimens and diabetes

The majority of clinics that the teenagers attended recommended four daily injections of insulin, in the hope that this would lead to increased flexibility of lifestyle, and better control of blood glucose levels. However, there was a marked difference in the number of daily insulin injections which the girls and boys interviewed gave themselves. Only one of the girls interviewed followed a regimen of twice daily injections, three injected themselves three times a day, whilst six of the girls injected themselves four times a day, which usually meant injecting themselves in public settings, such as at school. This reflected the fact that for them diabetes was seen as part of their social identities. For example, Alice is on four injections per day and said:

Alice: "I have to do one injection at school."

Int: "Do you mind that?"

Alice: "Well, I mean, I don't mind it any more. I used to, because other people sometimes find it a bit uncomfortable . . . I mean, it's not too bad now, people accept it, but they used to find it quite uncomfortable, especially the boys, because I just used to sit there and do it."

In contrast, of the 10 boys with diabetes, none had ever attempted to follow a regimen of four injections per day, four injected themselves three times a day and six chose a regimen of two daily injections. Phillip and Richard both explained why they chose to remain on two daily injections:

Phillip: "It's just that when I'm with my friends and I'm doing stuff with my friends it's [diabetes] not there, and I can keep it like that, and then when I get home I can do my insulin, and it's just there, at home."

Richard: "I'd have to keep vanishing every lunchtime, and I'm going to have to take an injection, a syringe into school which will probably get noticed, and there's not really many places to do it — I mean, the toilets have hardly got locks on the doors, half of them."

It seemed that in order to pass and to keep diabetes from their social identities, boys chose not to inject themselves in public settings, but tried as far as possible to keep diabetes contained within the private sphere, at home.

This enabled boys to manage their condition at home, and to pass in public. Boys also passed by keeping to what was often quite a strict routine, and by being adherent to their chosen regimen, which generally resulted in good control of their diabetes. For example, Julian explained:

> "I just do my injection in the morning and night, eat the same amount at about the same time every day, and forget about it."

In addition, the majority of these boys did not appear to have had any thoughts about not taking their insulin, and this again related to keeping diabetes invisible:

> Richard: "I don't see any point, no, I mean, it would cause more trouble. I mean, if you do an injection how long does it take, two minutes? Don't go and do an injection, how much feeling awful is that going to promote?"

Although the majority of boys with diabetes adhered to their chosen regimens, which generally resulted in good control, these 'strict' routines could impact on their day-to-day lives, giving them less flexibility. However, for these boys the most important factor appeared to be that the diabetes remained outside their social identities, and therefore invisible to others, which enabled them to pass. In contrast, although six of the girls with diabetes had chosen a regimen of four injections per day which should have resulted in improved blood sugar control, this did not necessarily follow. One of the reasons for this was the gendered impact of the focus upon diet in diabetes. Diet is one of two examples highlighted in this paper of how specific aspects relating to the treatment regimen of a chronic condition can interact with the social constructions of femininities and masculinities. The second example, exercise, was found to impact on the management of asthma and diabetes, and both will be discussed later in the paper.

Treatment regimens and asthma

The 10 girls interviewed all associated control of asthma with the correct taking of preventive medication. Nine of them claimed to take their preventer inhalers regularly, usually morning and evening, whilst one took it occasionally. These girls with asthma had learned from experience that they needed their preventer inhalers. For example, Carol, a 15-year-old who had had asthma for three years had only been taking her preventer inhaler as prescribed for the previous six months:

> "When I first started it was OK but then I forgot a couple of times, and then I couldn't be bothered to do it, to try and remember. I

thought, 'oh no, it's not worth it, I'm alright, you know, I don't need it'. But I've found out since I've been taking it that it's helped me ... I know if my asthma really affected me I wouldn't be able to go out with him [boyfriend], I won't be able to do the things I want to do, so I know I've got to take my inhaler to control it so I can carry on and do everyday things I want to do."

The regular taking of preventer inhalers indicates an incorporation of asthma as a part of both the personal and social identities of these girls. However, as with the girls with diabetes, this acceptance of asthma could also have negative effects, in that girls could lower their expectations for themselves. Here, Carol describes how she has learned to adapt her life to asthma:

"I realise now I've got to get on with it, because I can't get rid of it, it's not as easy as that, so I have to learn to live with it ... if I take it easy then I can do things — it can't — won't stop me from doing anything as long as I'm careful ... I won't give up, I still do some sport and hopefully, one day I will be able to run again. When I first got it, I said to my Mum, 'I'm not going to stop doing what I want, I don't care about asthma, it's not going to change my life', and it has, you don't realise how much effect it does have. When I look back I realise how stupid I was to just think I could carry on in life."

In contrast, the approach of seven of the 10 boys with asthma was typified by boys saying that they were growing out of their asthma, and so no longer needed regular preventive medication. It is worth noting that all of these boys had been identified by their GP or hospital consultant as having moderate or severe asthma, and at the time of interview a number had recently had severe attacks requiring hospitalisation. However, unlike the girls with asthma such as Carol, these boys were most unlikely to 'be careful', or to think that asthma might change their lives. All of the boys took their reliever inhaler if they felt they really needed it, although they would do this as 'invisibly' as possible, but only three took their preventer inhaler regularly. It was not that these boys denied that they had asthma, but more that they saw it — and made it — a separate, minor part of their lives, by thinking about it as little as possible, and by treating asthma as an episodic, acute illness rather than a chronic illness. Consequently boys felt that they did not have to rely on regular preventer inhalers, and in this way, boys were able to keep asthma outside their personal and social identities:

Paul: "It's not a case of, 'no, we don't have asthma so we don't have to take it' or anything, but it doesn't occur to us most of the time because I mean, I can't say that most of my life is ruled by my asthma attacks and that, so until recently I forgot I had asthma at all and then you get your attack and you think, 'oh', and then when you're over it you just forget about it."

Int: "You don't think of having asthma day-to-day?"

Paul: "No, it's not like diabetes where you have to take your injection every day. My uncle and grandma, they're taking their injections every day, and if they don't they get affected, but if I don't take my inhaler chances are I'll be alright."

Keith: "Because asthma just tends to be so episodic and you get lulled into a false sense of security when you don't display any symptoms."

Paul and Keith had both attended hospital within the past year for the treatment of severe asthma attacks. However, in contrast to the girls interviewed, this experience had not resulted in them taking preventer inhalers. The medication strategies the majority of boys with asthma employed appeared to have little in common with the boys with diabetes, the majority of whom kept to a strict routine with their regimen, and had no thoughts of not taking their insulin. However, this difference may relate more to the nature of the individual conditions and the treatment regimens. In terms of diabetes, not following treatment can have almost immediate effects, meaning that boys would no longer be able to pass. In contrast, most of the boys with asthma felt that there was a good chance nothing would happen if they omitted their preventive asthma therapy. In addition, whilst the taking of preventer inhalers may be seen positively for girls, in terms of the positive meanings that taking responsibility can have for femininities (Green and Hart, 1996), White et al. (1995) draw attention to the negative meanings sensitisation to bodily well-being and preventive medication may have for boys and men, threatening their place in masculine hierarchies. It seems that for these boys, control over their personal and social identities as 'normal, healthy males' was more important than controlling potential episodic occurrences of asthma. Despite this active self-regulation which might be seen as having a negative impact on the health of boys, there were other aspects of the treatment of asthma, such as the importance of exercise, which generally had a beneficial effect for boys. The gendered impact of both exercise and diet on the management of asthma and diabetes will now be discussed.

The gendered impact of exercise

The value of exercise in helping to control both asthma and diabetes may be seen to particularly advantage teenage boys, for whom the institution of sport is important, serving to construct and reconstruct masculinities (White et al., 1995). In this study, as Miller et al. (1993) found, there was a pronounced emphasis on the importance of sport and exercise for boys with asthma and diabetes, with boys' self-assessments of their health very much linked to the amount of sport they played. For example, Jasvir told me:

> "Every Tuesday I go to the swimming pool, and Wednesdays and Fridays I do weight training, and if I can't keep to those actual days, I'll make it another day... to look good and feel good I have to go and do it, I feel better (diabetes)."

In contrast, many of the girls participated in little sport or exercise. Along with diet, this was another issue about which girls frequently expressed guilt, and was often seen by them as a major cause of their perceived unhealthiness:

> Becky: "No, I don't think I'm healthy but I think that's to do with the fact that I don't do enough sport and I don't eat a healthy enough diet, and that makes me feel guilty (diabetes)."

> Joanna: "Asthma makes you unhealthy — you can't run as fast, can't do much exercise, aerobics makes you red-faced, it's better not to bother — but then I feel guilty."

Exercise was also used by boys with diabetes to control their blood sugar levels in contrast to many of the girls, who tended to give themselves more insulin. For example, Scott said:

> "If I go too high [blood glucose level] what I would do is, like, I would jog on the spot or something. I do a lot of jogging or running. I run round the house because it's usually at night that it happens. It never happens during the day, and so I run round the house and just use up the energy and then I'm OK."

> Int: "So you wouldn't give yourself more insulin?"

> Scott: "No, I control it myself. I wouldn't want to give more insulin in case it [blood glucose level] goes down too low. Now I know a safe remedy I'd rather just like wear it off, rather than give myself more insulin."

The gendered impact of diet

Diet is seen as critical in the control of blood glucose, and in this study was found to have a gendered impact in terms of the control of diabetes. In contrast to boys, who rarely mentioned diet, girls often adapted their diets in ways which resulted in sub-optimal control of their diabetes, as assessed by themselves. For example, Clare said:

> Clare: "No, it [diabetes control] could be a lot better, but I don't keep to my diet properly, like, if I want to eat something I shouldn't, say, if I'm going out, I'll just put a bit more [insulin] in."

Girls overwhelmingly mentioned poor diet as the key reason for their sub-optimal control of diabetes, and this was usually combined with feelings of guilt and negative health evaluations:

> Jemma: "I'm on a diet now because I'm eating too much and I want to lose weight. I'm conscious of how much I weigh, and even though I eat, I know I shouldn't be eating so I feel terrible guilty and go and eat some more because I feel guilty, and it's a vicious circle, so I'm not healthy at all."

Because of societal expectations about body image and shape, teenage girls are generally more concerned about diet and weight than boys (Miller et al., 1993), and it seems that the emphasis on food and weight in the treatment of diabetes can bring additional problems for girls, because of the ways in which contemporary femininities are constructed.

Exercise and diet are two examples of how aspects of the treatment of diabetes and asthma can have a gendered impact because of the ways in which femininities and masculinities are socially constructed. These particular aspects had a generally positive impact for the teenage boys interviewed, in terms of how they controlled and managed these conditions, and a generally negative impact for the teenage girls, supporting the findings of Miller et al. (1993). However, the interelation between gender and health is complex, and particular aspects of the social constructions of gender could have both positive and adverse effects. The paper will now explore one example of this, namely control of the body, which served to both advantage and disadvantage boys with asthma and diabetes.

Control of the body and the chronic condition

Earlier it was stated that chronic illnesses may particularly threaten dominant masculinity, with its emphasis on control (Seidler, 1998). In this study, boys were far more likely than girls to say that they could control their condition with their mind, although they described this in terms such as 'willpower' and 'being very strong mentally'. These feelings of control affected how boys managed their conditions, and their medication regimens. An example of the benefit of wanting to maintain control was seen in the previous section, when Scott preferred to manage a high blood glucose by controlling it himself using exercise. However, the importance for boys of maintaining control can be seen to have potentially positive and negative consequences, as Paul shows:

> "Asthma creeps up on you, it just creeps up on you . . . a lot of the time I know I'm having an attack, but if I'm playing football I'll say, 'now I'll ignore it and I'll play on', yes, and I'll fight through it. I'll say, 'look, I know what's happening, I'll take things slower', but you've just got to keep breathing and it goes away, it just goes because of my mental strength."

The positive effects for Paul could be the ability to perhaps control some of his potential asthma attacks. However, one of the potentially negative consequences had occurred in the month prior to his interview, when he had been rushed to hospital with a severe asthma attack. These feelings of control that boys described were also noted by Miller et al. (1993), although they only discussed this in terms of the beneficial effects this had for boys with cystic fibrosis. However, this study identified potentially serious adverse effects, as Paul illustrates. In addition, if these traditional assumptions of male identities such as feeling in control were not achieved, this could result in 'disparaged' or denigrated identities for boys (Charmaz, 1995).

'Disparaged' identities

There was a small but important minority of boys who for whatever reason did not appear to feel in control of their condition, and who were consequently unable to 'pass'. In relation to diabetes, this occurred when boys ignored their regimens as far as was possible. As previously described, three mothers who felt their sons' diabetes to be out of control were interviewed, although the boys themselves refused to be interviewed. One of these, Harry's mother, said:

> "He tells people he'll be dead soon anyway so it doesn't matter what he does, and that seems to be his whole attitude really . . . he just doesn't want to do it [follow treatment regimen], he doesn't want to know. As far as he's concerned, he hasn't got diabetes and he carries on as if he hasn't."

George's mother describes his reaction in the following way:

> "Within three months [of diagnosis] George had settled down into a routine of diet, exercise and injections, and was coping with bringing down his blood sugar — it didn't last long. At Christmas, George

became upset that he couldn't indulge his sweet tooth as he used to, and his blood sugar rose to levels never before seen. He refused to discuss his diabetes management with anyone, so I wrote to his consultant in desperation. By now he was saying things like, 'If I go blind [one of the possible consequences of poor blood sugar control] I'll just top myself'... I would have been devastated but not surprised if he had attempted to take his own life."

Although these young men were reported to have initially controlled their diabetes very well, they had then become angry about having the condition and had consequently stopped or reduced their treatment regimen. However, the symptoms which resulted meant that these boys were no longer able to pass in public as they had before. Mark was one of the few boys actually interviewed who did not feel in control of his condition. He told me that his health was 'just terrible', and he appeared to have given up hope of ever controlling his asthma:

"I've tried playing football with my friends but I can't play for long because I'm on the floor grabbing my chest and I can't breathe so they send me home... I can't beat it, if it will come it will come and every precaution I take, it will just come, it just finds a way, so I don't bother no more, there's no point... going up the stairs I'm just like my granddad, that's what I'm like with walking... I don't go outside no more 'cos of the fumes and all that."

The majority of boys in the study claimed to feel in control of their conditions. However, for the few boys who did not feel in control, this seemed to lead to disparaged or denigrated identities. This supports the work of Charmaz (1995) who argues that traditional assumptions of male identity can act as a 'double-edged sword', leading to a narrow range of credible behaviours for men, with an 'uneasy tension' between valued and disparaged identities. However, it should be noted that these boys were hard to identify through the usual channels of GPs, clinic nurses and hospitals, and even when they were located, mainly through their mothers responding to a letter in *Balance* magazine, they declined to be interviewed. This difficulty of access may be one of the reasons why the findings of this study differed from those of Miller et al. (1993), who found no boys with disparaged identities.

Discussion and conclusions

Young people in this study were found to manage asthma and diabetes in gendered ways, with the aim of projecting different, gendered identities. As Charmaz (1991, p. 5) states:

> ... having a chronic illness means more than learning to live with it. It means struggling to maintain control over the defining images of self and over one's life.

The majority of girls showed greater adaptation, incorporating their conditions and the associated treatment regimens into their social and personal identities. The social construction of femininities meant the conditions were not seen as the threat that they were for boys. In contrast, the majority of boys made every effort to keep asthma and diabetes out of their personal and social identities, attempting to pass (Goffman, 1963). This supports and extends the work of both Charmaz (1995) and Prout (1989), who draw attention to the stigmatising effects that illness can have for males of varying ages. This research also builds on Goffman's (1963) work by showing how gendered meanings of stigma can impact on strategies for dealing with chronic illness.

One of the benefits of exploring the management of two conditions is that if examined individually, the self-regulation of the treatment regimens of asthma and diabetes by boys would appear to have little in common. However, it seems that these different ways of managing have the common aim of minimising the potential threat asthma and diabetes pose to masculine identities. Whereas strict adherence to treatment regimens enabled boys with diabetes to pass and thus maintain valued identities (Charmaz, 1995), boys with asthma achieved this by seeing asthma as an acute, episodic condition which did not necessitate regular preventive medication. In addition, two aspects of the treatment regimens of diabetes and asthma, diet and exercise, impacted in gendered ways, having a generally positive effect for boys, helping them to pass.

The ways in which the social construction of femininities and masculinities impacted on the management of illness could be both beneficial and problematic. As with the research by Charmaz (1995) on older women, the girls in this study were found to show a greater adaptability to asthma and diabetes, but this could have detrimental effects, as girls sometimes lowered expectations for themselves. This, combined with the detrimental gendered effects of diet and exercise, could partly explain why the control of diabetes and asthma worsens for young women of this age.

For teenage boys, there appeared to be a narrow range of credible masculine behaviours when managing chronic illness (Charmaz, 1995). The majority of boys maintained a valued identity by passing, and by feeling in control of their body and their condition. However, for the small minority of boys who did not feel in control, and who were no longer able to pass, the impact of chronic illness led to disparaged identities (Charmaz, 1995). The results of this study indicate that boys at this stage in their lifecourse are more likely than girls to move between two extremes in terms of managing diabetes and asthma, with the majority managing well, and a small minority managing very poorly.

By focusing on both teenage girls and boys, it has been possible to consider some of the ways in which gender interacts differentially with two chronic conditions, asthma and diabetes. This is a complex two-way process, with aspects of the social constructions of contemporary femininities and masculinities impacting on the management of these conditions, and aspects of these conditions impacting in gendered ways upon the social constructions of gender. In other words, the interplay between health and gender can be conceptualised as both plural and reciprocal (Broom, 1999). Research comparing women and men of different ages and with different illnesses will enable the complexities of this interplay to be further explored.

Acknowledgements

I am very grateful to all of the people who participated in this study. Particular thanks go to Sara Arber who was the supervisor of my Ph.D. on which this paper is based, and who commented on an earlier draft of the paper. I also acknowledge the support of the Department of Health who funded my Ph.D.

References

Adams, S., Pill, R., Jones, A., 1997. Medication, chronic illness and identity: the perspective of people with asthma. Soc. Sci. Med. 45, 189–201.

Broom, D., 1999. The genders of health. Paper presented at "Gender, Health and Healing: reflections on the public-private divide" Conference, University of Warwick, 23–24 April.

Bury, M., 1991. The sociology of chronic illness: a review of research and prospects. Sociol. Health Illness 13, 455–468.

Bytheway, B., Furth, A., 1996. Asthma. In: Davey, B., Seale, C. (Eds.), Experiencing and Explaining Disease. Open University, Buckingham, pp. 81–112.

Cameron, E., Bernardes, J., 1998. Gender and disadvantage in health: men's health for a change. Sociol. Health Illness 20, 673–693.

Charmaz, K., 1990. 'Discovering' chronic illness: using grounded theory. Soc. Sci. Med. 30, 1161–1172.

Charmaz, K., 1991. Good Days, Bad Days: the Self in Chronic Illness and Time. Rutgers University Press, New Brunswick, NJ.

Charmaz, K., 1995. Identity dilemmas of chronically ill men. In: Sabo, D., Gordon, D. (Eds.), Men's Health and Illness: Gender, Power and the Body. Sage, London, pp. 266–291.

Connell, R., 1987. Gender and Power: Society, the Person and Sexual Politics. Stanford University Press, Stanford, CA.

Conrad, P., 1985. The meaning of medications: another look at compliance. Soc. Sci. Med. 20, 29–37.

Coppock, V., Haydon, D., Richter, I., 1995. The Illusions of 'Post-Feminism'. Taylor & Francis, London.

Donovan, J., Blake, D., 1992. Patient non-compliance: deviance or reasoned decision-making? Soc. Sci. Med. 34, 507–513.
Goffman, E., 1963. Stigma. Prentice Hall, Englewood Cliffs, NJ.
Green, J., Hart, L., 1996. Children's Views of Accident Risks: An Exploratory Study. South Bank University, London.
Gregg, I., 1983. Epidemiological aspects. In: Clarke, T., Godfrey, S. (Eds.), Asthma. Chapman and Hall Medical, London.
Klingelhofer, E., 1987. Compliance with medical regimens, self-management programs, and self-care in childhood asthma. Clin. Rev. Allerg. 5, 231–247.
Lofland, J., Lofland, L., 1984. Analyzing Social Settings: a Guide to Qualitative Observation and Analysis. Wadsworth, CA.
Mead, G., 1961. Mind, Self and Society. University of Chicago Press, Chicago.
Miller, R., Willis, E., Wyn, J., 1993. Gender and compliance in the management of a medical regimen for young people with cystic fibrosis. Paper presented at BSA Medical Sociology Conference, University of York, UK.
Nathanson, C., 1975. Illness and the feminine role: a theoretical review. Soc. Sci. Med. 2, 57.
Pond, N., Sturock, N., Jeffcoate, W., 1996. Age related changes in glycolated haemoglobin in patients with IDDM. Diabetic Med. 13, 510–513.
Prendergast, S., 1995. The spaces of childhood: psyche, soma and social existence: menstruation and embodiment at adolescence. In: Brannen, J., O'Brien, M. (Eds.), Childhood and Parenthood. Institute of Education, London, pp. 348–364.
Prout, A., 1989. Sickness as a dominant symbol in life course transitions: an illustrated theoretical framework. Sociol. Health Illness 11, 337–359.
Saltonstall, R., 1993. Healthy bodies, social bodies: men's and women's concepts and practices of health in everyday life. Soc. Sci. Med. 36, 7–14.
Seidler, V., 1998. Masculinity, violence and emotional life. In: Bendelow, G., Williams, S. (Eds.), Emotions in Social Life. Routledge, London, pp. 193–210.
Strauss, A., Corbin, J., 1990. Basics of Qualitative Research. Sage, London.
Sweeting, H., 1995. Reversals of fortune? Sex differences in health in childhood and adolescence. Soc. Sci. Med. 40, 77–90.
Verbrugge, L., 1997. Demography and older women's health. Paper presented at 'Gender and Health' Conference, Society for Social Medicine, London.
White, P., Young, K., McTeer, W., 1995. Sport, masculinity and the injured body. In: Sabo, D., Gordon, F. (Eds.), Men's Health and Illness: Gender, Power and the Body. Sage, London.
Williams, C., 1998. Mothers, young people and chronic illness: meanings, management and gendered identities. Ph.D. thesis. University of Surrey, Guildford.